Recognizing and Treating Breathing Disorders

Content Strategist: *Alison Taylor*
Content Development Specialist: *Carole McMurray*
Project Managers: *Anne Collett, Joanna Souch*
Designer/Design Direction: *Miles Hitchen*
Illustration Manager: *Jennifer Rose*
Illustrator: *Antbits Ltd*

Recognizing and Treating Breathing Disorders:
a multidisciplinary approach

Second edition

Leon Chaitow ND DO

Registered Osteopathic Practitioner and Honorary Fellow, School of Life Sciences, University of Westminster, London, UK

Dinah Bradley DipPhys NZRP MNZSP

Private Consultant, Respiratory Physiotherapist, Breathing Works, Remuera, Auckland, New Zealand

Christopher Gilbert PhD

Psychologist, Chronic Pain Management Program, Kaiser Permanente Medical Center, San Francisco, California, USA

With contributions by

Jim Bartley
Petr Bitnar
Aileen Chan
Tania Clifton-Smith
Rosalba Courtney
Jan van Dixhoorn

John C. Hannon
Gro K. Haugstad
Tor S. Haugstad
Alena Kobesova
Pavel Kolar
Laurie McLaughlin

Warrick McNeill
Suzanne Scott
Nilkamal Singh
Shirley Telles
Petra Valouchova
Eva Au Zveglic

Foreword by

David Peters MB ChB DRCOG, DM SMed MF Hom FLCOM, Clinical Director, Faculty of Science and Technology, University of Westminster, London, UK

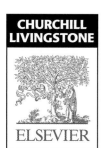

Edinburgh   London   New York   Oxford   Philadelphia   St Louis   Sydney   Toronto   2014

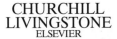

First edition 2002
Second edition 2014

ISBN 978-0-7020-4980-4
e-book ISBN: 978-0-7020-5427-3

British Library Cataloguing in Publication Data
A catalogue record for this book is available from the British Library

Library of Congress Cataloging in Publication Data
A catalog record for this book is available from the Library of Congress

Notices

Knowledge and best practice in this field are constantly changing. As new research and experience broaden our understanding, changes in research methods, professional practices, or medical treatment may become necessary. Practitioners and researchers must always rely on their own experience and knowledge in evaluating and using any information, methods, compounds, or experiments described herein. In using such information or methods they should be mindful of their own safety and the safety of others, including parties for whom they have a professional responsibility.

With respect to any drug or pharmaceutical products identified, readers are advised to check the most current information provided (i) on procedures featured or (ii) by the manufacturer of each product to be administered, to verify the recommended dose or formula, the method and duration of administration, and contraindications. It is the responsibility of practitioners, relying on their own experience and knowledge of their patients, to make diagnoses, to determine dosages and the best treatment for each individual patient, and to take all appropriate safety precautions.

To the fullest extent of the law, neither the Publisher nor the authors, contributors, or editors, assume any liability for any injury and/or damage to persons or property as a matter of products liability, negligence or otherwise, or from any use or operation of any methods, products, instructions, or ideas contained in the material herein.

 your source for books, journals and multimedia in the health sciences

www.elsevierhealth.com

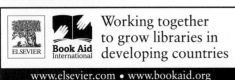

Working together to grow libraries in developing countries

www.elsevier.com • www.bookaid.org

The publisher's policy is to use paper manufactured from sustainable forests

Printed in India

Last digit is the print number: 15   14   13   12   11

Contents

Contents

Contributors

Jim Bartley, FRACS, FFPMANZCA
Associate Professor, Department of Surgery,
University of Auckland, Auckland, New Zealand

Petr Bitnar, DPT
Lecturer, Clinic of Rehabilitation and Sports Medicine, 2nd
Faculty of Medicine, Charles University, University Hospital
Motol, Prague, Czech Republic

Aileen Chan, RN, RM, BSc, PGDip(HIM), MHA, PhD
Assistant Professor, The Nethersole School of Nursing, The
Chinese University of Hong Kong, Shatin, Hong Kong

Tania Clifton-Smith, NZ Dip Phys MNZSP NZMTA ITEC (Lon)
Director, Breathing Works, Auckland, New Zealand

Rosalba Courtney, ND, DO, PhD
Osteopath, Breath and Body Clinic, Breathing Therapy and
Integrative Medicine, Avalon, NSW, Australia

Jan van Dixhoorn, MD, PhD
Center for Breathing Therapy, Amersfoort, Netherlands

John C. Hannon, DC
Certified Feldenkrais® Practitioner, Private Practice,
San Luis Obispo, CA, USA

Gro K. Haugstad, MHS, PhD
Oslo and Akershus University College, Institute of
Physiotherapy, Faculty of Health Science, Norway

Tor S. Haugstad, MD, PhD
Sunnaas National Rehabilitation Hospital, Dept of
Neurorehabilitation, Oslo, Norway

Alena Kobesova, MD, PhD
Assistant Academic Director, Lecturer, Clinic of Rehabilitation
and Sports Medicine, 2nd Faculty of Medicine, Charles
University, University Hospital Motol, Prague, Czech Republic

Pavel Kolar, PaedDr., PhD
Director, Clinic of Rehabilitation and Sports Medicine, 2nd
Faculty of Medicine, Charles University, University Hospital
Motol, Prague, Czech Republic

Laurie McLaughlin, PT, DSc, FCAMPT, CMAG
Owner and Director, ProActive Education, Oakville, ON,
Canada

Warrick McNeill, MCSP
Chartered Physiotherapist, Physioworks Chartered
Physiotherapists and Pilates Clinic, London, UK

Suzanne Scott, MA (Cantab), BSc
Suzanne Scott Pilates and Movement Practice,
The Scott Studio, Castle Cary, Somerset, UK

Nilkamal Singh, MD, PhD
Patanjali Research Foundation, India

Shirley Telles, MBBS, PhD
Patanjali Research Foundation, Patanjali Yogpeeth, Haridwar,
Uttarakhand 249405, India

Petra Valouchova, DPT, PhD
Lecturer, Clinic of Rehabilitation and Sports Medicine, 2nd
Faculty of Medicine, Charles University, University Hospital
Motol, Prague, Czech Republic

Eva Au Zveglic, BApplSci (Phty), MSc, MBBA, MCSP
Lead Cardiothoracic Physiotherapist,
BUPA Cromwell Hospital, London, UK

Foreword

As you have opened this book, you are probably a practitioner. Perhaps you have already come to rely on the previous version and are keen to get up to date. Welcome – you will not be disappointed. Or maybe something has made you curious about breathing and its power to support wellbeing, or on the other hand to send health into a tailspin. In which case prepare to have your clinical world expanded, for this is far more than a book about breathing pattern disorders. At its heart is a profoundly holistic approach to illness and disease as processes of adaptation, compensation and their failure. It is a book about making sense of that journey and getting it back on course.

21st Century medicine faces a pandemic of chronic, environmental-, stress- and lifestyle- mediated diseases. There is some urgency then for it to learn at least as much about building resilience as it has about 'fighting' disease. The editors and their expert authors shine some light on what that could mean in practical terms to clinicians, whatever their orientation. Indeed it is the breadth of this book that astonishes; inviting readers to make their own synthesis, it brings together views from diverse fields. Which of course it must, because breathing pattern disorders are whole person problems. And especially so in long-term conditions, where dysfunctional breathing can destabilise mind *and* muscles, mood *and* metabolism.

So it is a great loss to medicine that most doctors have yet to take this in. But sadder still is the bewilderment of so many patients; especially patients with complex long term conditions, co-morbidities, or perhaps most of all who have 'MUS'. Medically unexplained symptoms often become that much more explicable once the vicious mind-body cycle of over-breathing is understood. Leon Chaitow, and his co-editors, Dinah Bradley and Chris Gilbert, have done a great deal to address this widespread ignorance. Nor is it confined to doctors: in my experience too few physical therapists, psychotherapists and complementary practitioners have a good enough grasp on the part breathing pattern disorders can play for instance in chronic fatigue, persistent pain, fibromyalgia, and some aspects of anxiety or depression.

Yet breathing is par excellence the bridge between mind and body. Perhaps that is why it remains below the horizon of practitioners who feel their expertise must lie on one or other side of this divide. Thankfully, having overcome that false demarcation and learned to spot the problem, practitioners' ability to diagnose BPD can profoundly re-enable them and their patients. For once given the map BPD provides – and though ongoing support is often needed – they may at last get some traction on these downward spirals, and even reverse them.

The journeys are seldom easy, and rare is the practitioner who has all the knowledge and skills required to lead them. But, for the intrepid clinician-explorer this essentially multi-disciplinary book will provide much needed maps and signposts to the mind-body habits, beliefs, metabolic and structural distortions that keep the over-breathing tendency going. I recommend you read this book, use it and also share it with a few good colleagues, so that together you may help some of your most lost and puzzling patients find their way back.

Professor David Peters
Director, Westminster Centre for Resilience
University of Westminster
London

Preface

The second edition of this book has required a comprehensive revision of the original text – representing as it does changes in our understanding of the subject over the 12 years since it was first published.

What has changed in that decade?

The essentials of breathing function have remained the same, but our understanding of the processes involved, and what can go wrong, has advanced, and the revised text reflects that newly examined information.

As in the first edition, our emphasis is on function, dysfunction, and rehabilitation strategies – and not on pathology.

Just as poor posture is not a disease, so a poor breathing pattern is not a disease. However, an unbalanced breathing pattern (or breathing pattern disorder – BPD), which is frequently habitual, can contribute to the emergence and maintenance of multiple symptoms, just as poor posture can lead to pain and restriction.

One example of what is new in our understanding of what may aggravate or influence BPD emerged via research in 2009 by Lin & Peper. This showed what happened when students familiar with cell/mobile phone texting, were monitored during the sending and receiving of messages. Surface electromyography (SEMG) and skin conductance (SC) were used to measure changes on the palm of the non-texting hand, as well as the thorax and abdomen. The results indicated that all those tested showed significant increases in respiration rate, heart rate and skin-conductance (suggesting sympathetic arousal), as compared to baseline measures. 83% reported hand and neck pain during texting, and held their breath, as well as experiencing sympathetic arousal when receiving text messages. Most of those tested were unaware of these physiological changes.

The wider implications of these findings, in relation to breathing function/ dysfunction, can be speculated upon – but they do act as a reminder that while the essentials of respiration remain the same, potential influences on this function are to be found in many common environmental settings.

This is one reason for the decision to not only update the text, but to widely expand the therapeutic horizons in this second edition – as well as to marginally modify the title.

The new edition contains revised and expanded chapters that offer a general overview of BPD (Chapters 1 and 3), as well as chapters on the structure and function of breathing (Chapter 2.2), biochemistry (Chapter 4) and psychology/emotion (Chapter 5), in assessment and management settings, from osteopathic (Chapters 6.2, 7.2), physiotherapy (Chapters 6.3, 7.3) and psychological (Chapters 6.4, 7.4) perspectives.

We have also added chapters (many contributed by leading experts) that offer a variety of additional and pertinent views and options.

For example, in chapters 2.1 developmental kinesiology is evaluated – the way structural and functional development occurs in the early stages of life, and how this knowledge can be used in application of dynamic neuromuscular stabilization in both assessment (Ch 6.1) and management (Ch 7.1b) of breathing dysfunction.

A valuable addition is to be found in Chapter 2.3 which evaluates a topic largely absent from the first edition – nasal influences on breathing.

Chapter 6.5 introduces details of the use of key questionnaires (and other assessment methods) in management of BPD.

Chapter 6.6 provides an overview of the use of capnography in assessment settings, while Chapter 7.7 describes capnography in treatment contexts.

Chapter 7.1a provides valuable insights into indirect methods of regulating BPD.

Chapter 7.5 introduces details of the relationship between breathing and vocal dysfunction as it affects speech and singing – offering potential solutions to these widespread issues.

Breathing patterns, as these affect athletes, are analyzed from biomechanical, physiological and psychological perspectives, along with management protocols, in Chapter 7.6.

Breathing and chronic pain is discussed in Chapter 8.1 from a somatocognitive point of view.

A critical evaluation of the Buteyko system of breathing rehabilitation is offered in Chapter 8.2, while in Chapter 8.3 the Feldenkrais approach is detailed.

Breathing patterns in relation to Pilates are explained in Chapter 8.4, while Tai Chi/Qigong (chapter 8.5) and Yoga (Chapter 8.6) complete the selection of different potential therapeutic models that may impact respiration.

Chapter 9 provides a selection of self-help methods, exercises and suggestions, in addition to further questionnaires.

What we have set out to do, with the help of experts from a variety of backgrounds, is to offer as clear a picture as possible of how to understand, assess and manage breathing pattern disorders, based on current evidence and clinical practice.

Note that the methods outlined, particularly in the chapters on modalities (section 8), are not necessarily recommended for everyone with BPD characteristics. Also, many of the methods and techniques depend on the context of a particular discipline and/or specialized training. The descriptions are not meant to give complete directions, but should be useful for stimulating thinking about diverse approaches to breathing disorders, including facilitating referral to suitably trained practitioners.

The information provided is designed to offer options and insights – to be employed or disregarded, based on individual needs and indications.

Leon Chaitow
Dinah Bradley
Chris Gilbert

REFERENCE

Lin, I.M., Peper, E., 2009. Psychophysiological patterns during cell phone text messaging: a preliminary study. Appl Psychophysiol Biofeedback 34 (1), 53–57.

Acknowledgments

The compilation of this second edition was a truly international, inter-disciplinary, exercise – with authors scattered between New Zealand, Australia, Canada, Greece, Hong Kong, India, Czech Republic, Holland, Norway, USA and UK….with our wonderful editors and publisher, respectively in Scotland and England.

As editors – equally stretched between Greece, New Zealand and California - we owe a debt of gratitude to the many chapter contributors who have enhanced the book by bringing together a breathtaking (pun intended) range of disciplines, featuring their specialized knowledge, in order to focus attention on breathing dysfunction and its potential remedies. Our thanks to Professor David Peters for his insightful Foreword – emphasising as it does restoration of resilience as a primary objective.

Our profound thanks to everyone involved – and to each other!

Leon Chaitow
Dinah Bradley
Chris Gilbert

Disclaimer

The therapeutic and rehabilitation approaches described herein are designed for management of breathing pattern disorders – not for medical/pathological conditions, which require specialist knowledge and training. The editors strongly advise against application of the methods outlined in the book except by those qualified to do so. We trust clinical practitioners to know the limits of their discipline.

The Website

Besides the vast amount of information found within *Recognizing and Treating Breathing Disorders* 2e, the publishers have created a unique website – www.chaitowbreathingpattern.com – to accompany the volume. This site contains approximately 25 short videos illustrating many of the techniques described in the book. Where such a video clip exists, the text will be accompanied by a cursor arrow symbol . We hope that you will enjoy these short film sequences.

To access the site, go to www.chaitowbreathingpattern.com and follow the simple log-on instructions shown.

Glossary/ Acronyms/ Abbreviations

A alveolar (e.g. P_{AO_2})

a arterial (e.g. P_{aO_2})

ACh acetylcholine

anaerobic threshold highest oxygen consumption during exercise, above which sustained lactic acidosis occurs

ASI Anxiety Sensitivity Index

ASIS anterior superior iliac spine, an anatomical location

ATP adenosine triphosphate

BPD breathing pattern disorder

BPR breathing pattern retraining

BBT Buteyko breathing technique

BUL, BUM backward upward laterally, backward upward medially

C cervical (as in C7, or seventh cervical vertebra)

CAL chronic airway limitation (e.g. COPD)

capnography measurement of end-tidal CO_2 (from the nostril)

catecholamines collective term for compounds with a sympathomimetic action (e.g. adrenaline)

CHD coronary heart disease

CNS central nervous system

CO_2 carbon dioxide

COPD chronic obstructive pulmonary disease

CP controlled pause

CPAP continuous positive airways pressure

CT cervicothoracic

DNS Dynamic Neuromuscular Stabilization

dysphonia disorders of the voice

ECG electrocardiogram

EIA exercise induced asthma

EIH exercise induced hyperventilation

EMG electromyography

end-tidal CO_2 measure of CO_2 in exhaled air

ETCO$_2$ end-tidal CO_2 (normal 4–6%)

FVC forced vital capacity

FEV$_1$ forced expiratory volume in one second

GHJ Glenohumeral joint

Hb (haemoglobin) respiratory pigment in red blood cells, combines reversibly with O_2 (normal: men: 14.0–18.0 g/100 ml; women: 11.5–15.5 g/100 ml)

HVPT hyperventilation provocation test

HVT high velocity thrust, a manipulative method (also known as HVLA – high velocity low amplitude – thrust)

HRV Heart rate variability

hypercapnia increased blood CO_2 levels

hypocapnia P_{aCO_2} lower than usual

hypertonicity increased muscle tension, impairing normal muscle function

hyperventilation CO_2 removal in excess of CO_2 production, producing P_{aCO_2} < 4.6 kPa or 35 mmHg

hypoventilation CO_2 production in excess of CO_2 removal producing P_{aCO_2} > 6.0 kPa or 45 mmHG

IgE immunoglobulin E, an antibody involved in allergic reactions

IMT inspiratory muscle training

INIT integrated neuromuscular inhibition technique (a combination of different soft tissue approaches used to deactivate trigger points)

kPa kilopascal

kyphotic excessive curvature of upper back

L lumbar (as in L1, or first lumbar vertebra)

lordosis increased inward lumbar curve of the spine

LS lumbosacral

MARM Manual Assessment of Respiratory Movement (or Motion)

MP maximum pause

MV resting minute volume

NANC nonadrenergic noncholinergic

NO nitric oxide

NMT neuromuscular technique(s), a treatment method, or neuromuscular therapy, a therapeutic approach

μg microgram

mmHg millimetres of mercury

MET muscle energy technique, a treatment method

MFR myofascial release, a treatment method

MPI myofascial pain index (evaluation of the average current poundage required to evoke pain in an individual, on applied pressure, using a series of test points)

NQ Nijmegen Questionnaire

OMT osteopathic manipulative therapy (or treatment)

OA occipito-atlantal

OSA obstructive sleep apnoea

PEFR peak expiratory flow rate

PLB pursed-lips breathing

P_{aO_2} partial pressure of oxygen in the blood

P_{aCO_2} partial pressure of carbon dioxide in the blood

PETCO$_2$ measure of end-tidal CO_2 from exhaled air

pH relative alkalinity or acidity of body fluids

PIR post-isometric relaxation (an effect achieved in application of MET)

PRT positional release techniques

QL quadratus lumborum

QOL quality of life

REM rapid eye movement

RI reciprocal inhibition (an effect achieved in application of MET)

RIP respiratory induction plethysmography

RoBE Rowley Breathing pattern disorders self-efficacy scale

RSA respiratory sinus arrhythmia

RV residual value

SaO$_2$ saturation of haemoglobin with oxygen from arterial sampling

SCS strain/counterstrain (an osteopathic treatment method)

SEBQ self-evaluation of breathing questionnaire

SI(J) sacroiliac (joint)

SCM sternocleidomastoid (muscle)

SMT standardized Mensendieck test

somatocognitive therapy a hybrid treatment of physiotherapy and psychotherapy

SpO$_2$ noninvasive estimation of arterial oxyhaemoglobin by pulse oximetry

TFL tensor fasciae latae (muscle)

TL thoracolumbar

TMJ temporomandibular joint

torr mmHg

T thoracic (as in T1, or first thoracic vertebra)

TCM Traditional Chinese Medicine

TLC total lung capacity

VC vital capacity

VO$_2$ max volume of oxygen consumed while exercising at maximum capacity

VCD vocal cord/fold dysfunction

Vt tidal volume

Chapter | 1 |

What are breathing pattern disorders?

Leon Chaitow, Dinah Bradley, Chris Gilbert

The focus of this book is on normal versus abnormal respiratory patterns – referred to throughout the book as breathing pattern disorders (BPD) – and how best to restore normal function once an altered pattern has been established. This commonly requires the removal of causative factors, if identifiable, and, if possible, the rehabilitation of habitual, acquired dysfunctional breathing patterns. In order to achieve this most efficiently, some degree of structural mobilization to restore the machinery of breathing – the structural components – towards normality, is usually helpful.

If rehabilitation is attempted without taking account of etiological features, or of maintaining features – for example restricted rib articulations, shortened thoracic musculature, or psychosocial problems – results will be less than optimal.

An example of extreme breathing pattern alteration is hyperventilation. Acute, chronic, or acute on chronic hyperventilation, and its effects, occupy a major part of the book. It is also necessary to explore the widespread area of functional BPDs, in which normal patterning is clearly absent, even though symptomatic hyperventilation is not evident.

What is clearly evident is that hyperventilation syndromes/breathing pattern disorders (HVS/BPDs) are alive and thriving in the 21st century (Gardner 2004, Studer et al 2011). In the 5th century BC Hippocrates observed that breathing is the balancing force in maintaining mental and physical health: his words, 'The brain exercises the greatest power in human-kind – but the air supplies sense to it,' are as relevant today as they were 2500 years ago. More recently called 'a diagnosis begging for recognition' (Magarian 1982), these disorders are increasingly being recognized as major causes of ill health, though still remaining widely under-diagnosed and under-treated.

HISTORICAL BACKGROUND TO THE EXTREME OF BPD/HYPERVENTILATION

The first description of hyperventilation in Western medical literature dates back to the American Civil War, when a surgeon published a paper entitled 'On irritable heart: a clinical study of a form of functional cardiac disorder and its consequences' (Da Costa 1871). The series of 300 soldiers studied suffered breathlessness, dizziness, palpitations, chest pain, headache and disturbed sleep. The symptoms improved when the soldiers were removed from the front line, but their recovery was slow. Although Da Costa recognized the symptoms as functional in origin, he did not identify hyperventilation as the primary cause.

Physiologists Haldane & Poulton (1908) associated numbness, tingling, and dizziness with overbreathing. A year later, Vernon (1909) added an additional symptom, muscular hypertonicity. These symptoms occurred with respiratory alkalosis when patients were hyperventilating.

Kerr and colleagues (1937) introduced the term 'hyperventilation syndrome' (HVS) and pointed out the diversity and variability of symptoms in many systems of the body. Before these publications, a number of cardiologists following up Da Costa's syndrome had debated whether the heart was involved and coined phrases to fit in with their own views. Thomas Lewis (1940) used the terms 'soldier's heart' and 'effort syndrome' in relation to British soldiers in and after the First World War, whereas US cardiologists were reluctant to label the symptoms as cardiac or related to effort. They preferred the term 'neuro-circulatory asthenia'.

These arguments were largely settled when Soley & Shock (1938) found that all the manifestations of 'soldier's heart' and 'effort syndrome' could be induced by hyperventilation and consequent respiratory alkalosis. Since then, many names have been given to this complex set of symptoms – changing with the fads of the time. 'Designer jeans syndrome' (Perera 1988) was popular in the 1970s, and the current so-called Gulf and Balkan War syndromes include many of the same signs and symptoms. Broadly speaking, HVS/BPD was accepted as being of psychiatric origin in the USA and readily diagnosed, whereas in the UK physicians were reluctant to recognize it. A number of factors may have been operating. Most of the reports were in psychological and psychiatric literature, unnoticed by general practitioners and physicians. Influential UK cardiologist Paul Wood (1941) had reviewed Da Costa's syndrome and firmly placed it in the hands of the psychiatrists. Sadly there was little dialogue between the two specialties.

More recently, chest physician Lum (1977), writing from the Addenbrooke and Papworth hospitals in Cambridge, England, with physiotherapists Innocenti (1987) and Cluff (1984), who developed assessment and treatment programmes, has done much to enlighten the medical practitioners in the UK and re-ignite scientific interest and research into the condition. Since that time there has been a flowering of literature on the subject as more sophisticated and accessible research equipment has become available.

Despite such progress, there are still considerable numbers of cardiologists, general and specialist physicians, or general practitioners who are reluctant to diagnose or seek treatment for their patients with hyperventilation (Hornsveld & Garsson 1997). Endless, increasingly sophisticated tests are carried out. Alternatively, patients are referred to further specialists for symptoms related to other fields, or they are told 'nothing is wrong' with them. If hyperventilation as a causative factor is not considered and tested for, investigations may be protracted, diagnosis avoided, and the patient and the patient's file relegated to the 'too hard' basket. This puts patients at great risk of invalidism or of being labelled as malingerers. Medical historians have suggested, for example, that the chronic invalidism of Florence Nightingale and Charles Darwin in the 19th century was more likely chronic hyperventilation, rather than heart disease resulting from infections picked up in the Crimea and the Andes respectively, as was previously believed (Timmons & Ley 1994).

VARIETIES OF BPD AND ITS SYMPTOMS

There are a variety of symptoms, the most extreme of which is hyperventilation syndrome, which is defined as breathing in excess of metabolic requirements, reducing carbon dioxide (CO_2) concentrations of the blood to below normal. This alters the body's pH, increasing alkalinity, and so triggering a variety of adaptive changes that produce symptoms – described in more detail below. See also Figure 1.1, a flowchart which captures the consequences of BPD.

Other definitions worth noting are: (see Glossary)

- **Hypoventilation:** occurs when respiration is too shallow, and inadequate to perform the required gas exchange, leading to increased concentrations of CO_2 (hypercapnia) and respiratory or metabolic acidosis. This is commonly associated with morbid obesity (Resta et al 2004) or other pathologies such as diabetes, or in the terminal stages of respiratory disease.
- **Hypocapnia:** Deficiency of CO_2 in the blood resulting from hyperventilation, leading to respiratory alkalosis.
- **Hypoxia:** Reduction of oxygen (O_2) supply to tissue, below physiological levels, despite adequate perfusion of the tissue by blood. The extreme of hypoxia is anoxia.

There appears to be a spectrum of breathing patterns in the general population – with hyperventilation at the extreme end, and with ideal breathing at the other end. Altered patterns of breathing might emerge for a variety of

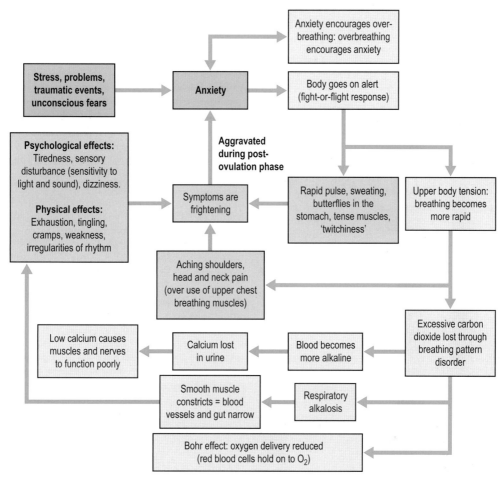

Figure 1.1 Stress–anxiety–breathing flow chart showing multiple possible effects and influences of breathing pattern disorders.

reasons, explored in this and subsequent chapters. Many people hyperventilate intermittently (in specific situations) and have a more rapid and upper-chest breathing pattern which, while not true hyperventilation, is also not an ideal pattern. That population of people who tend towards the dysfunctional end of the breathing pattern spectrum commonly experience fluctuating symptoms (fatigue for example) that have no obvious cause.

HOW COMMON IS HVS, AND WHO IS MOST AFFECTED?

De Groot (2011) reports that hyperventilation syndrome (HVS) is common in adults. The frequency in the general population is between 6% (Lum 1975) and 10% (Rice 1950). In a semirural general practice adult population,

8% of the patients who had no history of asthma demonstrated the presence of hyperventilation using the Nijmegen Questionnaire (see Ch. 6.5). Dysfunctional breathing was found to be seven times more prevalent in women (14%) than in men (2%) in this asthma study (Thomas et al 2005).

The level of dysfunctional breathing patterns in children is not known. However, in relation to 44 cases of paediatric hyperventilation, Enzer & Walker (1967) reported a ratio of females compared to males of 70%:30%. Between 1950 and 1975 The Mayo Clinic noted that the greatest number of cases of hyperventilation occurred in 13- to 15-year-old children, with no difference between boys and girls (Herman et al 1981). In Vancouver, Canada, 26.9% of children with a diagnosis of exercise-induced asthma, were found to have exercise-induced hyperventilation, and not asthma, with no difference between boys and girls (Seear et al 2005).

BPD is not a disease

The focus of this book is on understanding wide ranges of functional breathing pattern disorders (BPD) and their multiple effects. Although the impact of breathing dysfunction on health, wellbeing, energy and the potential to function normally can be profound, it is necessary to emphasize that BPDs are, as their title suggests, disorders, not diseases – although they may co-exist with diseases such as bronchiectasis or heart disease. There is no organic disease process.

This may be best appreciated by comparing BPD with poor posture. If someone habitually slouches – despite having the potential to stand and sit erect – this would not be classified as a 'disease'. Nevertheless, poor posture results in adaptive stresses and strains impacting the structures of the body, the muscles, ligaments and joints – and can result in aches, pain and restrictions. Poor posture might also compromise other systems – for example crowding and potentially modifying the behaviour of the organs housed in the abdominal and thoracic regions. Poor posture is therefore clearly not a disease, but a functional disorder that produces symptoms. Similarly, poor breathing habits, for all their multiple negative effects, are not regarded as pathological – unlike, for example, asthma, where there is usually evidence of actual pathology. And, just as poor posture can have negative influences on a variety of body areas and systems, so can BPD have aggravating effects on numerous functions. This is because breathing patterns can markedly modify the biochemistry of the body, producing profound influences on emotion, circulation, digestive function as well as on the musculoskeletal structures involved in the process of respiration. This is illustrated in Figure 1.1, which shows some of the multiple possible effects of BPD as a range of symptoms evolves, inevitably, from what is often no more than a 'pure habit'. As Lum (1975) noted:

> It has always seemed to me that hyperventilation is essentially a bad habit; a habit of breathing in such a way that the day to day level of CO_2 is relatively low. Given this basic bad habit, any physical or emotional disturbance may trigger off a chain reaction of increased ventilation, rapidly producing hypocapnic symptoms, alarm engendered by the symptoms, consequent sympathetic arousal resulting in increased ventilation and increased symptoms.

'The Great Mimic'

Having emphasized that BPDs are not a disease, they have been shown to be capable of producing symptoms that mimic real diseases.

For example:
- Pseudo-asthma – may be triggered by activity/exercise (Hammo 1999)
- Colon spasm or irritable bowel syndrome (IBS) (Ford et al 1995)
- Pseudo-angina – can be triggered by respiratory alkalosis, induced by hyperventilation.[1]

In the flowchart shown in Figure 1.1, starting from the upper centre, a link is seen between anxiety and overbreathing. Moving to the right we see several boxes highlighting sympathetic arousal ('fight or flight') that emerges from the anxiety/overbreathing background. The box on the right/middle of the chart describes a mechanical effect of overuse of accessory breathing muscles, leading to the likelihood of head, neck and shoulder pain/dysfunction. The arrows that then take us round the corner, to the bottom right of the chart, emphasize a key element of the BPD story – excessive loss of carbon dioxide (CO_2), with consequent alkalization of the bloodstream (i.e. pH rises). The long arrow that loops to the bottom left explains one of the direct effects of this CO_2/pH effect of BPD, as smooth muscles constrict, reducing blood flow to the organs, tissues and brain. Fatigue, as well as other symptoms, emerge as further compensations occur. To balance the pH, bicarbonate is excreted via the kidneys, leading to imbalances of calcium and magnesium in the system – with consequences including altered neural function, reduced pain threshold, and a variety of symptoms such as dizziness and cramps.

LUM'S PERSPECTIVE

As the catalogue of associated symptoms emerges from a background of BPD, self-confidence evaporates and secondary problems emerge. Avoidance behaviours and phobias may flourish along with feelings of extreme anxiety. Sighing and breathing discomfort are seen as signs of these understandable fears, when in fact habitual overbreathing is in and of itself a major cause of stress and anxiety (Lum 1975). Undoing years of suffering takes time and patience, as well as a good deal of detective work in identifying the source and effects of the original trigger ('stressor'), as in Figure 1.2.

Lum (1975) provided a simple adaption model (Fig. 1.2) in which stressors evoke hyperventilation, lowering CO_2 levels, leading to symptoms, including apprehension/anxiety, which involve release of chemicals involved in the fight-or-flight process, and which therefore reinforce arousal symptoms, leading to even greater hyperventilation.

---

[1]http://emedicine.medscape.com/article/153943-overview or http://bit.ly/Q4hLuB (Accessed June 2013)

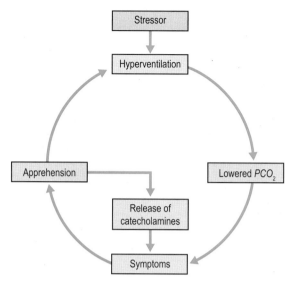

Figure 1.2 A vicious cycle.
From Lum 1975.

Breathing dysfunction (BPD) can therefore be seen to affect emotions. And while there are prescribed rituals to deal with well-understood major upheavals such as death, divorce or trauma, those who experience the frightening and worrying symptoms of chronically disordered breathing are often poorly understood. They suffer without the automatic social support given to more tangible life events or, sadly, are pigeon-holed as 'highly strung,' hypochondriacs or malingerers. It is time to make this disorder 'acceptable' – one that people are able to talk freely about and for which they are able to find effective help and treatment. An awareness and understanding of the multiple biomechanical, biochemical and psychosocial influences that can contribute to, or help maintain, BPD can offer the individual powerful resources in any rehabilitation process. These details are explained fully – with comprehensive validating support – in subsequent chapters. Included in these explorations of the causes, triggers and effects of BPDs are diagrams, lists, tables and flowcharts that summarize the sometimes complex explanatory material. A number of these carry a 'copyright-free' note, allowing them to be photocopied for use by practitioners, therapists and trainers, in order to assist their patients and clients.

Structure and function are intertwined and interdependent, in respiration as in most other body processes. Alterations in body use, such as habitually faulty posture, may interfere with thoracic and abdominal accommodation to the demands of continuous breathing. For example, shoulder and upper chest protrusions compress and limit thoracic expansion. Maintaining tense abdominal muscles limits accommodation to diaphragm movement and forces overuse of accessory breathing muscles.

Faulty breathing patterns can be due to a wide variety of reasons – from physical injury to bereavement, from a history of terror or abuse, to chronic sinusitis. Whether the cause is trivial or profound, the first step is to restore normal breathing function. If patients understand what is producing their sometimes frightening, often annoying symptoms, and that they are currently experiencing a range of symptoms (not just the one that worries them most), commitment to change is more likely.

The consequences of BPD can be seen to involve neurological, psychological, biochemical and biomechanical influences, adaptations and effects. And all because of a process (BPD) that is not pathological, and which, in most cases, is remediable by means of re-education and rehabilitation.

People seeking a diagnosis for their breathing pattern symptoms are frequently faced with the paradox of being told by their doctors, often after exhaustive tests showing that nothing is clinically wrong with them (i.e. 'no pathology'), to 'go away, have counseling, join a yoga class, relax.' (See Box 1.1.) But the symptoms continue, fuelled by habitual breathing dysfunction, and their bodies continue to signal distress. What can they do? Who can help?

To at least partially answer that question it is necessary to consider adaptation processes and how these impact on health, and a few examples are described below.

Adaptation

Travell & Simons (1992) discuss dysfunctional (paradoxical) breathing in their *Trigger Point Manual*:

> *In paradoxical respiration the chest and abdominal functions oppose each other; the patient exhales with the diaphragm, while inhaling via the thoracic muscles. Consequently a normal effort produces inadequate tidal volume, and the accessory respiratory muscles of the upper chest, including the scalenes, overwork, to exchange sufficient air. The muscular overload results from the failure to coordinate the different parts of the respiratory apparatus.*

Kolnes (2012) has noted that:

> *When breathing is withheld and/or highly costal, respiratory muscles are constantly being overactivated…the head is pulled forward, and the shoulders are hunched up and pulled forward…[and] a common observation is increased sway in the lower back, and the pelvis is tilted forward simultaneously as the back is overextended, resulting in a misalignment of the entire body. This may cause pain in the adjacent muscles of the back and pelvis. The possibility for free and deep breathing is inhibited in this position.*

Box 1.1 **When is overbreathing acceptable?**

While breathing patterns are commonly a source of a range of symptoms, there are situations and instances when rapid and shallow breathing is a response to psychological, physiological or pathological demands – or a combination of these.

- The complex connections between emotion and conditions such as anxiety and breathing are explored in depth in Chapter 5. Preparation for action stimulates overbreathing/hyperventilation when exertion seems imminent, because the raising of pH improves physiological readiness for action – provided that the exertion takes place.

- As illustrated in the flowchart (Fig. 1.1), breathing rapidly and shallowly (upper chest) leads to a reduction in acid levels in the blood (i.e. pH rises), tending towards a state of alkalosis. One of the effects of this pH change is to produce a degree of smooth muscle constriction – narrowing the 'tubes' of the body – including blood vessels. This is potentially life-saving if there happens to be intracranial bleeding, because hypocapnia (reduced carbon dioxide levels), encourages cerebral ischemia (Curley et al 2010).

- In conditions where the system is too acidic (metabolic acidosis), possibly as a result of liver or kidney disease, severe chronic obstructive pulmonary disease (COPD) or in toxaemia during advanced stages of pregnancy, hyperventilation may be an appropriate means whereby excess acid levels are reduced (Kellum 2007, Jensen et al 2008).

- In the latter stages of the menstrual cycle (post-ovulation) progesterone levels increase naturally. Since progesterone stimulates respiration, women with an existing tendency towards upper-chest overbreathing are more likely to hyperventilate (Ott et al 2006, Slatkovska et al 2006).

- Active exercise results in increased levels of acid products in the body (lactic, pyruvic, etc.), making it physiologically appropriate to hyperventilate when running (Hammo 1999). See also Chapter 7.6: Breathing pattern disorders and the athlete.

- Nasal congestion or obstruction can lead to alteration of the breathing pattern, as is fully explained in Chapter 2.3 (Bartley 2006).

- Conditions that involve chronic pelvic pain and abdominal splinting are commonly associated with breathing pattern disorders. The anatomical and structural connection between the pelvic floor and the diaphragm help to explain this association (Haugstad & Haugstad 2006). See Chapter 8.1.

- General levels of deconditioning (the opposite of aerobic fitness) lead to altered forms of energy production (anaerobic glycolysis) that encourages acidosis – hence a greater tendency to hyperventilation (Nixon & Andrews 1996, Smith & Taylor 2008).

- Individuals who are acclimatized to living at sea level, for example, who travel to cities such as Mexico City, Johannesburg or Denver – all around 2000 metres above sea level – are likely to hyperventilate (Harding & Mills 1983, Hodkinson 2011).

- Early wound repair requires fibroblasts to differentiate into myofibroblasts, as well as requiring increased collagen synthesis, so generating contractions to facilitate wound closure 'architecturally' (Falanga 2005, Ingber 2003). Hypoxia due to hyperventilation (HVS) – often associated with respiratory alkalosis–beneficially stimulates collagen synthesis, with TGF-β1 as a key feature (Jensen et al 2008).

In the context of misuse of the structures associated with breathing, it is useful to also consider overuse. Since we average between 10 and 14 cycles of inhalation/exhalation per minute during 'normal' breathing (~14 400 to 20 000 repetitions daily), and up to 30 cycles per minute (~40 000 + daily) when hyperventilating – there is an absolute certainty of repetitive overuse of the structures involved in breathing (Costanzo 2007, Sherwood 2006).

How well is the individual adapting?

A general sequence of progressive, adaptive dysfunctions, resulting from BPD, that evolve over time, has been described by Garland (1994). These adaptations follow from, or are commonly associated with, patterns involving hyperventilation or chronic upper-chest breathing:

- A degree of visceral stasis and pelvic floor weakness develops, together with an imbalance between increasingly weak abdominal muscles and increasingly tight erector spinae muscles. (See 'Janda's crossed syndromes' discussion in Chapter 2.2.)

- Fascial restriction occurs from the central tendon, via the pericardial fascia, all the way up to the basiocciput.

- The upper ribs will be elevated with sensitive costal cartilage tension on palpation. (See discussion of assessment and treatment of elevated and depressed ribs in Chapters 6.2 and 7.2.)

- The thoracic spine will be disturbed by virtue of the lack of normal motion of the articulation with the ribs, and sympathetic outflow from this area may be affected (see notes on assessment and treatment of thoracic spine restrictions in Chapters 6.2 and 7.2).

- Accessory muscle hypertonia, notably affecting the scalenes, upper trapezius and levator scapulae, will be palpable and observable. (See notes on assessment and treatment of these in Chapters 6.2 and 7.2.)
- Fibrosis will develop in these muscles, as will myofascial trigger points; Chapters 6.2 and 7.2.
- The cervical spine will become progressively rigid with a fixed lordosis being a common feature in the lower cervical spine.
- A reduction in the mobility of the 2nd cervical segment and second rib and disturbance of vagal outflow from this region is likely.
- Also worth noting in relation to breathing function and dysfunction are quadratus lumborum and iliopsoas, and transversus, all of which merge fibres with the diaphragm. Quadratus and psoas are postural muscles, with a propensity to shortening when stressed: the impact of such shortening, uni- or bilaterally, can be seen to have major implications for respiratory function, whether the primary feature of such a dysfunction lies in diaphragmatic or muscular distress. (Assessment and treatment methods for these muscles will be found in Sections 6 and 7.)
- Garland concludes his summary of evolving dysfunction with the elegant phrase: '*These changes run physically and physiologically against biologically sustainable patterns, and in a vicious circle, promote abnormal function, which alters structure, which then disallows a return to normal function.*'
- This is because as adaptation progresses, a point is reached where adaptive capacity is exhausted – and symptoms inevitably emerge involving pain, restriction and increasing levels of dysfunction.

Before focusing on localized dysfunctional patterns that have the potential to add to the patient's stress burden and to have a direct impact on breathing function, a brief diversion will be made to consider questions of assessment of the patient's adaptation status.

Has adaptation reached the point of exhaustion?

As adaptive processes progress, such as those described by Garland and others, above, compensation becomes increasingly difficult, until ultimately, as described in Selye's stress syndrome model (1980), exhaustion is reached and structures break down.

Since all therapeutic interventions add additional layers of adaptive demand, clinical thinking might include questions such as:

- How can we best evaluate this individual's potential for further compensation/decompensation, adaptation?

- Just how compromised is the patient's adaptive capacity?
- What potential for recovery remains?

BIOLOGICAL RHYTHMS AS A GUIDE

A chronically sick person can be described as being in a state of decompensation (Nixon & Andrews 1996) where adaptive processes are exhausted and compensation patterns have become pathological. As the adaptive capacities of the body are strained ever further, evidence of a breakdown of compensatory functions manifests as ill health and symptoms.

There are a number of ways in which it is possible to gain a 'snapshot' indication as to how well or how badly an individual is coping with the current load of stressors – whether these are biochemical, biomechanical or psychosocial, or a combination of these.

The more widely basic biological rhythms fluctuate throughout the day, (whether this represents blood pressure, heart rate, blood sugar levels, or anything else which is periodically measurable), the less well homeostatic functions are operating. This is an obvious method for eliciting evidence of homeostatic efficiency (Ringsdorf & Cheraskin 1980).

EVIDENCE OF FUNCTIONAL CHANGE WITH TREATMENT

Patients can be said to be capable of improvement if they are seen to improve by virtue of positive objective and subjective changes, over time, in response to therapeutic intervention and/or rehabilitation protocols.

For example if:

- Painful structures become less so
- Breathing function improves or normalizes
- Tight structures become looser
- Short structures lengthen
- Weak structures strengthen
- Posture and balance improve or normalize
- Muscle firing patterns approach normal
- Functional changes are reported – 'I can now walk 100 yards without too much breathlessness/difficulty', or 'I can now get dressed on my own without help'.

These features are the ones commonly measured, sometimes numerically ('give a score out of 10'), by use of questionnaires, body charts, and sometimes purely verbally. Some are objective and some subjective, and if signs of improvement are not realized as a therapeutic programme progresses, a review of the strategies involved is called for and shared care considered.

Patient categorization

Therapeutic objectives need to be realistic. It may be possible broadly to categorize patients into those who will recover either with or without intervention (keeping in mind the natural tendency toward normality reflected in recognition of homeostatic function, as discussed below). These individuals may be classified under the heading *fixable*.

Many patients are capable of improvement, although perhaps not to a point of complete symptom-free state. These individuals may be classified as *maintainable*.

The previous group is commonly distinguishable from patients whose condition is such that the best hope is a degree of *containment* – a holding together of an individual in decline, offering some respite from symptoms, perhaps, and an easing of the downward spiral.

Use of *fix*, *maintain* and *contain* categorizations allows for realistic plans of action to evolve. It should go without saying that there is, in such a model, a need for an inbuilt willingness to modify the assessment, and therefore to alter strategies, should new evidence emerge.

Homeostasis and heterostasis

The body is a self-healing mechanism. Broken bones mend and cuts usually heal, and most health disturbances – from infections to digestive upsets – get better with or without treatment (often faster without!), and, in a healthy state, there exists a constant process for normalization and health promotion. This is called *homeostasis*.

However homeostatic functions can become overwhelmed by too many tasks and demands as a result of any, or all, of a selection of negative impacts involving biochemical, psychosocial and/or biomechanical factors, as well as inborn features. Acquired habits involving poor posture and breathing dysfunction may well be part of this mix of adaptive stressors (see Fig. 1.3AB)

When adaptive capacity is exhausted the situation modifies from homeostasis to heterostasis, at which time help is needed – assessment and treatment (Selye 1952).

Treatment can take a number of forms, which are usually classifiable as involving one of three broad strategies:

1. Methods that aim to reduce the load impacting the body, reducing or removing as many of the undesirable adaptive factors as possible that might be overloading defence mechanisms.
2. Enhancing, improving, modulating the defence and repair processes via specific interventions or non-specific, constitutional methods.
3. Treating the symptoms, while making sure that nothing is being done to add further to the burden of the defence mechanisms.

Not all available therapeutic measures need to be employed, because once the load on the adaptation and repair processes has reduced sufficiently, a degree of normal homeostatic self-regulating function is automatically restored, and the healing process commences.

Therapy as a stress factor

A corollary to this perspective of therapy notes that, since almost any form of 'treatment' involves further adaptive demands, therapeutic interventions need to be tailored to the ability of the individual to respond to the treatment. Excessive adaptive demands made of an individual, already in a state of adaptive exhaustion, are likely to make matters worse.

A clinical rule of thumb adopted by one of the authors (LC) is that the more ill a patient is, the more symptoms that are being displayed, and the weaker is the evidence of vitality, the lighter, gentler, and more 'constitutional'

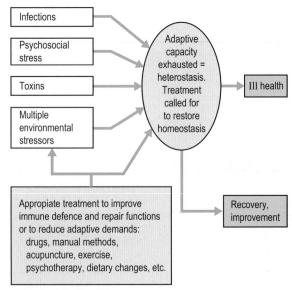

Figure 1.3B Heterostasis.

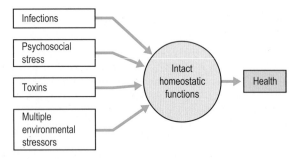

Figure 1.3A Homeostasis.

(whole person) the intervention needs to be. Whereas a robust, vital individual might well respond positively to several simultaneous therapeutic interventions, someone who is more frail might well collapse under such an adaptive therapeutic assault. For the frail patient, a single modification, or therapeutic change, might be called for, with ample time allowed for the individual to adapt to therapeutic measures. The 'art' of health care demands the employment of safe and appropriate interventions to suit the particular needs of each individual – taking full account of their ability to respond, and with ample time allowed for positive adaptive changes to manifest.

CONCLUSION

Disordered breathing patterns affect different patients in different ways. Some are more inclined to mental distress, fear, anxiety, and co-existing loss of self-confidence. Others may exhibit musculoskeletal and more physical symptoms, such as neck and shoulder problems, chronic pain and fatigue. See Figure 1.1 for a sense of the possible range of symptoms. Many have a combination of both mental and physical factors, so it is very useful to have a variety of therapeutic approaches available in order to match treatment to both symptom manifestation and underlying etiology. BPD in one person may call for breathing rehabilitation exercises accompanied by psychotherapy/counselling; in another, dietary modification and stress reduction could be merited; while in another, enhancement of immune function and structural mobilization using bodywork and exercise may be considered the most appropriate interventions. In all instances of BPD, however, breathing patterns will need to be at the heart of therapeutic interventions – replacing current habits with improved ones.

This book presents a variety of approaches derived from physiotherapy, osteopathy, psychology and other complementary approaches aimed at assessing and treating the common debilitating disorders caused by breathing pattern disorders.

The myriad symptoms related to hyperventilation and breathing pattern disorders at first glance may seem hard to relate to simply the rate and depth of breathing. A full explanation of this relationship is explained in subsequent chapters, particularly in Chapter 3 where clarification is offered as to how biochemistry transforms inappropriate breathing patterns to a diverse range of symptoms – including loss of balance, indigestion, paresthesias, visual disturbances and angina pain.

Ideally, the matching of breathing style to the individual's immediate circumstances is normally achieved smoothly and automatically, involving such diverse factors as immediate or anticipated energy requirements, expected physical activity, and required postural changes. However, psychological factors can also trigger a breathing pattern that might be appropriate to an emergency situation, when no such situation exists, with the mismatch having many negative consequences. The factors that might lead to this include conditioned reactions to past events, exaggerated expectations of danger, and habits manifesting inappropriately – leading to breathing becoming dysfunctional, interfering with the steady delivery of oxygen to the body and brain (and myriad other symptoms) – for strictly emotional reasons based on reactivated memories and erroneous expectations.

See Chapters 6.4 and 7.4 for further exploration of these issues.

Where next?

The overview of BPD that has been offered in this chapter, with its widespread influences and effects, emerging from a background of equally widespread etiological influences, demands that we return to the foundations of breathing in order to understand what is required for rehabilitation.

In the next chapters an insightful embryological and evolutionary perspective, relative to respiratory function, is followed by consideration of structural, biochemical and functional features, as well as a detailed evaluation of nasal physiology in relation to respiration.

REFERENCES

Bartley, J., 2006. Nasal congestion and hyperventilation syndrome. American Journal of Rhinology 19, 607–611.

Cluff, R.A., 1984. Chronic hyperventilation and its treatment by physiotherapy: discussion paper. Journal of the Royal Society of Medicine 77, 855–862.

Costanzo, L.S., 2007. Physiology, fourth ed. Lippincott Williams & Wilkins, Philadelphia.

Curley, G., et al., 2010. Hypocapnia and the injured brain: More harm than benefit. Critical Care Medicine 38 (5), 1348–1359.

Da Costa, J.M., 1871. On irritable heart: a clinical study of a form of

functional cardiac disorder and its consequences. American Journal of Medicine 61, 17–51.

De Groot, E.P., 2011. Breathing abnormalities in children with breathlessness. Paediatr Respir Rev 12 (1), 83–87.

Enzer, N.B., Walker, P.A., 1967. Hyperventilation syndrome in childhood. A review of 44 cases. J Pediatrics 70, 521–532.

Falanga, V., 2005. Wound healing and its impairment in the diabetic foot. Lancet 366, 1736–1743.

Ford, M., Camilleri, M., Hanson, R., 1995. Hyperventilation, central autonomic control, and colonic tone in humans. Gut 37, 499–504.

Garland, W., 1994. Somatic changes in hyperventilating subject. Presentation at International Society for the Advancement of Respiratory Psychophysiology Congress, Paris, 1994.

Gardner, W., 2004. Hyperventilation. Am. J. Respir. Crit. Care Med. 15, 2.

Haldane, J.S., Poulton, E.P., 1908. The effects of want of oxygen on respiration. Journal of Physiology 37, 390.

Hammo, A., 1999. Exercise-induced hyperventilation: a pseudo-asthma syndrome. Ann Allergy Asthma Immunol 82, 574–578.

Harding, R.M., Mills, F.J., 1983. Aviation medicine. Problems of altitude I: hypoxia and hyperventilation. British Medical Journal (Clinical research ed.) 286 (6375), 1408–1410.

Haugstad, G., Haugstad, T., Kirste, U., et al., 2006. Posture, movement patterns, and body awareness in women with chronic pelvic pain. J Psychosom Res 61 (5), 637–644.

Herman, S., Stickler, G., Lucas, A., 1981. Hyperventilation syndrome in children and adolescents: long-term follow-up. Pediatrics 67, 183–187.

Hodkinson, P.D., 2011. Acute exposure to altitude. Journal of the Royal Army Medical Corps, 157 (1), 85–91.

Hornsveld, H., Garsson, B., 1997. Hyperventilation syndrome: an elegant but scientifically untenable concept. The Netherlands Journal of Medicine 50 (1), 13–20.

Ingber, D.E., Tensegrity, I., 2003. Cell structure and hierarchical systems biology. J Cell Sci 116 (7), 1157–1173.

Innocenti, D.M., 1987. Chronic hyperventilation syndrome. Cash's textbook of chest, heart and vascular disorders for physiotherapists, fourth ed. Faber and Faber, London, pp. 537–549.

Jensen, D., Duffin, J., Lam, Y.-M., et al., 2008. Physiological mechanisms of hyperventilation during human pregnancy. Respiratory Physiology & Neurobiology 161 (1), 76–78.

Kerr, W.J., Dalton, J.A., Gliebe, P.A., 1937. Some physical phenomena associated with the anxiety states and their relation to hyper-ventilation. Annals of Internal Medicine 11, 961.

Kellum, J., 2007. Disorders of acid-base balance. Crit Care Med 35 (11), 2630–2636.

Kolnes, L.-J., 2012. Embodying the body in anorexia nervosa – a physio-therapeutic approach. Journal of Bodywork & Movement Therapies 16 (3), 281–288.

Lewis, T., 1940. The soldier's heart and the effort syndrome. Shaw, London.

Lum, L.C., 1975. Hyperventilation: the tip and the iceberg. J Psychosom Res 19, 375–383.

Lum, L.C., 1977. Breathing exercises in the treatment of hyperventilation and chronic anxiety states. Chest Heart and Stroke Journal 2, 6–11.

Magarian, G.J., 1982. Hyperventilation syndromes: infrequently recognized common expressions of anxiety and stress. Medicine 61, 219–236.

Nixon, P., Andrews, J., 1996. A study of anaerobic threshold in chronic fatigue syndrome (CFS). Biol Psychol 43, 264.

Ott, H., Mattle, V., Zimmermann, U.S., et al., 2006. Symptoms of premenstrual syndrome may be caused by hyperventilation. Fertility and Sterility 86 (4), 1001.e17–1001.e19.

Perera, J., 1988. The hazards of heavy breathing. New Scientist 3 Dec 1988, pp 46–49.

Resta, O., Bonfitto, P., Sabato, R., et al., 2004. Prevalence of obstructive sleep apnoea in a sample of obese women: Effect of menopause. Diabetes Nutr Metab 17, 296–303.

Rice, R.L., 1950. Symptom patterns of the hyperventilation syndrome. American J Medicine 8, 691–700.

Ringsdorf, Jr., W.m., Cheraskin, E., 1980. Another look at the 'ideal' serum cholesterol level? Arch Intern Med 140 (4), 580–581.

Seear, M., Wensley, D., West, N., 2005. How accurate is the diagnosis of exercise induced asthma among Vancouver schoolchildren? Arch Dis Child 90, 898–902.

Selye, H., 1952. The story of the adaptation syndrome. ACTA, Montreal, Canada.

Selye, H., 1980. Stress and holistic medicine. Fam Community Health 3 (2), 85–88.

Sherwood, L., 2006. Fundamentals of Physiology: A Human Perspective, Thomson Brooks/Cole, pp. 12–18.

Slatkovska, L., Jensen, D., Davies, G., et al., 2006. Phasic menstrual cycle effects on the control of breathing in healthy women. Respiratory Physiology & Neurobiology 154 (3), 379–388.

Smith, A., Taylor, C., 2008. Analysis of blood gases and acid-base balance. Surgery 26 (3), 86–90.

Soley, M.H., Shock, N.W., 1938. The aetiology of effort syndrome. American Journal of Medical Science 196, 840.

Studer, R., Danuser, B., Hildebrandt, H., et al., 2011. Hyperventilation complaints in music performance anxiety among classical music students. Journal of Psychosomatic Research, 70 (6), 557–564.

Thomas, M., McKinley, R.K., Freeman, E., et al., 2005. The prevalence of dysfunctional breathing in adults in the community with and without asthma. Prim Care Respir J 14, 78–82.

Timmons, B.H., Ley, R. (Eds.), 1994. Behavioral and psychological approaches to breathing disorders. Plenum, New York, p. 115.

Travell, J., Simons, D., 1992. Myofascial Pain & Dysfunction. Williams & Wilkins, Baltimore. Vol. 2 Lower Body.

Vernon, H.M., 1909. The production of prolonged apnea in man. Journal of Physiology 38, 18.

Wood, P., 1941. Da Costa's syndrome (or effort syndrome). British Medical Journal 1, 767.

Dynamic Neuromuscular Stabilization: developmental kinesiology: breathing stereotypes and postural-locomotion function

Pavel Kolar, Alena Kobesova, Petra Valouchova, Petr Bitnar

Breathing, like postural function, is an essential function of any living organism. However, ideal functional models or norms for either breathing or human postural patterns are not universally defined. Various authors and scientific articles define such basic 'functional norms' quite differently. Although, as Dr. Lewit states, function is as real as structure; physiology is as relevant as anatomy; function forms structure and structure serves function, and ideal functional stereotypes are to this day not unequivocally defined as anatomical norms tend to be. Specifically, from a clinical perspective, there is no consensus regarding whether a given individual's breathing pattern or posture can be assessed as ideal or incorrect. Two experienced clinicians will assess the same patient quite differently. They will select different additional examinations and they will differ in opinions regarding the primary etiology of symptoms and may, quite noticeably, differ in the selected treatment strategy. It can be quite difficult for an independent and knowledgeable observer to decide whose approach is correct.

Dynamic Neuromuscular Stabilization (DNS) is an approach based on developmental kinesiology and defines functional norms from a developmental perspective. Compared to many mammals, humans at birth are extremely anatomically and functionally immature – this includes the central nervous system (CNS) (Vojta 2004, Vojta & Schweizer 2009). Structural development is incomplete; e.g. a newborn does not present with definite spinal curvatures (Kapandji 1992, Lord et al. 1995), they are barrel-chested (Openshaw et al. 1984) and their foot structure is not fully formed (Volpon 1994). A newborn has an immature CNS and as a consequence immature muscle function, and postural-locomotor, breathing and sphincter functions.

Following birth, the trajectory of intrauterine development more or less continues and CNS maturation is a significant aspect of this development, including myelination, synaptogenesis, apoptosis and neurotransmitter activation. In conjunction with a certain level of CNS immaturity, a healthy infant presents with typical postural-locomotor patterns that are characteristic for a given age

(Hermsen-van Wanrooy 2006, Vojta 2004, Vojta & Schweizer 2009). Therefore, it can be said that movement patterns are genetically determined and specific only to humans. This includes the breathing pattern and functional norms of a human that depend on CNS control and on the quality of anatomical structures whose corresponding function they serve.

Functional norms are encoded within the CNS in the form of programmes and they are altered in different ways in pathological states.

DIAPHRAGM FUNCTION FROM A DEVELOPMENTAL PERSPECTIVE

In a human embryo, the origin of the diaphragm is concentrated in the cervical region, possibly as an extension of the rectus abdominis muscle (or the 'cervical portion' of the rectus cervicis muscle). During development, the diaphragm descends caudally and tilts forward. This development continues after birth and the diaphragm attains its definite position in an almost transverse plane between 4–6 months.

The muscular portion of the diaphragm has two main parts with different embryonic origins: costal and crural (Pickering & Jones 2002). They are formed by different types of fibres and have specific influence on the ribcage and purposeful movement; e.g. during vomiting or belching, the costal fibres are active while the crural fibres around the esophagus are inactive (Abe et al.1993). The dorsal mesesophagus and mesogastrium partially contribute to the development of the crural portion, which plays an important role in the sphincter function of the diaphragm (Langman 1981).

During ontogenetic development, the diaphragm initially participates in respiration (Murphy & Woodrum 1998). With completion of the neonatal developmental stage (the first 28 days of life), the diaphragm begins to contribute in both postural and sphincter functions. The non-respiratory functions of the diaphragm emerge as the postural anti-gravity role develops – the infant begins to prop up onto forearms and lifts the head when prone or in supine lifts the lower extremities (LE) above the mat (Hermsen-van Wanrooy 2006, Vojta 2004, Vojta & Schweizer 2009). This combined postural-respiratory function of the diaphragm is an important prerequisite for trunk stabilization followed by locomotor movement of the upper and lower extremities (Hemborg et al. 1985, Hodges & Gandevia 2000a, Hodges & Gandevia 2000b, Kolar et al. 2010).

The diaphragm of a healthy newborn is flat and positioned cranially (Devlieger et al 1991); the thorax short and cone-shaped (Openshaw et al. 1984). The posterior rib angles are ventral to the spinous processes, and neither the spinous nor the transverse processes have a definitive shape. The transverse processes exhibit a progressive posterior and inferior angulation with age and move down the thoracic spine. The facet joints angulate accordingly (Lord et al. 1995). The distances between the jugular fossa and the xyphoid process and between the xyphoid process and the pubic symphysis differ from an adult. The newborn has a 'short' thorax and a 'long' stomach. The thoracic cavity of the newborn is limited by the thymus and diaphragm excursion is limited by the large liver. Only breathing movements are realized by the activity of the diaphragm; it does not yet participate in postural and sphincter functions (Murphy & Woodrum 1998).

With CNS maturation, muscle co-activation develops when the neonatal stage is completed. Simultaneous and balanced activity of the agonists and the antagonists allows for active body posture within the gravitational field. An infant no longer only passively lies on the mat, but begins to lift the head and the extremities above the mat and stabilization, support and equilibrium functions develop (Hermsen-van Wanrooy 2006, Vojta 2004, Vojta & Schweizer 2009).

Simultaneous and symmetrical co-activation of the diaphragm, abdominal, back and pelvic muscles allows for the interconnection between breathing pattern and stabilization function (Hodges et al. 2007, Hodges & Gandevia 2000a, Kolar et al. 2009). This combined muscle function is relatively challenging and is only possible in a healthy CNS, which allows for perfect motor control (Assaiante et al. 2005, Hodges & Gandevia 2000a). A disturbance in CNS control causes not only a deficit in movement patterns, including the breathing pattern, but also structural deformities (Koman et al. 2004). A child with a developmental CNS dysfunction will never demonstrate an ideal skeletal anatomy.

Central motor programmes coordinate muscles that significantly influence growth plates. If muscle function is balanced and ensures a symmetrical pull in the area of the growth plates, it is very likely that the anatomical development will be correct. Muscle imbalance during ontogenesis results in less than ideal skeletal development. In extreme cases (e.g. cerebral palsy), various deformities can be observed in extremity joints (e.g. coxa valga antetorta neurogenes) and the thorax (Koman et al. 2004). Respiratory function will then be modified not only as a result of less than ideal CNS control but also as a result of an abnormal shape and position of the spine, ribs, clavicles and other structures.

In a physiologically normal situation, at 3 months the stabilization quality of muscle synergies increases, the cervical and thoracic spine straightens and development of lower costal breathing begins. At 4½ months, when the differentiation of extremity function occurs in the form of support and stepping (grasping) movements, the differentiation function of the muscles of the trunk and the abdominal cavity continues. A child begins to use one upper extremity (UE) and one lower extremity for support and the opposite UE and LE for stepping. This differentiated function allows for active grasp and later for crawling and ambulation (Hermsen-van Wanrooy 2006, Vojta 2004).

Trunk muscles must serve as a support base for extremity function within the framework of such movement patterns. Through intra-abdominal pressure regulation, they contribute to spinal stabilization and, at the same time, ensure respiratory function and influence other visceral functions (food intake, peristalsis, defecation, vomiting, etc.). At 4½ months, the infant also begins to coordinate breathing with vocalization.

In the 6-month-old, costal breathing is fully established. While the combined activity of the lumbar portion of the diaphragm continues to develop, during breathing, it must simultaneously stabilize the proximal insertion of the psoas muscle which pulls in a distal direction when the child supports on the palms and proximal thighs. Also, control mechanisms for both striated- and smooth-muscle esophageal regions are incompletely developed in neonates, participating in reflux mechanism in newborns and infants (Staiano et al. 2007). The combined sphincter function of the esophagus and the diaphragm fully matures in the first 6 months of life.

DEFINITION OF AN IDEAL RESPIRATORY PATTERN FROM A DEVELOPMENTAL PERSPECTIVE

The motor function of the thorax is important for breathing and for postural (stabilization) function. Two types of thoracic movements are distinguished. The first is related to the movement of the spine, the second occurs in the costovertebral joints independently of the movements of the spine. Clinical distinction of such movements plays a fundamental role in the assessment of the quality of respiratory and stabilization functions.

With spinal flexion, the ribs descend and the intercostal spaces narrow. With spinal extension, the entire process is reversed and the thorax positions cranially. The rib cage also moves during thoracic rotation (Kapandji 1992). In a physiologically normal situation, the thorax should be able to move independently of the thoracic spine and vice versa, i.e. the thoracic spine segments straighten without co-movement from the thorax. A disturbance in this function has a marked kinesiological or pathokinesiological significance. This movement, or the positioning of the neutral 'lower' alignment of the thorax with a simultaneous straightening of the spine, depends on the costovertebral articulations, or rib movements. In good health, this posture is observed as early as in a 4½-month-old infant.

During breathing, the ribs elevate and descend around an axis leading from the centre of the head of the rib obliquely and dorsolaterally to the costotransverse joint (Kapandji 1992). The ribs also move with muscle

activation during trunk stabilization; therefore, independently of breathing.

Given that the top seven pairs of ribs are attached anteriorly to the sternum by cartilage, their movement is always linked to movement of the sternum. In a normal pattern, the sternum moves anteriorly (Fig. 2.1.1A) rather than cranially (Fig. 2.1.1B), which can be observed in an accessory (upper chest) breathing pattern.

With diaphragm and intercostal muscle activation, the thoracic cavity enlarges anteriorly and, at the same time, laterally as a result of rib curvature. During exertion, the lateral 'opening' of the lower ribs is also accentuated by the contraction of the diaphragm and by its pressure against the internal organs (Fig. 2.1.2). Breathing and stabilization movements are small in the area of the manubrium and first ribs and are greatest in the area of the longest ribs (especially the rib pairs 7 and 8). In a physiologically normal pattern, the sternum moves in an anterior-posterior (Fig. 2.1.1A) direction, which is allowed for by rotation at the sternoclavicular joint. In a non-physiological breathing pattern, involving mainly vertical (craniocaudal) sternal movement (Fig. 2.1.1B), the movement in the sternoclavicular joint is substituted by movement in the acromioclavicular joint during breathing and also during postural stabilization. This alters the position of the clavicles, which become more horizontal. This situation occurs typically in incorrect positioning of the thorax as a result of dominant accessory muscles, especially during their shortening.

Therefore, the initial alignment of the thorax is essential for physiologically balanced breathing and postural stabilization of the trunk. The neutral position, in which breathing and stabilization should occur without excessive activation of accessory muscles (i.e. sternocleidomastoids, scalenes, pectorales) (Lewit 2010) is considered an alignment of the thorax in which the clavicles form a 25–30-degree angle from the horizontal while the thoracic spine is erect, though great individual variation occurs (Todd 1912).

The alignment of the rib cage should ideally correspond to the position of the pelvis (Fig. 2.1.3A, 2.1.3C). The surmise is that when the thoracic spine is erect, the rib cage is positioned parallel to the pelvis and the centrum tendineum of the diaphragm is on a horizontal plane. Such alignment of the thorax allows for the centrum tendineum to act in a caudal direction, as a piston against the pelvic floor (Fig 2.1.3A, 2.1.3C). From a developmental perspective, this harmony and the above-described alignment of the pelvis and the thorax to one another should already be ensured at the age of 4½ months. This is the time when stabilization of the thorax, spine and pelvis in the sagittal plane is completed as a basic prerequisite to locomotor function of the extremities. In later stages, when the child attains quadruped, sitting and standing positions, the child uses the ideal breathing pattern described above, activates the same stabilizing muscle

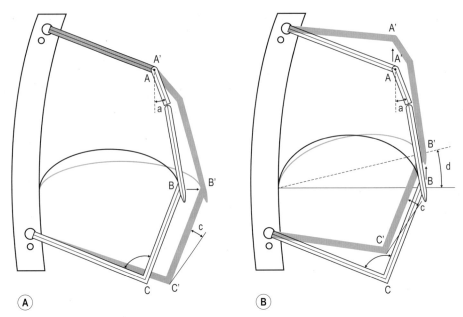

Figure 2.1.1 A Optimal 'diaphragmatic' breathing: position of the ribs in transverse plane remains more or less the same during respiratory cycle; widening of the intercostal spaces and lower chest cavity occurs (distance C–C'); movement of the sternum is mainly ventro-dorsal (distance B–B', 'a' angle); with inspiration the diaphragm descends caudally and flattens while maintaining its position in sagittal plane. **B** Accessory breathing pattern: cranial movement of the whole chest occurs with every inspiration (A–A' distance, B–B', C–C' distance); insufficient widening of the lower chest and intercostal spaces (distance C–C') and cranial movement of the xyphoid (distance B–B'); diaphragmatic excursion is smaller and as the chest lifts the diaphragm goes into a more oblique position ('d' angle) without the ideal flattening.

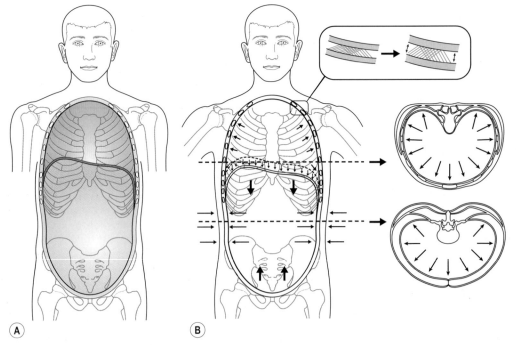

Figure 2.1.2 During exercise or any postural activity, eccentric activity of the stabilizing muscles occurs except for diaphragm and pelvic floor which activate in a concentric manner. The diaphragm descends in a caudal direction, pressurizing intra-abdominal content from above, pelvic floor activates against; muscles of the chest and abdominal wall activate eccentrically like a belt, thus intra-abdominal pressure is increased, stabilizing the spine. Comparing the resting state (**A**), to that of exertion/postural tasks (**B**) the chest and abdominal cavity expand proportionally in ventral, dorsal and lateral directions.

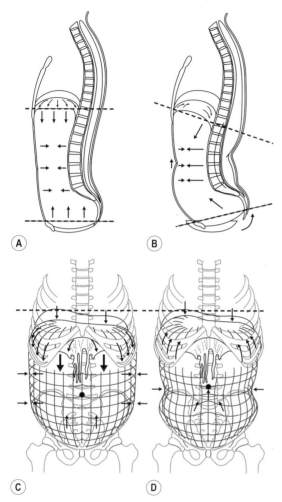

Figure 2.1.3 A, C Physiologically balanced coordination between the diaphragm, abdominal muscles and the pelvic floor. **A** Proper alignment between diaphragm and pelvic floor – their axis is almost horizontal and parallel. **C** During postural activities the abdominal cavity expands, diaphragmatic costal attachments are stabilized (small arrows), and the centrum tendineum descends (large arrows). **B, D** Pathological coordination between the diaphragm, abdominal muscles and the pelvic floor. **B** Common type of postural disturbance: anterior pelvic tilt, cranial 'inspiratory' position of the chest, diaphragm and pelvic axis oblique: this malposition does not allow for ideal postural coordination and optimal intra-abdominal pressure regulation, and results in substitutive hyperactivity of the paraspinal muscles. **D** Abnormal muscle coordination during postural activities: abdominal wall 'hollowing', diaphragmatic costal attachments are not stabilized, inversion function of the diaphragm (arrows), and the centrum tendineum remains in a cranial position.

co-activation during exertion and the same mutual alignment between the pelvis and the thorax while the spine is erect.

POSTURE AND POSTURAL FUNCTION OF THE DIAPHRAGM

The function of the diaphragm is usually analyzed from the perspective of vital functions, such as breathing and metabolism. Much less work focuses on its postural function (Hodges & Gandevia 2000a, Hodges & Gandevia 2000b, Kolar et al. 2009, Kolar et al. 2012). Within the context of posture, individual authors analyze the function of the diaphragm from the perspective of symmetrical (balance) functions (Caron et al. 2004), while others focus on assessment in standing (Butler et al. 2001, Caron et al. 2004) or sitting (Takazakura et al. 2004). However, the term *posture* is much broader.

Posture is understood to be an active maintenance of body segments against the action of external forces, from which gravity has the greatest impact. Posture, however, is not a synonym to erect standing or sitting, but rather a component of any position (i.e. straight head position of an infant in prone or LE lifting against gravity in supine), especially of every movement with locomotion. Posture is the main prerequisite for locomotion. Sherrington wrote: 'Posture follows movement like a shadow' (Sherrington 1931). If any movement is broken down into phases, short time segments of a given motion are obtained, or 'frozen phases' (Janda 1972), from which posture can be derived. This involves joint alignment in a static position, which is a component of movement.

Postural stabilization is the active (muscle) maintenance of body segments within the gravitational field and against the activity of external forces, controlled by the CNS. In a static scenario (i.e. sitting, standing), relative joint stability is ensured through muscle activity. This stability allows for resistance against the gravitational force in a given position. Postural stabilization, however, is a component of all movements. During every movement of a body segment that requires force production (i.e. lifting or holding an object, extremity movement against or without resistance, push-off effort, ball throw), a necessary contractile muscle force is always generated to overcome the resistance. It is then transferred to force moments in a segmental pulley system within the human body and elicits reaction muscle forces within the entire muscular system. The biological purpose of this reaction is to enforce the individual movement segments (joints) to achieve the most stable 'punctum fixum' and for the joint segments to resist external forces. The strength of the interconnection between the segments can be, to a certain extent, altered and several anatomical segments in this chain can be interconnected into one unit. The desired strength of the interconnections is achieved by coordinated activity of the agonists, antagonists and other muscle groups. For movement, the trunk needs to be stabilized and, at the same time, sufficient freedom of movement needs to be allowed for in the joints of the extremities. Coordination of concentric, isometric and especially eccentric muscle activity is required to achieve this goal.

No purposeful movement (including extremities) can be executed without stabilization at the insertion of the muscles performing a given movement (in other words, the segment to which the muscles performing the movement attach, needs to be stabilized). For example, hip flexion cannot be performed without stabilization of the spine and the pelvis. A stabilized spine and pelvis ensure stabilization of the hip flexor tendons (rectus femoris, iliopsoas, sartorius) (Fig. 2.1.4) and protect the segment

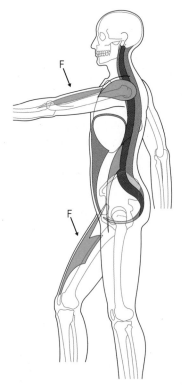

Figure 2.1.4 The muscles stabilizing the shoulder, pelvic girdle and spine. Under normal physiological conditions, the stabilizers: in grey – the diaphragm, the pelvic floor, all the sections of the abdominal wall and spinal extensors – automatically activate prior to purposeful movement (e.g. hip flexion provided by the muscles in blue: m. iliopsoas, rectus femoris, sartorius) to establish a stable base ('feed-forward mechanism'). In normal subjects, the stabilizing function of the trunk (in grey) muscles control shear of lumbar segments during hip flexion. Well-balanced activity between the deep neck flexors and spinal extensors is necessary for stabilization in the cervical and upper thoracic region. F, force (extremities activate against gravity or other force).

in this way from being overexerted during movement (Kolar et al. 2010, Kolar et al. 2012).

Movement in the segment (in this case, a hip joint) then includes spinal extensors, abdominal muscles, diaphragm, pelvic floor, etc., which prevent movement in the insertional region of the flexors. The activity of the stabilizing muscles generates activity in other muscles that are insertional related. These muscles then ensure stabilization in other segments. This mechanism leads to functionally interlinked stabilization of the entire trunk during movement. Segmental stabilization is biomechanically interconnected and depends on coordinated muscle activity controlled by the CNS. From the perspective of ontogenesis, these principles are already fully utilized at 5 months of age. The coordination of trunk stabilization, or the quality of stabilizing muscle coordination, which a child forms within the first few months of life, is then used for the rest of their life. It is therefore essential for early ontogenetic development to occur in an ideal pattern rather than for a child to encode a pathological pattern from the beginning.

The fact that breathing accompanies each movement also influences postural function. Breathing movements are an integral component of postural functions. Breathing influences not only body posture but, through its rhythmical activity, also neuron excitability (Rekling et al 2000). With a few exceptions, an inspiration triggers excitation of most muscles while expiration is inhibitory. These findings are often used during rehabilitation treatment (Lewit 2010).

It has been empirically found and later experimentally demonstrated that the diaphragm is tonically activated when lifting objects (Hemborg et al.1985). From a kinesiology perspective, it is important that the diaphragm contracts prior to activation of the upper and lower extremity muscles (or any locomotion). Various authors (Hodges et al 1997, Kolar, et al 2012) state that stabilization of the pelvis and lumbar spine is ensured prior to any actual movement of the extremities. The CNS has to anticipate purposeful movement and automatically position the body to achieve the desired outcome.

Hodges and Gandevia (2000a) observed EMG activity of the diaphragm and muscles of the shoulder girdle during alternating movements of the upper extremities (UEs). EMG activity of the diaphragm occurs approximately 20 ms prior to activation of UE movement without taking into consideration the phase of the breathing cycle, therefore including expiration. As a result, the diaphragm shortens (shown by an ultrasound) and the transdiaphragmatic pressure P_{di} (the difference between the intra-pleural and intra-abdominal pressures) increases. This muscle synergy stabilizes the trunk and forms a foundation that is a prerequisite for all movement activities (Hodges et al 1997).

Since stabilization function is integrated in nearly all movements, the effects of internal forces are recognized not only due to their quantity, but also from their marked stereotypical repetition. If they elicit non-physiological, unbalanced loading, it is only a matter of time as to when problems will emerge, including morphological changes. It is also important that while a targeted movement is freely controlled, the reactive stabilization functions occur automatically and without volitional control, therefore, without awareness. A number of studies document coordinated synergy of the diaphragm, transverse abdominis, pelvic floor and the multifidus muscles during postural activity (Hodges & Gandevia 2000b). However, this synergy is not under full volitional control and modifiable. Therefore, the diaphragm, controlled by the CNS, assists in ensuring postural body control. The activity of motor neurons of the phrenic nerve is organized in such a way that the diaphragm simultaneously contributes to respiration as well as body stabilization and other nonventilatory behaviours (Mantilla & Sieck 2008).

The motor activity of the diaphragm has three components: tonic, phasic coordinated with a breathing cycle and phasic coordinated with movements of the trunk and/or the extremities (Hodges & Gandevia, 2000a). The dome of the diaphragm flattens during inspiration and during the trunk's postural stabilization function, or independent of breathing (Fig. 2.1.3C). The degree of flattening depends on the quality of the breathing pattern and postural function (Kolar et al 2012) (Fig. 2.1.5, Fig. 2.1.6).

In a physiologically normal situation, during postural activity related to breathing, diaphragm excursion and its flattening are more accentuated when compared to breathing at rest (Kolar et al 2010). By its caudal descent, or flattening during inspiration and during postural exertion, the diaphragm increases pressure on the internal organs (works as a piston) and the increased intra-abdominal pressure acts against the abdominal and pelvic floor musculature. The activity of the abdominal muscles stabilizes the diaphragm's insertions to the ribs (see Fig. 2.1.2B, Fig. 2.1.3A and Fig 2.1.3C).

During inspiration and postural activation, an eccentric expansion of the abdominal wall occurs so that the volume of the abdominal and thoracic wall increases (Fig. 2.1.2). When the abdominal wall adequately expands, its volume is maintained isometrically. In an ideal scenario, this 'eccentric-isometric' muscle activity is proportional to the degree of exerted muscle work and to the demands of the motion. If a greater muscle activity is needed, the diaphragm flattens; however, its excursions during breathing are smaller. Therefore, the diaphragm in this situation favours postural function. During significant exertion, a person usually holds their breath to increase postural stabilization and the diaphragm is primarily activated for its stabilization function.

The flattening of the dome of the diaphragm leads to changes in the volume and shape of the rib cage and

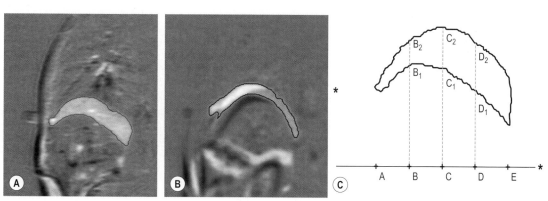

Figure 2.1.5 A Subtracted magnetic resonance image of the diaphragm excursions in the most caudal (inspiratory) and cranial (expiratory) diaphragm positions during tidal breathing in a healthy person. **B** A subtracted image of the diaphragm excursions in the most caudal (inspiratory) and cranial (expiratory) diaphragm positions during tidal breathing in a patient with chronic low back pain. Note more cranial and domed position of the diaphragm compared to healthy individual. **C** Schematic description of three diaphragmatic points (B, C and D) used for diaphragm excursion calculations. The following six distances (in mm) were obtained by measuring the distance between the horizontal baseline in both expiratory and inspiratory diaphragm positions. Diaphragm excursion points: B_1 to D_1 were derived from the inspiratory diaphragm positions obtained from MRI images; B_2 to D_2 were derived from expiratory diaphragm positions obtained from respective MRI images. The inspiratory diaphragm position is designated by points B_1, C_1 and D_1. The expiratory diaphragm position is designated by points B_2, C_2 and D_2. Total diaphragm excursion is designated by the distance from the lower to the upper curve along points B_1 to B_2, C_1 to C_2, and D_1 to D_2. *Reproduced with permission from: Kolár P, Šulc J, Kyncl M, et al. Postural function of the diaphragm in persons with and without chronic low back pain. J Orthop Sports Phys Ther 2012;42(4):352–362, Epub 21 December 2011. doi:10.2519/jospt.2012.3830.*

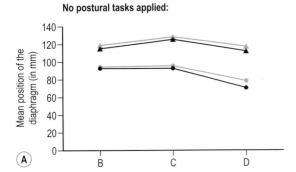

No postural tasks applied:

(A)

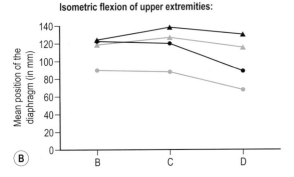

Isometric flexion of upper extremities:

(B)

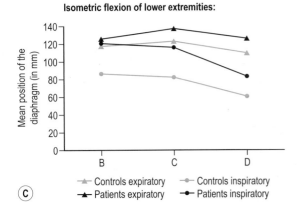

Isometric flexion of lower extremities:

Controls expiratory   Controls inspiratory
Patients expiratory   Patients inspiratory

(C)

Figure 2.1.6 A Inspiratory and expiratory positions of the diaphragm during tidal breathing for patient and control groups. Position and shape of the diaphragm is similar in both groups. (B, C, D points in the graphs correspond with the points in Fig. 2.1.5C). **B** Inspiratory and expiratory positions of the diaphragm during tidal breathing with isometric flexion of the upper extremity in the patient and control groups. Note a higher (more cranial) position of the diaphragm and a reduced diaphragm excursion in the patient group (black lines are higher and the distance between the black lines is smaller than the distance between the blue lines). In addition, a steeper slope in the middle-posterior diaphragm in the patient group occurs. **C** Inspiratory and expiratory positions of the diaphragm during tidal breathing with isometric flexion of the lower extremity in the patient and control groups. Cranial position and reduced diaphragm excursion as well as steeper slope in the posterior (lumbar) section of the diaphragm is even more pronounced in a patient group during lower extremity activation. *Reproduced with permission from: Kolar P, Sulc J, Kyncl M, et al. Postural function of the diaphragm in persons with and without chronic low back pain. Orthop Sports Phys Ther. 2012 Apr;42(4):352–62. Epub 2011 Dec 21.*

wall expands in a cylindrical fashion in all directions. This requires synchronized eccentric activity of all muscles inserting into the thorax and muscles of the abdominal wall (see Fig. 2.1.2B, Fig 2.1.3A and Fig. 2.1.3C). Only the pelvic floor and diaphragm work concentrically against the content of the abdominal cavity.

During normal inspiration and also during stabilization related to the flattening of the dome of the diaphragm, the pectorales, scalenes, sternocleidomastoids, all abdominal muscles, quadratus lumborum, spinal extensors and hip external rotators must accommodate the expansion of the thoracic, abdominal and pelvic cavities by their eccentric activity (Fig. 2.1.7). Once the dome of the diaphragm fully flattens in coordination with the eccentric activity of the muscles of these cavities, an isometric or stabilization contraction of these muscles occurs allowing for movement of the extremities. The eccentric activity of the muscles inserting into the thorax and pelvis also increases their excitability. This allows for a greater stabilizing force of the trunk. This pattern is quite obvious in power lifters, sumo wrestlers, Samurai fighters and other athletes who need to produce maximal force, as well as, technical precision during their performance. The quality of the described stabilization of muscle coordination is essential for prevention of overloading and for the onset of secondary vertebrogenic pain syndromes. A similar postural respiratory pattern can be elicited during Vojta's reflex locomotion and can also be observed during physiologically normal ontogenesis after the 4th month of life (Vojta & Schweizer 2009).

abdominal cavity. The thoracic cavity expands anteriorly and, as a result of rib curvature, also laterally (Fig. 2.1.2). During normal movement, the sternum moves anteriorly with movement occurring in the sternocostal joints (Fig 2.1.1A). The content of the abdominal cavity is non-compressible (with the exception of approximately 100–300 ml of air). This means that, during inspiration or during postural activity of the diaphragm, the organs of the abdominal cavity shift caudally and the abdominal

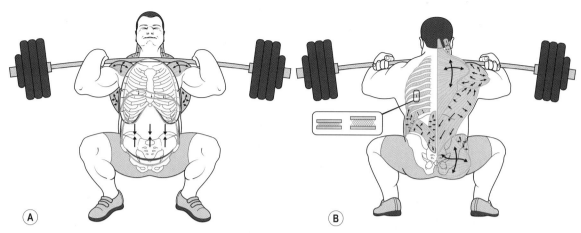

Figure 2.1.7 Eccentric activation of the stabilizers during postural tasks. The timing is important: stabilizing muscles must first activate eccentrically, expanding the trunk's volume, and then hold the stabilizing activation isometrically (or even concentrically). Only the diaphragm and the pelvic floor muscles are concentrically activated from the start.

PATHOLOGICAL RESPIRATORY POSTURAL PATTERN

During non-respiratory or strictly postural activity, the diaphragm does not change its shape in a typical fashion. It does contract and flatten, but non-homogenously (the diaphragm does not activate as one muscle but rather its individual parts can be active at different times). This pattern also differs in healthy individuals and in patients with chronic low back pain. Dynamic MRI demonstrated that patients with chronic low back pain and abnormal morphological findings in the lumbar spine, show greater flattening of the lumbar portion of the diaphragm when compared to a healthy population (Kolar et al 2012) (see Figs. 2.1.5 and 2.1.6).

From clinical experience, it is known that a marked individual difference exists in the extent of respiratory and non-respiratory movements of the diaphragm. Individuals who do not demonstrate sufficient ability to contract the diaphragm during trunk stabilization pose a greater risk of low back pain (O'Sullivan et al 2002). Chronic abnormal loading of the spine as a result of imbalance of internal muscle forces acting on the spine during postural stabilization is seen as the main reason.

Smaller flattening of the dome of the diaphragm during postural activity and also an imbalance in its activation are seen as the main components of insufficient stabilization of the diaphragm (Boyle et al 2010). In this situation, the diaphragm loses its function as a piston (see Figs 2.1.3B and 2.1.3D). The reason for a smaller flattening of

the diaphragm can either be weakness of the diaphragm, which has been demonstrated by measuring maximal respiratory muscle strength during inspiration in patients with chronic back pain, disrupted intra-muscular coordination or abnormal coordination of the diaphragm and other postural-respiratory muscles (Kolar et al 2012, Boyle et al 2010).

In a pathological scenario (see Figs 2.1.3B and 2.1.3D), during postural activity, an inverse (paradoxical) function of the diaphragm can be observed, during which the centrum tendineum is in a fixed alignment and no stabilization in the area of the lower ribs occurs. During diaphragm activation, the lower ribs are elevated cranially and the intercostal spaces narrow as a result of stretching the diaphragm's insertions to the ribs.

Through the sternum, the cranial movements are transferred to the upper ribs that are also elevated by activity of the accessory inspiratory muscles (Fig. 2.1.1B). In such individuals, hypertrophy of the paravertebral muscles (Fig 2.1.3B) of the lower thoracic and upper lumbar spine can often be observed, where they over-activate in challenging situations as a compensatory mechanism for posturally insufficient function of the diaphragm. In addition, in such individuals, the postural activity of the diaphragm is disproportional to the lumbar portion, which is mainly being utilized (Fig. 2.1.6). An abnormal stabilization function always goes hand in hand with a dysfunctional breathing pattern. Cranial movement of the ribcage with an inward drawing of the lateral intercostal spaces during inspiration is a typical pathological movement (Fig 2.1.3D).

VISCERAL AND SPHINCTER FUNCTIONS OF THE DIAPHRAGM

The visceral and sphincter functions of the diaphragm are additional and often forgotten functions of the diaphragm. The diaphragm influences the internal organs in two important ways; first, during the diaphragm's pressure on the internal organs within the breathing and postural functions as described above and, second, during the diaphragm's interplay with the lower esophageal sphincter (LES).

The diaphragm is a true visceral muscle, especially its crural portion. This portion phylogenetically develops in amphibians as a ring-like muscle around the esophagus. During evolution, this musculature merges with the developing diaphragm giving rise to the crural portion of the diaphragm. This is supported by ontogenesis and embryonic development of the human diaphragm because the crural portion develops from esophageal structures, specifically the mesesophagus (Langman 1981).

The diaphragm is also a skeletal muscle partially innervated by the vagus nerve. It is particularly the crural portion of the diaphragm that is innervated from the nucleus of the vagus nerve (Young et al 2010). Given this innervation, the crural portion of the diaphragm is in perfect co-activation with swallowing, during which the crural portion needs to relax to allow for the transport of the bolus to the stomach. In contrast, with an increasing intra-gastric pressure, activation of the crural portions needs to occur as well as an increased pressure at the LES region, which prevents the return of the stomach content to the esophagus (Liu et al 2005). Therefore, the diaphragm is actually two muscles in one anatomical unit (Pickering & Jones 2002) with three main functions: respiratory, postural and visceral.

Pressure activity of the diaphragm and the effect on internal organ function

Visceral movement and peristalsis

During a breathing cycle, a rhythmic compression of the abdominal cavity occurs and leads to a cyclical movement of the internal organs. During inspiration, almost all internal organs of the abdominal and retroperitoneal areas shift several centimetres in a caudal direction (Xi et al 2009). This organ movement and the pressure activity of the diaphragm partially contribute to the transport of food and digestive juices. In this way, the diaphragm assists in digestive processes and significantly contributes to peristalsis and food propulsion.

Birth

The size of the fetus influences the position of the diaphragm, which gradually shifts cranially during pregnancy (fetal growth). The diaphragm, as a result of pressure and a change in position, becomes functionally less active, which leads to an increased activity of the accessory inspiratory muscles. This can lead to overuse, hypertonus and pain, especially in the cervical region. Decreased diaphragm function is also manifested by sphincter dysfunction (see below). Therefore, reflux episodes significantly increase in pregnant women, which can lead to an onset of gastro-esophageal reflux disease (GERD) (Rey at al 2011). In contrast, the pressure action of the diaphragm is an important force (with an optimal vector) necessary for fetal progression and expulsion during the second phase of delivery.

Defecation

Similarly to postural trunk stabilization, correct co-activation (timing, synergy) between the diaphragm, abdominal musculature (especially transverse abdominis) and the pelvic floor is essential during defecation. Therefore, postural dysfunction also presents in problems with defecation (constipation). Weakness of an abdominal brace resulting in limited defecation propulsion is one of the most frequent disturbances in patients with constipation. Deficit in co-activation can also be seen in dyssynergic defecation (Rao 2008), in which a paradoxical contraction of the pelvic floor and drawing in of the abdominal wall and the lower ribs (inversion function of the diaphragm – see above, Fig. 2.1.3D) occur during a defecation attempt. This dysfunction serves as an example of a deficit in co-activation of abdominal and pelvic floor musculature with the diaphragm playing an important role.

Vomiting

The diaphragm also plays an important role during vomiting, when an interesting functional division of the sternal and crural portions of the diaphragm can be observed. The process occurs as follows. Initially, the entire diaphragm is activated (sternal and crural portions) and presses on the stomach, which significantly increases the intra-gastric pressure. Then, the crural portion is inhibited, but the sternal portion continues in large rhythmical contractions and the gastric contents are pumped into the esophagus. During vomiting, the posterior aspect of the diaphragm is inhibited (which opens the cardium) and the anterior aspect generates the force with such vector to allow retrograde movement of the vomitus back to the esophagus and the mouth.

The diaphragm's role as a lower esophageal sphincter

The lower esophageal sphincter (LES) is an essential structure preventing movement of the stomach content back into the esophagus. It prevents, in this way, the onset of GERD. The incidence of GERD continues to grow (Sonnenberg 2011) and the disease manifests itself by many associated symptoms, including heartburn, regurgitation, retrosternal pain, etc. with subsequent complications of esophagitis, bronchial asthma, Barret's esophagus and esophageal cancer. The LES is formed by two components: the circular musculature of the esophagus and the crural portion of the diaphragm, which forms an anatomical loop in the LES region. The crural portion of the diaphragm has specifically been shown to be the main component of LES (Mittal et al 1987). Diaphragm dysfunction is viewed as one of the essential causes of GERD (Pandolfino et al 2007).

The diaphragm is considered to be an external esophageal sphincter and, for example, during the respiratory cycle will demonstrate regular pressure fluctuations (pressure increase during an inspiratory phase) in the LES region, which can be verified by manometric observation. Since the diaphragm is simultaneously a respiratory and postural muscle, a dysfunction in these areas reflects also in sphincter dysfunction, which is an important component in the diagnosis and treatment of GERD. Many patients with GERD, therefore, demonstrate not only sphincter dysfunction, but also a combined respiratory-postural dysfunction, which is manifested by a tendency toward spinal pathologies, altered postural activity and stabilization (especially in the lumbar, cervical and thoracolumbar regions) and an altered breathing pattern, in which the activity of the accessory inspiratory muscles dominates over the diaphragm. Decreased occlusion pressures (the force of respiratory muscles) during inspiratory as well as expiratory manoeuvres (PI_{max} and PE_{max}) was the dominant finding in our sample of patients with GERD. In short, it can be stated that patients with GERD are also 'respiropathics' as far as the force of the respiratory musculature is concerned (Bitnar et al 2010a).

During a normal inspiratory manoeuvre (PI_{max}), a pressure decrease is observed in the thoracic portion of the esophagus as a result of intrathoracic underpressure. In contrast, a large increase in pressure is observed in the abdominal portion of the esophagus (LES region) caused by contraction of the diaphragmatic crura. In patients with GERD, this increase is smaller and the sphincter is weaker. Also, in patients with a significant reflux, a paradoxical reaction of the diaphragm can almost be observed during PI_{max} manoeuvres, in which the crural portion of the diaphragm does not contract during maximum inspiration. Rather, the crural portion paradoxically weakens, which is manometrically observed by a paradoxical decrease in pressure in the sphincter and an expansion of the gastro-esophageal junction (Bitnar et al 2010b).

In patients with GERD, however, in addition to the diaphragm's (or respiratory musculature) strength, it is important to also monitor the quality of the breathing pattern (breathing mechanics) because an incorrect respiratory pattern is the most common dysfunctional pattern in patients with such disease. It is important that a therapeutic change in breathing pattern with facilitation of diaphragmatic breathing led to correction of LES hypotonus, which can also be observed during manometric examination (Bitnar at al 2010a, Bitnar at al 2010b, Smejkal et al 2010).

Breathing pattern correction is then the basic therapeutic intervention within conservative treatment in patients with GERD. During breathing alteration, or during facilitated abdominal (diaphragmatic) breathing, the LES pressure significantly increases, which is caused by activation of the diaphragmatic crura without a change in respiratory volumes (the amount of air ventilated). This has been demonstrated by spirometry (Bitnar at al 2010a, Bitnar at al 2010b, Smejkal et al 2010). This means that a change in the quality of the breathing pattern (with greater participation of the diaphragm and lesser activation of the accessory inspiratory muscles) positively influences the ability of the LES. This qualitative change leads to restoration of the anti-reflux barrier.

REFERENCES

Abe, T., Kusuhara, N., Katagiri, H., et al., 1993. Differential function of the costal and crural diaphragm during emesis in canines. Respir Physiol. 91 (2–3), 183–193.

Assaiante, C., Mallau, S., Viel, S., et al., 2005. Development of postural control in healthy children: a functional approach. Neural Plast. 12 (2–3), 109–118.

Bitnar, P., Smejkal, M., Dolina, J., et al., 2010a. Diaphragm function monitoring in the lower esophageal sphincter area. Available at: http://www.rehabps.com/REHABILITATION/Literature_Research_files/Bitnar%20LES_GER.jpg (Accessed June 2013)

Bitnar, P., Smejkal, M., Dolina, J., et al., 2010b. Diaphragm function in GERD patients: PFT assessment with extended esophageal manometry. Available at: http://www.rehabps.com/REHABILITATION/Literature_Research_files/Bittnar%20GER_2_1.pdf (Accessed June 2013)

Boyle, K.L., Olinick, J., Lewis, C., 2010. The value of blowing up a balloon.

N Am J Sports Phys Ther. 5 (3), 179–188.

Butler, J.E., McKenzie, D.K., Gandevia, S.C., 2001. Discharge frequencies of single motor units in human diaphragm and parasternal muscles in lying and standing. J Appl Physiol. 90 (1), 147–154.

Caron, O., Fontanari, P., Cremieux, J., et al., 2004. Effects of ventilation on body sway during human standing. Neurosci Lett. 366 (1), 6–9.

Devlieger, H., Daniels, H., Marchal, G., et al., 1991. The diaphragm of the newborn infant: anatomical and ultrasonographic studies. J Dev Physiol. 16 (6), 321–329.

Hemborg, B., Moritz, U., Löwing, H., 1985. Intra-abdominal pressure and trunk muscle activity during lifting. IV. The causal factors of the intra-abdominal pressure rise. Scand J Rehab Med. 17, 25–38.

Hermsen-van Wanrooy, M., 2006. Baby moves. Baby Moves Publications, New Zealand.

Hodges, P.W., Butler, J.E., McKenzie, D.K., et al., 1997. Contraction of the human diaphragm during rapid postural adjustments. J Physiol. 505 (Pt 2), 539–548.

Hodges, P.W., Gandevia, S.C., 2000a. Changes in intra-abdominal pressure during postural and respiratory activation of the human diaphragm. J Appl Physiol. 89, 967–976.

Hodges, P.W., Gandevia, S.C., 2000b. Activation of the human diaphragm during a repetitive postural task. J Physiol. 522 (Pt 1), 165–175.

Hodges, P.W., Sapsford, R., Pengel, L.H., 2007. Postural and respiratory functions of the pelvic floor muscles. Neurourol Urodyn 26 (3), 362–371.

Janda, V., 1972. What is the typical upright posture in man? Cas Lek Cesk. 111 (32), 748–750. Czech.

Kapandji, I.A., 1992. The Physiology of the joints, second ed. Churchill Livingstone, Edinburgh, London, New York.

Kolar, P., Neuwirth, J., Sanda, J., et al., 2009. Analysis of diaphragm movement, during tidal breathing and during its activation while breath holding, using MRI synchronized with spirometry. Physiol Res 58, 383–392.

Kolar, P., Sulc, J., Kyncl, M., et al., 2012. Postural function of the diaphragm in persons with and without chronic low back pain. J Orthop Sports Phys Ther. 42 (4), 352–362.

Kolar, P., Sulc, J., Kyncl, M., et al., 2010. Stabilizing function of the diaphragm: dynamic MRI and synchronized spirometric assessment. J Appl Physiol. 109 (4), 1064–1071.

Koman, L.A., Smith, B.P., Shilt, J.S., 2004. Cerebral palsy. Lancet 363 (9421), 1619–1631.

Langman, J., 1981. Body cavities and serous membranes. In: Langman, J. (Ed.), Medical embryology, fourth ed. William and Wilkins Co, Baltimore, pp. 147–148 (Chapter 11).

Lewit, K., 2010. Manipulative Therapy. Churchill Livingstone, Edinburgh.

Liu, J., Puckett, J.L., Takeda, T., et al., 2005. Crural diaphragm inhibition during esophageal distension correlates with contraction of the esophageal longitudinal muscle in cats. Am J Physiol Gastrointest Liver Physiol. 288 (5), G927–G932.

Lord, M.J., Ogden, J.A., Ganey, T.M 1995. Postnatal development of the thoracic spine. Spine 20 (15), 1692–1698.

Mantilla, C.B., Sieck, G.C., 2008. Key aspects of phrenic motoneuron and diaphragm muscle development during the perinatal period. J Appl Physiol. 104 (6), 1818–1827.

Mittal, R.K., Rochester, D.F., McCallum, R.W., 1987. Effect of the diaphragmatic contraction on lower oesophageal sphincter pressure in man. Gut. 28 (12), 1564–1568.

Murphy, T., Woodrum, D., 1998. Functional development of respiratory muscles. In: Polin, R.A., Fox, W.W. (Eds.), Fetal and neonatal physiology, vol. 1. WB Saunders Company, Philadelphia, pp. 1071–1084.

Openshaw, P., Edwards, S., Helms, P., 1984. Changes in rib cage geometry during childhood. Thorax. 39 (8), 624–627.

O'Sullivan, P.B., Beales, D.J., Beetham, J.A., et al., 2002. Altered motor control strategies in subjects with sacroiliac joint pain during the active straight-leg-raise test. Spine (Phila Pa 1976). 27 (1), E1–E8.

Pandolfino, J.E., Kim, H., Ghosh, S.K., et al., 2007. High-resolution manometry of the EGJ: an analysis of crural diaphragm function in GERD. Am J Gastroenterol. 102 (5), 1056–1063.

Pickering, M., Jones, J.F., 2002. The diaphragm: two muscles in one. J Anat. 201 (4), 305–312.

Rao, S.S., 2008. Dyssynergic defecation and biofeedback therapy. Gastroenterol Clin North Am. 37 (3), 569–586.

Rekling, J.C., Funk, G.D., Bayliss, D.A., et al., 2000. Synaptic control of motoneuronal excitability. Physiol Rev. 80 (2), 767–852.

Rey, E., Rodríguez-Artalejo, F., Herraiz, M.A., et al., 2011. Atypical symptoms of gastro-esophageal reflux during pregnancy. Rev Esp Enferm Dig. 103 (3), 129–132.

Smejkal, M., Bitnar, P., Dolina, J., et al., 2010. The importance of the diaphragm in the etiology and the possibility of its use in the treatment of GERD. Available at: http://www.rehabps.com/REHABILITATION/Poster_GR.html (Accessed June 2013)

Sherrington, C., 1931. Hughlings Jackson Lecture on quantitative management of contraction for 'lowest-level' co-ordination. Br Med J. 1 (3657), 207–211.

Sonnenberg, A., 2011. Effects of environment and lifestyle on gastroesophageal reflux disease. Dig Dis. 29 (2), 229–234.

Staiano, A., Boccia, G., Salvia, G., et al., 2007. Development of esophageal peristalsis in preterm and term neonates. Gastroenterology. 132 (5), 1718–1725.

Takazakura, R., Takahashi, M., Nitta, N., et al., 2004. Diaphragmatic motion in the sitting and supine positions: Healthy subject study using a vertically open magnetic resonance system. J. Magn. Reson. Imaging. 19 (5), 605–609.

Todd, T.W., 1912. The Descent of the Shoulder After Birth. Anat. Anz. 12, 257.

Vojta, V., 2004. Die zerebralen Bewegungsstörungen im Säuglingsalter: Frühdiagnose und Frühtherapie. Thieme.

Vojta, V., Schweizer, E., 2009. Die Entdeckung der idealen Motorik. Richard Pflaum Vlg GmbH.

Volpon, J.B., 1994. Footprint analysis during growth period. J Pediatr Orthop 14 (1), 83–85.

Xi, M., Liu, M.Z., Li, Q.Q., et al., 2009. Analysis of abdominal organ motion using four-dimensional CT. Ai Zheng. 28 (9), 989–993.

Young, R.L., Page, A.J., Cooper, N.J., et al., 2010. Sensory and motor innervation of the crural diaphragm by the vagus nerves. Gastroenterology. 138 (3), 1091–1101.

Chapter | **2.2** |

The structure and function of breathing

Leon Chaitow, Dinah Bradley, Chris Gilbert

THE STRUCTURE–FUNCTION CONTINUUM

Nowhere in the body is the axiom of structure governing function more apparent than in its relation to respiration. Any prolonged modifications of function – such as that involving the inappropriate breathing patterns displayed during hyperventilation – inevitably induces structural changes, for example involving the accessory breathing muscles and thoracic articulations. Ultimately, the self-perpetuating cycle of functional change creating structural modification, leading to reinforced dysfunctional tendencies can become complete, from whichever direction dysfunction arrives. For example: structural adaptations can prevent normal breathing function, and abnormal breathing function ensures continued structural adaptation stresses, and predictable changes, for example involving the scalene muscles (Hill & Eastwood 2011).

Restoration of normal function requires restoration of adequate mobility to the structural component and, self-evidently, maintenance of any degree of restored biomechanical integrity requires that function (how the individual breathes) should be normalized through re-education and training.

MULTIPLE INFLUENCES: BIOMECHANICAL, BIOCHEMICAL AND PSYCHOLOGICAL

The area of respiration is one in which the interaction between biochemical, biomechanical and psychosocial features is dramatically evident. Inappropriate breathing can result directly from structural, biomechanical causes, such as a restricted thoracic spine or rib immobility, or shortness of key respiratory muscles.

Causes of breathing dysfunction can also have a more biochemical etiology, possibly involving an allergy or infection which triggers narrowing of breathing passages and subsequent asthmatic-type responses. Acidosis resulting from conditions such as kidney failure will also directly alter breathing function as the body attempts to reduce acid levels via elimination of CO_2 through the means of hyperventilation.

The link between psychological distress and breathing makes this another primary cause of many manifestations of dysfunctional respiration. Indeed, it is hard to imagine examining a person suffering from anxiety or depression without breathing dysfunction being noted.

Other catalysts that may impact breathing function include environmental factors (altitude, humidity, etc.). Even factors such as where an individual is born may contribute to subsequent breathing imbalances:

> *People who are born at high altitude have a diminished ventilatory response to hypoxia that is only slowly corrected by subsequent residence at sea level. Conversely, those born at sea level who move to high altitudes retain their hypoxic response intact for a long time. Apparently therefore ventilatory response is determined very early in life.*

> West 2000

How we breathe and how we feel are intimately conjoined in a two-way loop. Feeling anxious produces a distinctive pattern of upper-chest breathing which modifies blood chemistry, leading to a chain reaction of effects, inducing anxiety, and so reinforcing the pattern which produced the dysfunctional pattern of breathing in the first place.

Even when an altered pattern of breathing is the result of emotional distress, it will eventually produce the structural and biomechanical changes as described below. This suggests that when attempting to restore normal breathing – by means of re-education and exercise for example – both the psychological initiating factors and the structural compensation patterns need to be addressed. (The psychological effects of breathing dysfunction are covered in greater detail in Chapter 5.)

Objectives and methods

A perspective needs to be held in which function and structure are kept in mind as dual, interdependent features, so intimately bound to each other as to ensure that changes in one inevitably lead to, or derive from, the other. When breathing function is being assessed, a complex set of functions, all of which have structural linkages, are being observed. If a pattern of breathing has been disturbed for any length of time, clinical experience suggests that normalization of the muscles and joints associated with the breathing process frequently require primary attention, before normal patterns of use can be restored. In some instances however, even where structural changes are well established, a reformed breathing pattern alone may reverse changes – for example involving the accessory breathing muscles – allowing enhanced thoracic biomechanics to manifest (Yamaguti et al 2012). In treatment/ rehabilitation of BPD, a multi-track approach is recommended, in which musculoskeletal mobilization accompanies rehabilitation of breathing patterns, together with a greater understanding and awareness of the role of respiration.

The causes of dysfunctional breathing patterns will be seen to possibly involve etiological features which may in nature be largely biomechanical (for example post-surgical or postural factors), biochemical (including allergic or infection factors), or psychosocial (chronic emotional states such as anxiety, depression and anger). Etiology may also involve combinations of these factors, or established pathology may be the cause. In many instances, altered breathing patterns, whatever their origins, are maintained by nothing more sinister than pure habit (Lum 1994).

Where pathology provides the background to altered breathing patterns, the aim of this book is not to explore these disease states (e.g. asthma, cardiovascular disease) in any detail, except insofar as they impact on breathing patterning (for example where nasal airway obstruction causes mouth breathing). The changes this text is concerned with are largely functional in nature, rather than pathological, although the impact on the physiology of the individual of an altered breathing pattern such as hyperventilation can be profound, possibly resulting in severe health problems ranging from anxiety, depression and panic attacks, to fatigue and chronic pain (Timmons & Ley 1994, Cenker et al 2010).

It is axiomatic that in order to make sense of abnormal respiration, it is essential to have a reasonable understanding of normality. As a foundation for what follows, this chapter outlines the basic characteristics of normal breathing. The biochemical and alveolar processes involved in respiration (as distinct from the biomechanical process of breathing), are covered in later chapters.

The upper airway

To enter the air sacs of the lungs, air journeys through a series of passages: nose, nasopharynx, oropharynx, laryngeal pharynx, larynx, trachea, bronchi and bronchioles. Disease and dysfunction can affect any of these segments and cause abnormal breathing patterns, and it is important to recognize and treat any such conditions before attempting to correct abnormal patterns such as hyperventilation.

The nose

The nose is an intriguing characteristic facial feature, taking on a variety of shapes and sizes, and changing with age. It is a complex structure with a number of vital functions. This is explored in detail in Chapter 2.3.

Pathological states affecting the airways

Before considering the etiology of breathing pattern disorders, the possibility of pathology playing a part in their etiology needs to be considered. Corrin & Nicholson (2011) make a useful distinction between two forms of pathological influence:

> The function of the airways is to conduct gas in and out of the lungs and all airway diseases are liable to impede this, resulting in 'obstructive lung disease', as opposed to the 'restrictive lung disease' that is caused by many diseases of the lung parenchyma.

Acute causes of breathing disorder may involve smoking (Sorheim et al 2010), environmental, infectious or industrial pollutants, affecting the mucous membranes of the trachea and bronchi specifically, and breathing function generally. Chronic obstruction of the nose and oropharynx can arise from a deviated nasal septum, exuberant distorted conchae, enlarged adenoids, hay fever, cluster headaches, nasopharyngeal tumours, or Wegener's granulomatosis. Obstruction increases the resistance to airflow, necessitating intercostal breathing and a switch to mouth breathing. The patient should be referred back to a general practitioner, or to an ear, nose, and throat surgeon, or perhaps an allergist. In obese people, redundancy and laxity of the mucosal folds can give rise to laryngeal obstruction and cause sleep apnoea or the obstructive sleep syndrome. Tumours of the vocal chords can cause laryngeal obstruction. In acromegaly, where there is a pituitary tumour overproducing growth hormone, the vestibular folds enlarge and tend to obstruct breathing. A previous tracheotomy can give rise to a tracheal stenosis. Chronic, inadequately treated asthma causes spasm of the

bronchioles, producing an expiratory wheeze and breathlessness. Lung tumours are another cause of breathlessness, while emphysema and heart disease are more common causes.

The therapist who concentrates on psychological causes and on correcting abnormal breathing patterns in these patients is unlikely to succeed, since the major factor is not psychological but physical, is often life-threatening, and requires precise diagnosis and treatment. Such patients should be referred to an appropriate specialist – a general physician or an expert in respiratory diseases.

A large body of individuals who display BPD do however have what have been termed somatoform or 'bodily distress' syndromes, presenting with physical symptoms that are not readily explained by well-recognized medical illness. Fink & Schroder (2010) note that a range of such functional conditions exist, that includes hyperventilation as a major symptom, commonly coexisting in individuals who have been diagnosed with chronic fatigue syndrome, fibromyalgia, irritable bowel syndrome, noncardiac chest pain and other pain syndromes. Chapters 5, 6.4 and 7.4 explore this topic in depth. In such cases psychological interventions may be useful.

Postural considerations

It is a truism worth repeating that in order to appreciate dysfunction, a clear picture of what lies within normal functional ranges is needed. For normal breathing to occur, a compliant, elastic, functional state of the thoracic structures, both osseous and soft tissue, is a requirement. If restrictions are present which reduce the ability of the rib cage to appropriately adapt in response to muscular activity and altered pressure gradients during the breathing cycle, compensating changes are inevitable, always at the expense of optimal function.

In manual medicine, practitioners and therapists need to have the opportunity to evaluate and palpate normal individuals, with pliable musculature, mobile joint structures, and sound respiratory function, so that dysfunction can be more easily appreciated, assessed and identified. Apart from standard functional examination, it is also important that practitioners and therapists acquire the ability to assess by observation and touch, relearning skills familiar to former generations of 'low-tech' health care providers. Assessment approaches will be outlined in Section 6.

Is there such a thing as an optimal breathing pattern?

If structural modifications result from, and reinforce functional imbalances, it is of some importance to establish whether an optimal, ideal, state is a potential clinical reality.

Optimal breathing involves:

- Since the objective of breathing is to meet the metabolic demands of the body, oxygen (O_2) and carbon dioxide (CO_2) need to be efficiently moved into and out of the lungs (Abernethy et al 1996).
- During quiet breathing, respiratory efficiency is achieved as the diaphragm descends into the abdominal cavity during inhalation, increasing the vertical dimensions of the thorax as the ribs rise and move laterally, to expand the transverse dimensions of the thorax.
- The diaphragm relaxing, and returning to its domed position on exhalation follows this sequence, as the abdomen and chest wall return to their starting positions.
- In good health, meeting the metabolic demands of the body optimally requires a steady, rhythmical pattern with a respiratory rate of 10–14 breaths per minute; involving a ratio of inspiration to expiration of $1:1.5$–2.
- Ideally the least amount of mechanical effort from the respiratory musculature should be involved (Jones et al 2003).
- If such an optimal pattern is disrupted, abnormal and potentially inefficient respiratory mechanics may become the new norm – with the emergence of a breathing pattern disorder.

Since breathing function is largely dependent for its efficiency on the postural and structural integrity of the body, the question might be rephrased as: 'Is there an optimal postural state?' This topic was briefly highlighted in Chapter 1, and is considered further here.

Is there an ideal posture?

Kuchera & Kuchera (1997) describe what they consider an ideal posture:

Optimal posture is a balanced configuration of the body with respect to gravity. It depends on normal arches of the feet, vertical alignment of the ankles,

and horizontal orientation (in the coronal plane) of the sacral base. The presence of an optimum posture suggests that there is perfect distribution of the body mass around the centre of gravity...Structural and functional stressors on the body, however, may prevent achievement of optimum posture. In this case homeostatic mechanisms provide for 'compensation' in an effort to provide maximum postural function within the existing structure of the individual. Compensation is the counterbalancing of any defect of structure or function.

This succinct description of postural reality highlights the fact that there is hardly ever an example of an optimal postural state, and, by implication, of optimal respiratory function. However, there can be a well-compensated mechanism (postural or respiratory) that functions well despite moderate asymmetry and compensations. This is probably the reality normally observed in most symptom-free people. Examples of useful structural and functional assessment methods are to be found in Sections 6 and 7.

Janda's crossed syndromes (Janda 1983)

Upper crossed syndrome (Fig. 2.2.1)

The upper crossed syndrome involves the following basic imbalance:

Pectoralis major and minor Upper trapezius Levator scapulae Sternomastoid	} All tighten and shorten
while	
Lower and middle trapezius Serratus anterior and rhomboids	} All weaken

As these changes take place they alter the relative positions of the head, neck, and shoulders, as follows:

- The occiput and C1/2 hyperextend, with the head translating anteriorly. Weakness of the deep neck flexors develops along with increased tone in the suboccipital musculature

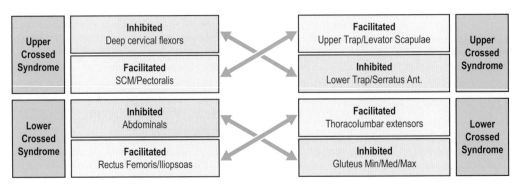

Figure 2.2.1 Upper and lower crossed syndromes.

- The lower cervical segments down to the 4th thoracic vertebra will be stressed as a result
- Rotation and abduction of the scapulae occur as the increased tone in the upper fixators of the shoulder (upper trapezius, levator scapula, for example) results in shortening, inhibiting the lower fixators such as serratus anterior and the lower trapezii
- An altered direction of the axis of the glenoid fossa develops resulting in stabilization of the humerus by additional levator scapula and upper trapezius (plus supraspinatus) activity
- Breathing function is negatively influenced because of the crowded and slumped upper body positioning.

The results of these changes include greater cervical segment strain, the evolution of trigger points in the stressed structures, and referred pain to the chest, shoulders and arms. Pain mimicking angina may be noted, as well as a decline in respiratory efficiency.

The solution, according to Janda, is to identify the shortened structures – as described in Chapter 6.2, and to release (stretch and relax) these, followed by re-education towards more appropriate function – as described in Chapter 7.2.

A similar pattern can be observed in the lower trunk, the lower crossed syndrome, in which:

Hip flexors	
Iliopsoas, rectus femoris	All tighten
TFL, short adductors	and shorten
Erector spinae group of the trunk	
while	
Abdominal and gluteal muscles	All weaken
Additional stress commonly appears in the sagittal plane in which:	
Quadratus lumborum	Tightens
while	
Gluteus maximus and medius	Weaken

As a result, adaptive demands will focus on the lumbodorsal junction, the diaphragm, and the thorax.

When this 'lateral corset' becomes unstable the pelvis is held in increased elevation, accentuated when walking, resulting in L5–S1 stress in the sagittal plane. One result is low back pain. The combined stresses described produce instability at the lumbodorsal junction, an unstable transition point at best.

POSTURE AND BREATHING

As detailed below, alterations in posture profoundly influence breathing function. It is also well established that altered breathing patterns, such as hyperventilation, have immediate negative effects on postural stability and balance (David et al 2012).

Among the more profound links between human posture and breathing is the involvement – in a key role, in both – of the diaphragm.

Smith et al (2006) explain that in the absence of disease, the diaphragm and transversus abdominis simultaneously control both respiration and posture (contributing to 'core stability'). They note, however, that in chronic respiratory disease, as well as during hypercapnia (Hodges et al 2001) postural activation of these muscles is impaired, leading to a compromised breathing pattern, as well as loss of stabilization of the spine. It has been noted that a similar poorly adapted state may occur in the pelvic floor muscles, particularly in women with incontinence, in whom pelvic floor muscle activity is insufficient (Deindl et al 1994). Reduced efficiency of the diaphragm, transversus abdominis and multifidus – as well as the pelvic floor muscles – are therefore capable of impairing the mechanical stability of the spine, negatively affecting its strength and flexibility. Respiration is seen to be essential to the proper functioning of these muscles (Kolnes 2012, Smith et al 2006).

Kolnes (2012) observes that in cases involving chronic upper-chest (costal) patterns of breathing, the respiratory muscles are constantly over-activated (see notes on the scalenes (Chiti et al 2008), later in this chapter). This results in the head being 'pulled forward, the shoulders hunched up and pulled forward'. Additionally, a common observation is increased extension of the lower back posture, with the pelvis simultaneously tilted anteriorly 'resulting in a misalignment of the entire body'.

There are many other obvious associations between postural deviation and breathing pattern changes, for example, as Correa & Berzin (2008) have explained:

> *Enlarged tonsils and adenoids, allergic rhinitis and chronic respiratory problems cause a mouth breathing syndrome (MBS), which may be associated with compensatory adaptation of natural head posture, as well as whole body posture in children.*

Neiva et al (2009) confirm that children who are mouthbreathers, are prone to altered respiratory function, and commonly exhibit: 'forward head posture, a reduced physiological cervical lordosis, protrusion of the shoulders, elevation and abduction of the scapulas.' These adaptive changes usually involve forward head posture, a low and forward tongue position and increased activity of the accessory muscles of respiration (sternocleidomastoid, scalenes and pectorals) that tend to hypertrophy over time (Correa & Berzin 2008, Hall & Brody 2005). This pattern is perpetuated by the decreased activity of the diaphragm and hypotonicity of the abdominal musculature that weaken due to inactivity (Lima et al 2004).

Deliberate alteration of posture also affects respiratory function. For example it has been shown that breathing efficiency is likely to be compromised in cyclists due to the posture adopted when riding. Specifically, time trial

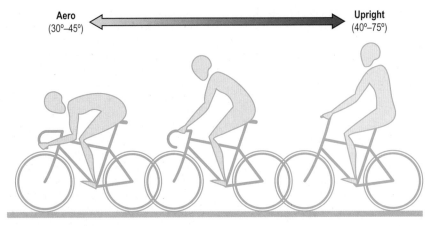

Figure 2.2.2 Rider seating position showing different seating positions on a bicycle, altering posture and respiratory biomechanics.

cyclists adopt a crouched aerodynamic position (Fig 2.2.2) to minimize their frontal area in order to maximize speed, with negative impact on respiration – and possibly performance! (Faria, Parker & Faria 2005). This intermingling of regions (pelvis and thorax) and conditions (hyperventilation and pelvic dysfunction) is confirmed by Lee et al (2008), who summarize the possible interactions:

> *Nonoptimal strategies for posture, movement and/or breathing create failed load transfer, which can lead to pain, incontinence and/or breathing disorders.*

Key et al (2010) have observed and catalogued a number of variations within the patterns of compensation/adaptation associated with chronic postural realignment involved in what Janda (1987) described as crossed syndromes.

In Figure 2.2.3 the major features include:

- Flexors tend to dominate
- Loss of extension throughout spine
- Thoracolumbar junction hyperstabilized in flexion.

In Figure 2.2.4 the major features include:

- Trunk extensors shortened
- Thoracolumbar region hyperstabilized in extension
- Poor pelvic control
- Decreased hip extension
- Abnormal axial rotation.

A frequent association exists between lower-crossed postural patterns and upper-crossed patterns, as shown in Figure 2.2.5.

In Figure 2.2.5 the major features include:

- Shortening of cervicothoracic extensors
- Shortening of scalenes, sternomastoid, pectorals
- Inhibition of deep neck flexors and lower fixators of the scapulae.

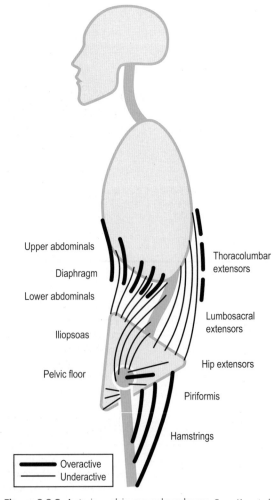

Figure 2.2.3 Anterior pelvic crossed syndrome. *From Key et al 2008 Figure 1; after Janda et al 2007.*

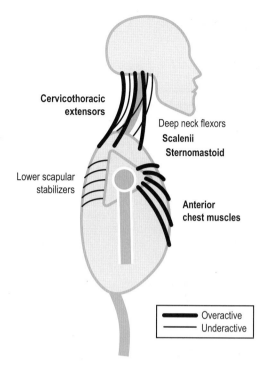

Figure 2.2.5 Shoulder crossed syndrome.

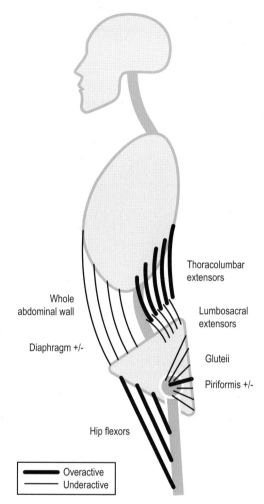

Figure 2.2.4 Posterior pelvic crossed syndrome. *From Key 2010, Key et al 2008 Figure 7.*

respiratory changes – while in others altered breathing patterns (for example open mouth breathing) appear to initiate postural changes. This highlights the essential co-dependency of structure and function, and the absolute requirement for attention to be offered in both spheres: for example breathing rehabilitation exercises may need to be accompanied by biomechanical interventions, as required – possibly alongside exploration of psychogenic issues – if necessary.

The likely outcome of these examples of postural adaptations would include altered thoracic biomechanical features and inevitable dysfunctional breathing patterns.

For example, Key et al (2010) report that, in relation to what they term the posterior pelvic crossed syndrome, characterized by 'a posterior [pelvic] shift with increased anterior sagittal rotation or tilt', together with an anterior shunt/translation of the thorax, among many other stressful modifications, there will inevitably be poor diaphragmatic control and altered pelvic floor muscle function.

In some of these examples of posture-breathing involvement the postural features (for example deliberate modification as in cycle racing, or the chronic changes seen in the crossed-syndrome patterns) appear to determine the

Further structural considerations

Kuchera & Kuchera (1997) have connected gravitational strain with changes of muscle function and structure that lead predictably to observable postural modifications and functional limitations:

> *Postural muscles, structurally adapted to resist prolonged gravitational stress, generally resist fatigue. When overly stressed, however, these same postural muscles become irritable, tight, shortened*

> Janda 1987

The antagonists to these postural muscles demonstrate inhibitory characteristics described as 'pseudoparesis' (a functional, non-organic, weakness) or 'myofascial trigger points with weakness' when they are stressed.

Observable changes such as those illustrated in Figures 2.2.3 and 2.2.4 (upper and lower crossed syndromes), emerge through overuse, misuse and abuse of the structures responsible for normal posture, leading to changes in which some muscles shorten and tighten while others are inhibited and weaken and/or lengthen. Common dysfunctional postural patterns emerge with inevitable modification of optimal function, including breathing function.

Observation and functional assessments – as described in Chapter 6.2 – provide indications of local dysfunction as well as more widespread, global influences that may be negatively influencing breathing function, with therapeutic choices described in the chapters in Section 7.

The thoracic cylinder

The thoracic cage can be thought of as a cylindrical structure housing most major organs – lungs, heart, liver, spleen, pancreas and kidneys. The functions associated with the thorax (or with muscles attached to it) include respiration, visceral activity, stabilization and movement (and therefore posture) of the head, neck, ribs, spinal structures and upper extremity. See Figures 2.2.6 and 2.2.7.

Lung volume, intra-abdominal pressure and back pain

Grewar & McLean (2008) note that respiratory dysfunctions are commonly seen in patients with low back pain, pelvic floor dysfunction and poor posture. Additional evidence exists connecting diaphragmatic and breathing pattern disorders, with various forms of pelvic girdle dysfunction – including sacroiliac pain (O'Sullivan & Beales 2007). Similarly Carriere (2006) noted that disrupted function of either the diaphragm, or the PFM may alter the normal mechanisms for regulating intra-abdominal pressure.

Lung volume is determined by changes in the vertical, transverse, and anteroposterior diameters of the thoracic cavity, therefore movements that increase any of these three diameters (without reducing the others) should increase respiratory capacity, under normal circumstances (i.e. if the pleura are intact). See Box 2.2.1.

Individuals with LBP have been shown to perform lifting tasks with more inhaled lung volume than individuals without LBP. These findings are consistent with the theoretical link between breath control, intra-abdominal pressure, and lumbar segmental control (Hagins & Lamberg 2011).

Interactive processes exist in which breathing patterns can be seen to influence intra-abdominal pressure that directly relate to spinal stability.

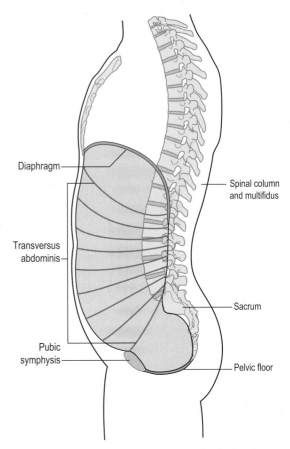

Figure 2.2.6 Lateral view of the abdominal cylinder. The abdominal cylinder contains the abdominal and pelvic viscera, bounded above by the diaphragm, including its crura and therefore by extension the psoas muscles via fascial connections, that blend with the pelvic floor and the obturator internus muscles. Forming the anterior, lateral and posterior boundaries of the cylinder, are the deep abdominal muscles including transversus abdominis and its associated fascial connections, the deep fibres of multifidus, the intercostals, the thoracolumbar vertebral column (T6–12 and all associated ribs, L1–L5) and osseous components of the pelvic girdle (innominates, sacrum and femora). The lumbopelvic cylinder comprises 85 joints – all of which require stabilization during functional tasks, including respiration. *With thanks to Diane Lee.*

THE BIOMECHANICS OF BREATHING

Inhalation and exhalation involve expansion and contraction of the lungs themselves, and this takes place:

- By means of a movement of the diaphragm, which lengthens and shortens the vertical diameter of the thoracic cavity. This is the normal

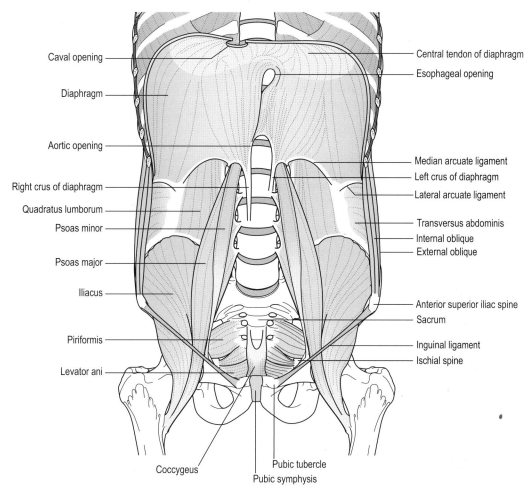

Caval opening

Diaphragm

Aortic opening

Right crus of diaphragm

Quadratus lumborum

Psoas minor

Psoas major

Iliacus

Piriformis

Levator ani

Central tendon of diaphragm

Esophageal opening

Median arcuate ligament

Left crus of diaphragm

Lateral arcuate ligament

Transversus abdominis

Internal oblique

External oblique

Anterior superior iliac spine

Sacrum

Inguinal ligament

Ischial spine

Coccygeus

Pubic tubercle

Pubic symphysis

Figure 2.2.7 Anteroposterior view of the abdominal cylinder. *With thanks to Josephine Key.*

means of breathing at rest. This diameter can be further increased when the upper ribs are raised during forced respiration, where the normal elastic recoil of the respiratory system is insufficient to meet demands. This brings into play the accessory breathing muscles, acting rather like a reserve tank, including sternocleidomastoid, the scalenes and the external intercostals.

- Movement of the ribs into elevation (inhalation) and depression (exhalation) alters the diameters of the thoracic cavity, increasing the vertical dimension by the actions of the diaphragm and scalenes. The transverse dimension is increased with the elevation and rotation of the lower ribs ('bucket handle' rib action) involving the diaphragm, external intercostals and levatores costarum. Elevation of the sternum is provided by upwards pressure due to spreading of the ribs ('pump handle' rib action), and the action of sternocleidomastoid and the scalenes.

The biomechanical structures that comprise the mechanism with which we breathe include the sternum, ribs, thoracic vertebrae, intervertebral discs, costal joints, muscles and ligaments. Structural and functional aspects of all of these have been summarized below (see Figs 2.2.9 to 2.2.11).

Put simply, the efficiency of breathing/respiration depends upon the production of a pumping action carried out by neuromuscular and skeletal exertion. The effectiveness of the pumping mechanism may be enhanced or retarded by the relative patency, interrelationships and efficiency of this complex collection of structures and their activities:

- On inhalation, air enters the nasal cavity or mouth and passes via the trachea to the bronchi, which

Box 2.2.1 **Lung volumes and capacities**

- Total lung capacity (TLC) is the amount of air the lung can contain at the height of maximum inspiratory effort. All other lung volumes are natural subdivisions of TLC.
- Residual volume (RV) is the amount of air remaining within the lung after maximum exhalation. Inhaled at birth, it is not exhaled until death because the rib cage prevents total lung collapse. The volumes and capacities within these two limits are described in Figure 2.2.8.
- Lung volumes are measured in a variety of ways. From simple hand-held peak expiratory flow (PEF) meters used by patients with asthma to record air flow resistance, to sophisticated laboratory equipment to establish both static and exercise lung capacities, volumes, and pressures, accurate information can be gained as to lung health or otherwise. For instance, vital capacity (VC) may be greatly reduced by limited expansion (restrictive disease) or by an abnormally large tidal volume (chronic obstructive pulmonary disease or during asthma attacks). During vigorous exercise, tidal volume (Vt) may increase to half the VC to maintain adequate alveolar ventilation. Limitation of exercise capacity is often the first sign of early lung disease that limits VC (Berne & Levy 1998, p. 530).

Respiratory function (breathing) therefore demonstrably depends on the efficiency with which the structures constituting the pump mechanisms operate. At its simplest, for this pump to function optimally, the thoracic spine and the attaching ribs, together with their anterior sternal connections and all the soft tissues, muscles, ligaments, tendons and fascia, need to be structurally intact, with an uncompromised neural supply.

Without an efficient pump mechanism all other respiratory functions will be suboptimal. Clearly, a host of dysfunctional patterns can result from altered airway characteristics, abnormal status of the lungs, and/or from emotional and other influences. However, even if allergy or infection is causal in altering the breathing pattern, the process of breathing can be enhanced by relatively unglamorous nuts-and-bolts features such as the normalization of rib restrictions or shortened upper fixator muscles.

The major structural components of the process of breathing are outlined below. These notes discuss the fascia, the joints of the thoracic cage – including spinal and rib structures – and the musculature and other soft tissues of the region. Functional influences on these structures (e.g. gait and posture) are evaluated insofar as they impact on the efficiency of the respiratory process.

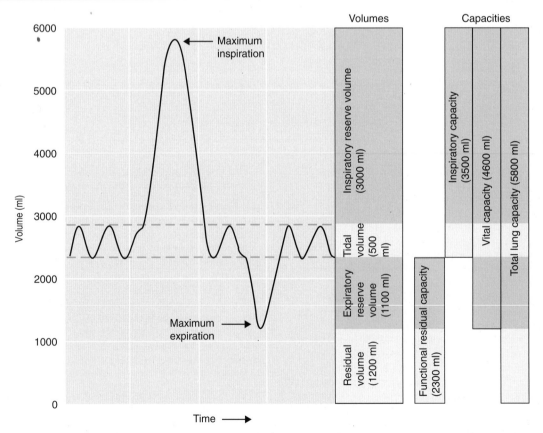

Figure 2.2.8 Lung volumes and capacities as displayed by a time versus volume spirogram. Values are approximate. The tidal volume is measured under resting conditions. *Reproduced from Beachey 1998.*

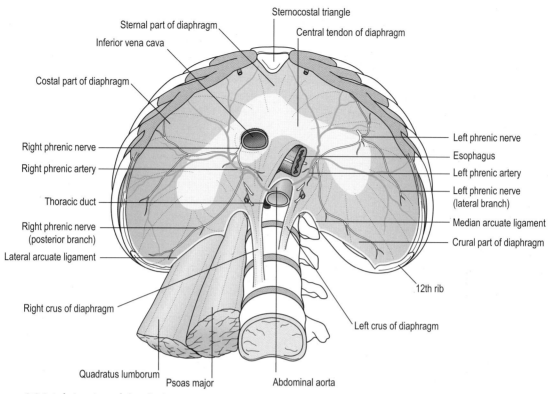

Figure. 2.2.9 Inferior view of the diaphragm.

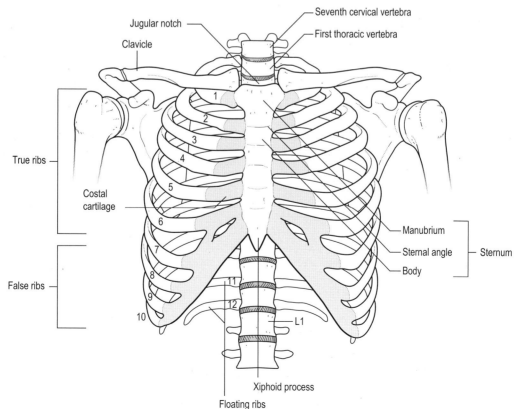

Figure 2.2.10 Anterior view of the thoracic cage. *Reproduced from Seeley et al 1995.*

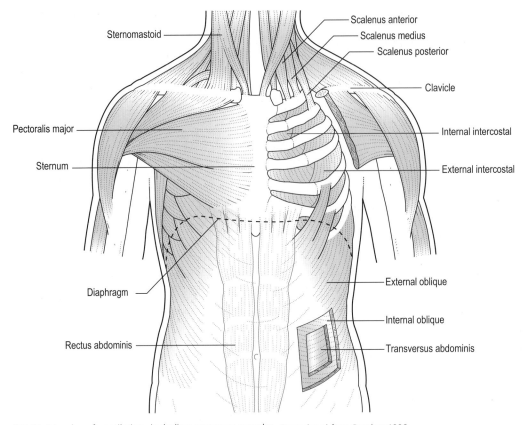

Figure 2.2.11 Muscles of ventilation, including accessory muscles. *Reproduced from Beachey 1998.*

separate to form four lobar bronchi and subsequently subdivide into ever narrower bronchi until 'At the 11th subdivision, the airway is called a bronchiole' (Naifeh 1994).

- Normal nasal function is described in Chapter 2.3.
- The structure of the trachea and bronchi includes supporting rings which are made up of varying proportions of cartilage – for rigidity – and elastic muscle. While the wider and more cephalad trachea has a larger proportion of cartilage, the narrower and more caudad bronchioles are almost entirely elastic.
- Gas exchange takes place in the alveoli (air sacs), situated toward the end of the bronchioles, mainly in the alveolar ducts. These air sacs have fine membranous walls surrounded by equally thin-walled capillaries which allow gas exchange to occur.
- In order for the lungs to expand and contract, the thoracic cavity lengthens and shortens due to the rise and fall of the diaphragm as the ribs elevate and depress to produce an increase and decrease in the anteroposterior diameter of the rib cage. Any

restrictions imposed by joint or soft tissue dysfunction will retard the efficiency of this pumping process.
- Some of the thoracic activities described are under muscular control, whereas others result from elastic recoil (D'Alonzo & Krachman (1997)). If the accessory breathing muscles become shortened or fibrotic they negatively influence the efficiency of these processes. See notes on muscular influences later in this chapter.

The muscles of respiration

The extrinsic thoracic musculature is responsible for positioning the torso, and therefore the placement in space of the shoulders, arms, neck and head. The intrinsic thoracic muscles move the thoracic vertebrae or the rib cage (and possibly the entire upper body) and/or are associated with respiration.

The deeper elements of the thoracic musculature represent a remarkable system by means of which respiration occurs. Some of these muscles also provide rotational components which carry similar, spiralling, lines of oblique tension from the pelvis (external and internal obliques) through the entire torso (external and internal intercostals), almost as if the ribs were 'slipped into' this supportive web of continuous muscular tubes. Rolfer Tom Myers (1997) describes the physical continuity which occurs between these muscles (obliques and intercostals). Above the pelvic crest this myofascial network creates a series of crossover (X-shaped) patterns:

The obliques tuck into the lower edges of the basket of ribs. Between each of the ribs are the internal and external intercostals, which taken all together form a continuation of the same 'X', formed by the obliques. These muscles, commonly taken to be accessory muscles of breathing, are seen in this context to be perhaps more involved in locomotion [and stability], helping to guide and check the torque, swinging through the rib cage during walking and running.

Myers 1997

Richardson and colleagues (1999) describe research into the behaviour of the abdominal muscles during quiet breathing. They found that the abdominal musculature was activated towards the end of exhalation, and noted that: 'Contraction of the abdominal muscles contributes towards the regulation of the length of the diaphragm, end-expiratory lung volume and expiratory airflow'.

With a voluntary increase in exhalation force, all the muscles of the abdomen contract simultaneously. However, when increased exhalation force occurs involuntarily, transversus abdominis is recruited before the other abdominal muscles (rectus abdominis, obliquus externus abdominis), producing enhancement of inspiratory efficiency by increasing the diaphragm's length and permitting an elastic recoil of the thoracic cavity.

Like the erector system of the posterior thorax, the abdominal musculature plays a significant role in positioning the thorax and in rotating the entire upper body. It is also now known to play a key part in spinal stabilization and intersegmental stability, particularly transversus abdominis (Hodges 1999). The rectus abdominis, external and internal obliques and transversus abdominis are also involved in respiration due to their role in positioning the abdominal viscera as well as depression of the lower ribs, assisting in forced expiration (especially coughing).

Role of intercostal musculature

Stone (1999) amplifies the generally understood role of the intercostal muscles and their functions:

For many years the intercostals were attributed with a very complex biomechanical effect, such that the internal intercostals were considered expiratory muscles and the external intercostals inspiratory muscles.

Kapandji 1974

Stone continues by explaining that the processes involved are far more complicated and that they relate to air and fluid movement within the thoracic cavity:

During inspiration and expiration there are cascades of action within the intercostal muscles, which start at one end of the rib cage and progress to the other to produce the required changes in rib cage shape.

De Troyer & Estenne (1988) showed that during inhalation the external intercostals are activated from superior to inferior, while during forced exhalation the internal intercostals are activated from inferior to superior. The implication is that, on inhalation, stabilization of the upper ribs is required, involving scalenes (De Troyer 1994) to allow the sequential intercostal contraction wave to progress inferiorly. In contrast, during forced exhalation the lower ribs require stabilization – by quadratus lumborum – to allow the superiorly directed wave to occur. Muscular imbalances (shortness, weakness, etc.) could therefore impact on normal breathing function. (Assessment and treatment of muscular imbalances are discussed in Sections 6 and 7.)

- The muscles and other soft tissues associated with respiration are listed in Box 2.2.2 and are detailed and discussed fully in Chapters 6.2 (assessment) and 7.2 (treatment).
- The different ways of characterizing muscles are summarized in Box 2.2.3.

Additional muscular and fascial influences and connections

- The soft tissue links between the thoracic region and the pelvic region include major structures such as quadratus lumborum, transversus abdominis, and psoas, which merge with the diaphragm and therefore have the potential to influence breathing function.
- The internal and external obliques (usually described as trunk rotators) also merge with the diaphragm and lower ribs and can have marked influences on respiratory function. It is worth reflecting that this works in reverse, and that diaphragmatic and respiratory dysfunction is bound to affect these associated muscles.
- The primary inspiratory muscles are the diaphragm, the more lateral external intercostals, parasternal internal intercostals, scalene group and levatores costarum, with the diaphragm providing 70–80% of the inhalation force (Simons et al 1998).

35

Box 2.2.2 **Muscles of breathing**

Muscles of inhalation

Primary

Diaphragm
Parasternal (intercartilaginous) internal intercostals
Upper and more lateral external intercostals
Levatores costarum
Scalenes

Accessory

Sternocleidomastoid
Upper trapezius
Serratus anterior (arms elevated)
Latissimus dorsi (arms elevated)
Serratus posterior superior
Iliocostalis thoracis
Subclavius
Omohyoid

Muscles of exhalation

Primary

Elastic recoil of lungs, diaphragm, pleura and costal
  cartilages

Accessory

Interosseous internal intercostals
Abdominal muscles
Transversus thoracis
Subcostales
Iliocostalis lumborum
Quadratus lumborum
Serratus posterior inferior
Latissimus dorsi

- These muscles are supported, or their role is replaced, by the accessory muscles during increased demand (or dysfunctional breathing patterns): sternocleidomastoid (SCM), upper trapezius, pectoralis major and minor, serratus anterior, latissimus dorsi, serratus posterior superior, iliocostalis thoracis, subclavius and omohyoid (Kapandji 1974, Simons et al 1998).
- Page (1952) observed:

  'There is direct continuity of fascia from the apex of the diaphragm to the base of the skull. Extending through the fibrous pericardium upward through the deep cervical fascia and the continuity extends not only to the outer surface of the sphenoid, occipital and temporal bones but proceeds further through the foramina in the base of the skull around the vessels and nerves to join the dura'.

An obvious corollary to this vivid description of the continuity of the fascia is that distortion or stress affecting any one part of the structure will have repercussions on other parts of the same structure. For example, if the position of the cervical spine in relation to the thorax alters (as in a habitual forward-head position), or if the position of the diaphragm alters relative to its normal position (as in a slumped posture), the functional efficiency of the breathing mechanisms may be compromised.

- Myers (1997) has described what he terms the 'deep front line' – fascial connections linking the osseous and soft tissue structures which highlight clearly how modifications in posture involving spinal and/or other attachment structures will directly modify the fascia which envelops, supports, and gives coherence to the soft tissues of the breathing mechanism:
  - the anterior longitudinal ligament, diaphragm, pericardium, mediastinum, parietal pleura, fascia prevertebralis and the scalene fascia connect the lumbar spine (bodies and transverse processes) to the cervical transverse processes and via longus capitis to the basilar portion of the occiput
  - other links in this chain involve a connection between the posterior manubrium and the hyoid bone, via the subhyoid muscles and the fascia pretrachealis, between the hyoid and the cranium/mandible, involving the suprahyoid muscle as well as the muscles of the jaw linking the mandible to the face and cranium.

In considering function and dysfunction of the respiratory system, fascial continuity should be kept in mind, since evidence of a local dysfunctional state (say of a particular muscle, spinal segment, rib, or group of ribs) can be seen to be capable of influencing (and being influenced by) distant parts of the same mechanism, as well as other areas of the body, via identifiable fascial connections.

Chapter 6.2 contains details of assessment of the key respiratory structures (muscles, ribs, thoracic spine) while Chapter 7.2 describes various methods of osteopathic soft-tissue treatment of those structures found to be dysfunctional and affecting respiratory function.

THORACIC SPINE AND RIBS

The posterior aspect of the thorax is represented by a mobile functional unit, the thoracic spinal column, through which the sympathetic nerve supply emerges:

Box 2.2.3 **Muscle characterizations**

Richardson and colleagues (1999) have categorized muscles capable of controlling one joint or one area of the spine as being 'monoarticular'. These could also be referred to as 'local' muscles. They also describe 'multijoint' muscles which are capable of moving several joints at the same time. These muscles are also phylogenetically the oldest. They can be referred to as 'global' muscles. This nomenclature allows clinical disciplines to communicate with other basic science disciplines in order to facilitate research and learning.

Other muscle categorization models include 'postural/phasic' (Janda 1983), and 'mobilizer/stabilizer' (Norris 1999). There are relative advantages in being able to describe and see the way the body works using these models.

Dual roles of specific muscles

Research shows that many of the muscles supporting and moving the thorax and/or the spinal segments (including erector spinae) prepare to accommodate for subsequent movement as soon as arm or shoulder activity is initiated, with deep stabilizing activity from transversus abdominis, for example, occurring milliseconds before unilateral rapid arm activity (Hodges & Richardson 1997). Stabilization of the lumbar spine and thorax has been shown to depend, to a large extent, on abdominal muscle activity (Hodges 1999). Transversus abdominis is categorized as a local, stabilizing structure. Richardson and colleagues (1999) note that the direct involvement of this muscle in respiration – where it contributes to forced exhalation – leads to a potential conflict with its role as a spinal stabilizer. They have identified a clear linkage between dysfunction of transversus abdominis and low back pain. Interestingly, the dysfunctional pattern seems to have less to do with strength or endurance capabilities than with motor control. Since the muscle acts to stabilize the spine, dysfunction is bound to contribute to spinal imbalance; however, the impact on respiration is less clear.

Richardson and colleagues also highlight the importance, in postural control, of the diaphragm. In a study which measured activity of both the costal diaphragm and the crural portion of the diaphragm, as well as transversus abdominis, it was found that contraction occurred in all these structures when spinal stabilization was required (in this instance during shoulder flexion). 'The results provide evidence that the diaphragm does contribute to spinal control and may do so by assisting with pressurization and control of displacement of the abdominal contents, allowing transversus abdominis to increase tension in the thoracolumbar fascia or to generate intra-abdominal pressure.' The involvement of the diaphragm in postural stabilization suggests that situations might easily occur where such contradictory demands are evident, where postural stabilizing control is required at the same time that physiological requirements create demands for greater diaphragmatic movement: 'This is an area of ongoing research, but must involve eccentric/concentric phases of activation of the diaphragm' (Richardson et al 1999).

Just what the impact is on respiratory function of transversus abdominis and of the diaphragm when dual stabilizing and respiratory roles occur is an open question; the impact would doubtless be strongly influenced by the relative fitness and health of the individual.

Confusion of nomenclature is currently a feature of muscle categorization. The basic fact is that some muscles behave differently from others, some tending to shortness with others tending to weakness and possibly lengthening. What labels are attached is a matter of convenience and debate. In this book the widely used Jull & Janda (1987) terminology will be employed (i.e. postural and phasic).

- The degree of movement in all directions (flexion, extension, side flexion, and rotation) allowed by the relatively rigid structure of the thorax is less than that available in the cervical or lumbar spines, being deliberately limited in order to protect the vital organs housed within the thoracic cavity.
- In most individuals the thoracic spine has a kyphotic (forward-bending) profile which varies in degree from individual to individual.
- The thoracic spinous processes are especially prominent, and therefore easily palpated.
- The transverse processes from T1 to T10 carry costotransverse joints for articulation with the ribs.

The thoracic facet joints, which glide on each other and restrict and largely determine the range of spinal movement, have typical plane-type synovial features, including an articular capsule.

Facet orientation

Hruby and colleagues (1997) describe a useful method for remembering the structure and orientation of the facet joints (of particular value when using mobilization methods, see Ch. 7.2):

The superior facets of each thoracic vertebrae are slightly convex and face posteriorly (backward), somewhat superiorly (up), and laterally. Their angle of declination averages 60° relative to the transverse plane and 20° relative to the coronal plane. Remember the facet facing by the mnemonic 'BUL' (backward, upward, and lateral). This is in contrast to the cervical and lumbar regions where the superior facets face backwards, upwards, and medially ('BUM'). Thus, the superior facets [of the entire spine] are BUM, BUL, BUM, from cervical, to thoracic to lumbar.

Discs

The disc structure of the thoracic spine is similar to that of the cervical and lumbar spine. The notable difference is the relative broadness of the posterior longitudinal ligament that together with the restricted range of motion potential of the region, makes herniation of thoracic discs an infrequent occurrence. Degenerative changes due to osteoporosis and ageing, as well as trauma, are relatively common in this region and may impact directly on respiratory function as a result of restricted mobility of the thoracic structures.

Structural features of the ribs

(see Fig. 2.2.10)

The ribs are composed of a segment of bone and a costal cartilage. The costal cartilages attach to the costochondral joint of most ribs (see variations below), depressions in the bony segment of the ribs.

Ribs 11 and 12 do not articulate with the sternum ('floating ribs'), whereas all other ribs do so, in various ways, either by means of their own cartilaginous synovial joints (i.e. ribs 1–7, which are 'true ribs') or by means of a merged cartilaginous structure (ribs 8–10, which are 'false ribs').

The head of each rib articulates with its thoracic vertebrae at the costovertebral joint. Ribs 2–9 also articulate with the vertebrae above and below by means of a demifacet. Ribs 1, 11 and 12 articulate with their own vertebrae by means of a unifacet.

Typical ribs (3–9) comprise a head, neck, tubercle, angles and shafts and connect directly, or via cartilaginous structures, to the sternum.

The posterior rib articulations allow rotation during breathing, while the anterior cartilaginous elements store the torsional energy produced by this rotation. The ribs behave like tension rods and elastically recoil to their previous position when the muscles relax. These elastic elements reduce with age and may also be lessened by intercostal muscular tension.

Rib articulations, thoracic vertebral positions and myofascial elements must all be functional for normal breathing to occur. Dysfunctional elements may reduce the range of mobility, and, therefore, lung capacity.

Atypical ribs

Atypical ribs and their key features include:

- Rib 1, which is broad, short and flat, is the most curved. The subclavian artery and cervical plexus are anatomically vulnerable to compression if the 1st rib becomes compromised in relation to the anterior and/or middle scalenes, or the clavicle.
- Rib 2 carries a tubercle which attaches to the proximal portion of serratus anterior.

- Ribs 11 and 12 are atypical due to their failure to articulate anteriorly with the sternum or costal cartilages.

Rib dysfunction and appropriate treatments are discussed in Chapter 7.2.

Structural features of the sternum

(see Figs 2.2.10 and 2.2.12)

There are three key subdivisions of the sternum:

1. The manubrium (or head) which articulates with the clavicles at the sternoclavicular joints. The superior surface of the manubrium (jugular notch) lies directly anterior to the 2nd thoracic vertebra. The manubrium is joined to the body of the sternum by means of a fibrocartilaginous symphysis, the sternal angle (angle of Louis), which lies directly anterior to the 4th thoracic vertebra (Fig. 2.2.11).
2. The body of the sternum provides the attachment sites for the ribs, with the 2nd rib attaching at the sternal angle. This makes the angle an important landmark when counting ribs.
3. The xyphoid process is the 'tail' of the sternum, joining it at the xyphisternal symphysis (which fuses in most people during the fifth decade of life), usually anterior to the 9th thoracic vertebra.

Posterior thorax

In regional terms, the thoracic spine is usually divided into (White & Panjabi 1978): upper (T1–4), middle (T5–8), lower (T9–12):

- The total range of thoracic flexion and extension combined (between T1 and T12) is approximately 60° (Liebenson 1996)
- The total range of thoracic rotation is approximately 40°
- Total range of lateral flexion of the thoracic spine is approximately 50°.

Neural regulation of breathing

This autonomic nervous system (ANS) enables the automatic unconscious maintenance of the internal environment of the body in ideal efficiency, including both respiratory and heart rates, as the ANS adjusts to the various demands of the external environment, be it sleep with repair and growth, quiet or extreme physical activity and stress. The nerves that innervate the smooth muscle of the alimentary canal cause propulsion of food, while the nerves to exocrine glands initiate secretion of digestive juices. The system is also concerned with the emptying of the bladder and with sexual activity.

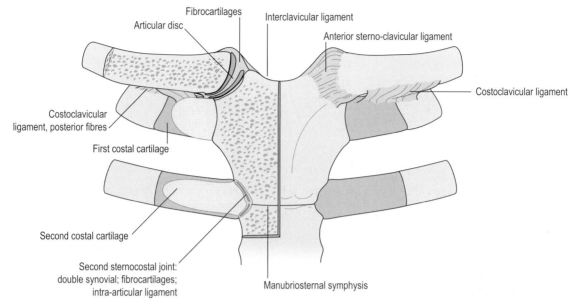

Figure 2.2.12 Manubrium sternum. *Reproduced with kind permission from Williams et al 1995.*

Innervation of the smooth muscles in the walls of the arterioles varies their caliber, permitting the maintenance of blood pressure and the switching up and down of various parts of the circulation according to whether digestion, growth and repair, heat conservation or loss, or strong muscular activity are required. The maintenance of an adequate circulation also depends on the heart rate, the strength of the cardiac muscle contraction thereby varying the cardiac output.

Respiratory centres in the most primitive part of the brain, the brainstem, unconsciously influence and adjust alveolar ventilation to maintain arterial blood oxygen and carbon dioxide pressures (PCO_2) at relatively constant levels in order to sustain life under varying conditions and requirements.

There are three main neural influences:

1. The **dorsal respiratory group** is located in the distal portion of the medulla. It receives input from peripheral chemoreceptors and other types of receptors via the vagus and glossopharyngeal nerves. These impulses generate inspiratory movements and are responsible for the *basic rhythm of breathing*.
2. The **pneumotaxic centre** in the superior part of the pons transmits inhibitory signals to the dorsal respiratory centre, controlling the *filling phase of breathing*.
3. The **ventral respiratory group**, located in the medulla, causes either inspiration or expiration. It is inactive in quiet breathing but is important in stimulating abdominal expiratory muscles during levels of high respiratory demand.

The *Hering-Breuer reflex* prevents overinflation of the lungs and is initiated by nerve receptors in the walls of the bronchi and bronchioles sending messages to the dorsal respiratory centre, via the vagus nerves. It 'switches off' excessive inflation during inspiration, and also excessive deflation during exhalation.

Chemical control of breathing

The central role of respiration is to maintain balanced concentrations of oxygen (O_2) and carbon dioxide (CO_2) in the tissues. Increased levels of CO_2 act on the central chemosensitive areas of the respiratory centres themselves, increasing inspiratory and expiratory signals to the respiratory muscles. O_2, on the other hand, acts on peripheral chemoreceptors located in the carotid body (in the bifurcation of the common carotid arteries) via the glossopharyngeal nerves, and the aortic body (on the aortic arch) which sends the appropriate messages via the vagus nerves to the dorsal respiratory centre.

Voluntary and neural control of breathing

The lungs are entirely governed by autonomic sensory and motor nerves, there being no voluntary motor control over airway smooth muscles. It is known that respiration influences autonomic rhythms, however it is also true that autonomic challenges are able to modify respiration (Naschitz et al 2006).

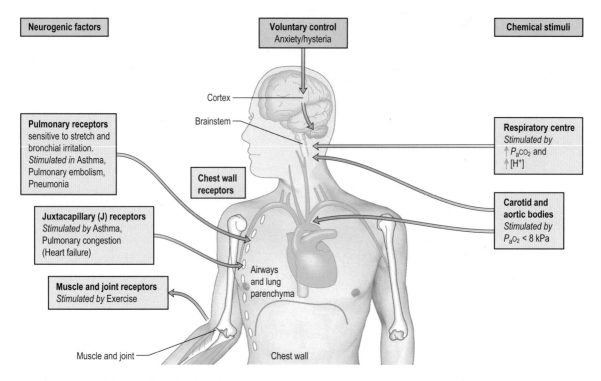

Figure 2.2.13 Multiple neurological and biochemical influences on respiration.

Automatic breathing can be overridden by higher cortical conscious input (directly, via the spinal neurons which drive the respiratory muscles) in response to, for instance, fear or sudden surprise. Speaking requires voluntary control to interrupt the normal rhythmicity of breathing, as does singing and playing a wind instrument. There is evidence that the cerebral cortex and thalamus also supply part of the drive for normal respiratory rhythm during wakefulness (cerebral influences on the medullary centres are withdrawn during sleep). Breathing pattern disorders (BPDs) and hyperventilation syndromes (HVSs) probably originate from some of these higher centres (Timmons & Ley 1994, p. 35). See Figure 2.2.13.

Breathing originates in the brainstem, which consists of the medulla and the pons, as well as a central pattern generator that has outputs to respiratory muscles, modulated by various sensory afferent inputs. Efferent impulses leave via the phrenic and intercostal nerves to produce contraction of the diaphragm and intercostal muscles. Other nerves travel to the accessory muscles (e.g. larynx) to synchronize their contractions with phases of breathing. See Figure 2.2.14.

NANC system

Researchers have recognized a 'third' nervous system regulating the airways called the *nonadrenergic noncholinergic*

(NANC) system, containing inhibitory and stimulatory fibres; nitric oxide (NO) has been identified as the NANC neurotransmitter (Snyder 1992).

- NANC inhibitory nerves cause calcium ions to enter the neuron, mediating smooth muscle relaxation and bronchodilation.
- NANC stimulatory fibres – also called C-fibres – are found in the lung supporting tissue, airways, and pulmonary blood vessels, and appear to be involved in bronchoconstriction following cold air breathing and in exercise-induced asthma (Beachey 1998, p. 30).

Where next?

This chapter has summarized the main structural features of breathing function. Details of assessment and treatment of dysfunctional soft tissues, and other biomechanical changes, relating to breathing pattern disorders (BPD) will be found in various chapters in Sections 6, 7 and 8.

In the next chapter, nasal influences on breathing are outlined followed by descriptions of the major patterns of dysfunctional breathing. This is followed by chapters on biochemical and psychological relationships with BPD.

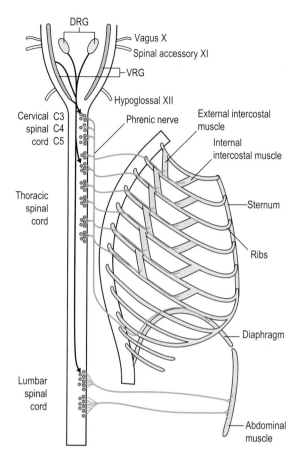

Figure 2.2.14 Location of the spinal motor neurons that control respiratory muscles. The cell bodies of motor neurons that activate the diaphragm are located in C3–C5. Their axons collect in the phrenic nerve. Cell bodies of motor neurons controlling the intercostal muscles are located in the thoracic spinal cord. The abdominal muscles are controlled by motor neurons whose cell bodies are in the lower thoracic and upper lumbar spinal cord. All of these motor neurons receive inputs from controlling centres in the medulla. DRG, dorsal respiratory group in the medulla; VRG, ventral respiratory group. *Adapted from Hlastala M.P., Berger A.J., 2001. Physiology of Respiration, Oxford University Press.*

REFERENCES

Abernethy, A., Mackinnon, L., Neal, R.J., et al., 1996. The biophysical foundations of human movement. Human Kinetics Publishers, Melbourne.

Beachey, W., 1998. Respiratory care anatomy and physiology. Mosby, St Louis.

Berne, R.M., Levy, M.N., 1998. Physiology. Mosby, St Louis.

Carriere, B., 2006. Interdependence of posture and the pelvic floor. In: Carriere, B., Markel Feldt, C. (Eds.), The pelvic floor. Thieme, New York, pp. 68 & 76.

Cenker, E., Cem, O., Ayse, B., et al., 2010. Anxiety and depressive disorders in patients presenting with chest pain to the emergency department: a comparison between cardiac and non-cardiac origin. The Journal of Emergency Medicine. 39 (2), 144–150.

Chiti, L., Biondia, G., Morelot-Panzinia, C., et al., 2008. Scalene muscle activity during progressive inspiratory loading under pressure support ventilation in normal humans. Respiratory Physiology & Neurobiology 164, 441–448.

Correa, E., Berzin, F., 2008. Mouth Breathing Syndrome: Cervical muscles recruitment during nasal inspiration before and after respiratory and postural exercises on Swiss Ball. International Journal of Pediatric Otorhinolaryngology 72, 1335–1343.

Corrin, B., Nicholson, A. (Eds.), 2011. Chapter 3 – Diseases of the conductive airways. In: Pathology of the Lungs, third ed. pp. 91–134.

D'Alonzo, G., Krachman, S., 1997. Respiratory system. In: Ward, R. (Ed.), Foundations for osteopathic medicine. Williams and Wilkins, Baltimore.

David, P., Laval, D., Terrien, J., et al., 2012. Postural control and ventilatory drive during voluntary hyperventilation and carbon dioxide rebreathing. Eur J Appl Physiol. 112 (1), 145–154.

Deindl, F.M., Vodusek, D.B., Hesse, U., et al., 1994. Pelvic floor activity patterns: Comparison of nulliparous continent and parous urinary stress incontinent women. A kinesiological

EMG study. British Journal of Urology 73, 413–417.

De Troyer, A., 1994. Do canine scalene and sternomastoid muscles play a role in breathing? Journal of Applied Physiology 76, 242–252.

De Troyer, A., Estenne, M., 1988. Functional anatomy of the respiratory muscles. Clinics in Chest Medicine 9, 175–193.

Faria, E.W., Parker, D.L., Faria, I.E., 2005. The science of cycling. Factors affecting performance – part 2. Sports Medicine 35 (4), 313–337.

Fink, P., Schroder, A., 2010. One single diagnosis, bodily distress syndrome, succeeded to capture 10 diagnostic categories of functional somatic syndromes and somatoform disorders. Journal of Psychosomatic Research 68 (5), 415–426.

Grewar, H., McLean, L. 2008. The integrated continence system: A manual therapy approach to the treatment of stress urinary incontinence. Man. Ther. 13, 375–386.

Hagins, M., Lamberg, E., 2011. Individuals with low back pain breathe differently than healthy individuals during a lifting task. J Orthop Sports Phys Ther 41 (3), 141–148.

Hall, C., Brody, L., 2005. Therapeutic exercise: moving towards function, second ed. Williams & Wilkins, Lippincott.

Hodges, P., 1999. Is there a role for transversus abdominis in lumbo-pelvic stability? Manual Therapy 4 (2), 74–86.

Hodges, P., Richardson, C., 1997. Feedforward contraction of transversus abdominis is not influenced by direction of arm movement. Experimental Brain Research 114, 362–370.

Hodges, P.W., Heijnen, I., Gandevia, S.C., 2001. Postural activity of the diaphragm is reduced in humans when respiratory demand increases. Journal of Physiology (Cambridge) 537, 999–1008.

Hruby, R., Goodridge, J., Jones, J., 1997. Thoracic region and rib cage. In: Ward, R. (Ed.), Foundations for osteopathic medicine. Williams and Wilkins, Baltimore.

Hill, K., Eastwood, P., 2011. Effects of loading on upper airway and respiratory pump muscle motoneurons. Respiratory Physiology & Neurobiology, 179 (1), 64–70.

Janda, V., 1983. Muscle function testing. Butterworths, London.

Janda, V., 1987. Muscles and motor control in low back pain – assessment and management. In: Twomey, L. (Ed.), Physical therapy of the low back, first ed. Churchill Livingstone, pp.253–278.

Janda, V., Frank, C., Liebenson, C., 2007. Evaluation of muscular imbalance. In: Liebenson, C. (Ed.), Rehabilitation of the spine: a practitioner's manual, second ed. Lippincott Williams & Wilkins, Philadelphia.

Jones, A., Dean, E., Chow, C., 2003. Comparison of the oxygen cost of breathing exercises and spontaneous breathing in patients with stable chronic obstructive pulmonary disease. Physical Therapy 83 (5), 424–431.

Jull, G., Janda, V., 1987. Muscles and motor control in low back pain. In: Twomey, L., Taylor, J. (Eds.), Physical therapy for the low back. Clinics in physical therapy. Churchill Livingstone, New York.

Kapandji, I., 1974. The physiology of the joints, second ed. Churchill Livingstone, Edinburgh, Vol 3.

Key, J., Clift, A., Condie, F., et al., 2008. A model of movement dysfunction provides a classification system guiding diagnosis and therapeutic care in spinal pain and related musculo-skeletal syndromes: a paradigm shift. Journal of Bodywork & Movement Therapies 12 (2), 105–120.

Key, J., 2010. The Pelvic Crossed Syndromes: A reflection of imbalanced function in the myofascial envelope; a further exploration of Janda's work. Journal of Bodywork and Movement Therapies, 14 (3), 299–301.

Kolnes, L.-J., 2012. Embodying the body in anorexia nervosa – a physiotherapeutic approach. Journal of Bodywork and Movement Therapies 16 (3), 281–288.

Kuchera, M., Kuchera, W., 1997. General postural considerations. In: Ward, R. (Ed.), Foundations for osteopathic medicine. Williams and Wilkins, Baltimore.

Lee, D., Lee, L.J., McLaughlin, L., 2008. Stability, continence and breathing: The role of fascia following pregnancy and delivery. Journal of Bodywork and Movement Therapies 12, 333–348.

Liebenson, C., 1996. Rehabilitation of the spine. Williams and Wilkins, Baltimore.

Lima, L., Barauna, M., Sologurem, M., 2004. Postural alterations in children with mouth breathing assessed by computerized biophotogrammetry. J. Appl. Oral Sci. 232–237.

Lum, L.C., 1994. Hyperventilation syndromes: physiological considerations in clinical management. In: Timmons, B. (Ed.), Behavioural and psychological approaches to breathing disorders. Plenum Press, New York.

Myers, T., 1997. Anatomy Trains. Journal of Bodywork and Movement Therapies 1 (2), 91–101.

Naifeh, K.H., 1994. Basic anatomy and physiology of the respiratory system and the autonomic nervous system. In: Timmons, B.H., Ley, R. (Eds.), Behavioral and psychological approaches to breathing disorders. Plenum Press, New York.

Naschitz, J., Mussafia-Priselac, R., Kovalev, Y., 2006. Patterns of hypocapnia on tilt in patients with fibromyalgia, chronic fatigue syndrome, nonspecific dizziness, and neurally mediated syncope. Am J Med Sci 31 (6), 295–303.

Neiva, P., Kirkwood, R., Godinho, R., 2009. Orientation and position of head posture, scapula and thoracic spine in mouth-breathing children. International Journal of Pediatric Otorhinolaryngology 73, 227–236.

Norris, C.M., 1999. Functional load abdominal training. Journal of Bodywork and Movement Therapies 3 (3), 150–158.

O'Sullivan, P., Beales, D., 2007. Changes in pelvic floor and diaphragm kinematics and respiratory patterns in subjects with sacroiliac joint pain following a motor learning intervention: A case series. Manual Therapy 12, 209–218.

Page, L., 1952. Academy of Applied Osteopathy Yearbook. Carmel, California.

Richardson, C., Jull, G., Hodges, P., et al., 1999. Therapeutic exercise for spinal segmental stabilization in low back pain. Churchill Livingstone, Edinburgh.

Seeley, R.R., Stephens, T.D., Tate, P., 1995. Anatomy and physiology, third ed. McGraw-Hill, New York.

Simons, D., Travell, J., Simons, L., 1998. Myofascial pain and dysfunction: the trigger point manual, second ed. Williams and Wilkins. Baltimore, Vol. 1.

Smith, M.D., Russell, A., Hodges, P.W., 2006. Disorders of breathing and continence have a stronger association with back pain than obesity and physical activity. Australian Journal of Physiotherapy 52, 11–16.

Snyder, S.H., 1992. Nitric oxide: first in a new class of neurotransmitters? Science 257, 494.

Sorheim, I.-C., Johannessen, A., Gulsvik, A., et al., 2010. Gender differences in COPD: are women more susceptible to smoking effects than men? Thorax 65, 480–485.

Stone, C., 1999. The science and art of osteopathy. Stanley Thornes, Cheltenham.

Timmons, B., Ley, R. (Eds.), 1994. Behavioral and psychological approaches to breathing disorders. Plenum Press, New York.

West, J.B., 2000. Respiratory physiology: the essentials. Lippincott Williams and Wilkins, Philadelphia.

White, A., Panjabi, M., 1978. Clinical biomechanics of the spine. J B Lippincott, Baltimore.

Williams, P.L., Bannister, L.H., et al. (Eds.), 1995. Gray's anatomy, thirty eighth ed. Churchill Livingstone, New York.

Yamaguti, W.P., Claudino, R., Neto, A., et al., 2012. Diaphragmatic breathing training program improves abdominal motion during natural breathing in patients with chronic obstructive pulmonary disease: a randomized controlled trial. Archives of Physical Medicine and Rehabilitation 93 (4), 571–577.

Chapter | **2.3** |

Nasal influences on breathing

Jim Bartley

INTRODUCTION

Many of the interactions between the upper and lower respiratory tracts remain poorly understood. Important, well-known nasal functions include the filtering, warming and humidifying of inspired air before inhalation into the lungs (Sahin-Yilmaz & Naclerio 2011). Olfactory nerves within the nose also provide us with our sense of smell. Smell, an early and fundamental sense, is linked to the limbic system and our emotions (Soudry et al 2011). Nasal breathing (as opposed to mouth breathing) increases circulating blood oxygen and carbon dioxide levels, slows the breathing rate and improves overall lung volumes (Swift et al 1988, Tanaka et al 1988). Many lower respiratory tract diseases, such as asthma and chronic obstructive pulmonary disease, are associated with both breathing pattern disorders as well as significant upper respiratory disease (Krouse et al 2007, Hurst 2009). Improved medical management of nasal and sinus disease can lead to corresponding improvements in lower respiratory tract function (Krouse et al 2007).

NASAL ANATOMY AND PHYSIOLOGY

The internal nose is comprised of two nasal cavities, situated on either side of the midline of the face, each with a roof, a floor and medial and lateral walls. The two cavities are separated medially by the septum, which is comprised of cartilage and bone. The lateral nasal wall is uneven owing to three horizontal scroll shaped elevations called the superior, middle and inferior turbinates (Sahin-Yilmaz & Naclerio 2011). After inhaled air has passed through the external nostrils, it enters narrow slit-like areas termed the nasal valves. The resistance of the nasal valves is regulated principally by erectile tissue (the purpose of which is explained later in the chapter) within the inferior turbinates and nasal septum (Cole 2003).

The narrow nasal valves initially accelerate the inspired air creating turbulence. The nasal passages then widen, airflow slows and particulate matter is deposited on the surrounding surfaces (Cole 2003). Turbulence minimizes the presence of any air boundary layer that would exist with laminar flow and maximizes interaction between the airstream and the nasal mucosa. The turbulent inspired air then travels over the turbinates. The turbinates and septum consist of narrow slit-like spaces that present a large mucosal surface area to the airflow. The inferior turbinates, which are the largest of the turbinates, are responsible for the majority of the humidification, heating and filtering of air inhaled through the nose. The smaller middle turbinates project downwards over the openings of the maxillary, frontal and anterior ethmoid sinuses. Most inhaled airflow travels between the inferior and middle turbinates.

The internal nose not only provides around 90% of the respiratory system air-conditioning requirements, but also recovers around 33% of exhaled heat and moisture (Elad et al 2008).

In the posterior part of the nose (nasopharynx), lymphoid tissue called the adenoids may be present. This tissue is often present during early childhood, but regresses usually by about the age of seven. Enlarged adenoidal tissue can contribute to nasal obstruction in both children and adults. When air reaches the posterior part of the nose, airflow is directed to the lower airways. The right-angled nature of the bend in the nasopharynx also means that any residual particulate matter will be deposited on the posterior wall.

Ciliated pseudostratified columnar epithelium lines the majority of the inside of the nasal cavities; olfactory epithelium extending down from the roof of the nose lines the remainder. Cilia (fine hairs) beating at about 1000 times per minute, in synchronized patterns within a liquid sol layer on the airway surfaces, transport a superficial gel layer of mucus at a rate of 3 to 25 mm/minute towards the nasopharynx, where it is later cleared by swallowing or expectoration. The 10- to 15-μm deep mucus layer, which is negatively charged and slightly acidic (pH 5.5–6.5), through entrapment in the sticky mucus of the gel layer, provides the first line of defence against microbes, particles and airborne pollutants. Antimicrobial peptides: defensins, cathelicidin, and larger antimicrobial proteins such as lysozyme, lactoferrin and secretory leukocyte protease inhibitor are also present in the airway secretions (Rogan et al 2006). Oscillatory compressive stresses (as opposed to a constant airway pressure) increase adenosine triphosphate (ATP) release onto the airway surfaces. This activates apical purinoceptors, increasing liquid secretion and accelerating mucociliary clearance. For optimal function nasal and lung mucosal epithelia need exposure to oscillatory stresses. The beneficial effects of physical and deep-breathing exercises upon respiratory tract health may also be due to the action of oscillatory physical air pressures improving airway hydration and mucus clearance (Button et al 2008).

The lining of the nose contains a rich blood supply. Erectile tissue in the nose (inferior and middle turbinates and septum) undergoes a cycle of periodic congestion and decongestion. This 'nasal cycle' results in alternating patent and congested passages within the two nasal cavities for periods ranging from 1–7 hours. This time span is made up from combinations of discrete recurrent cycles spanning 1–1½ hrs. The nasal cycle usually goes unnoticed, since the total nasal airflow resistance remains unaffected. This nasal cycle, which is part of an overall body cycle, is controlled by the hypothalamus. Sympathetic dominance on one side causes nasal vasoconstriction of the ipsilateral turbinate, while parasympathetic dominance on the other causes nasal vasodilatation of the contralateral turbinate. Increased airflow though the right nostril is correlated to increased left brain activity and enhanced verbal performance, whereas increased airflow through the left nostril is associated with increased right brain activity and enhanced spatial performance (Shannahoff-Khalsa 1993). Brain wave cycles during sleep are also synchronized to this nasal cycle (Shannahoff-Khalsa 1993). The purpose of the nasal cycle is unknown, however the periodic congestion and decongestion of nasal venous sinusoids may provide a mechanism for the generation of plasma exudate – this mechanism is an important component of respiratory defence (Eccles 1996).

The paranasal sinuses are pneumatic or air-filled extensions of the nasal cavity. The frontal sinuses are situated superior to the orbits, the maxillary sinuses inferior to the orbits, the ethmoid sinuses medial to the orbits and the sphenoid sinuses posterior to the ethmoid sinuses. Although various theories have been proposed, the functions of the sinuses remain unknown. Hypotheses include: lightening the skull to maintain proper head balance, imparting resonance to the voice, contributing to facial growth and nitric oxide (NO) production (Selimoglu 2005). NO is a gas that is produced by the nose and paranasal sinuses. NO concentrations within the maxillary sinus are bacteriostatic against *Staphylococcus aureus*. NO may have a role in the sterilization of incoming air, and it also improves ventilation-perfusion in the lungs (Selimoglu 2005).

NASAL RESISTANCE

The nose provides a resistance to breathing that is twice that of the open mouth (Swift et al 1988). This increased resistance to inspiration and expiration appears to have a number of physiological benefits. Nasal breathing increases total lung volume (Swift et al 1988). The corresponding increase in functional residual capacity (volume of air present in the lungs present after passive expiration) is thought to improve arterial oxygen concentrations. In a study of arterial PaO_2 (partial pressure of oxygen: the measurement of oxygen in arterial blood) levels before and after jaw wiring (this forced patients to breathe through their noses), PaO_2 level increased by nearly 10% (Swift et al 1988). End tidal pCO_2 levels, which are considered to be a reliable indirect measure of the CO_2 partial pressure in the arterial blood, also increase with nasal breathing. This may be due to an increase in dead space (Tanaka et al 1988). Nasal resistance is also inversely related to end tidal pCO_2 levels (Bartley 2006). People who are anxious typically have lower arterial pCO_2 levels and are thus more likely to present complaining of nasal congestion (Bartley 2006). During exercise, nasal breathing causes a reduction in FEO_2, indicating that on expiration the percentage of oxygen extracted from the air by the lungs is increased, and an increase in FECO$_2$, indicating an increase in the percentage of expired air that is carbon dioxide (Morton et al 1995). This equates to more efficient oxygen extraction and carbon dioxide excretion. Nasal breathing also increases the timing of the expiratory phase of the respiratory cycle (Ayoub et al 1997). Increasing the expiratory phase of the respiratory cycle is known to increase the body's relaxation response (Cappo & Holmes 1984).

SMELL AND THE LIMBIC SYSTEM

Evolutionary theory teaches that in primitive life forms, the olfactory brain was probably a layer of cells above the brainstem that registered a smell and then simply categorized it. New layers of the olfactory brain then developed into what was initially called the rhinencephalon (nose brain) or limbic system (Le Doux 2003). About 100 million years ago, after the development of the limbic system, the mammalian brain had another growth spurt. Further brain layers were added on the limbic system to form the neocortex. The neocortex makes us human, giving us the advantages of rational thought, planning, memory and strategy (Le Doux 2003). Our limbic system, which has been called our 'emotional brain', coordinates the stress 'fight-or-flight' response. As part of this response not only does the heart rate increase, but the respiratory rate also goes up; the limbic system is able to override normal pCO$_2$ homeostasis (Plum 1992).

Aromas have also been used throughout history for their medicinal and mood-altering properties. The physiological evidence suggests that lavender and rosemary fragrances have direct effects on human memory and mood (Moss et al 2003). Fragrances such as lavender have a role in stress reduction (Setzer 2009).

LOWER RESPIRATORY TRACT DISEASE

The upper and lower respiratory tracts communicate with each other through a number of mechanisms. An inflammatory stimulus to the nasal mucosa results in lung inflammation and vice versa. These mechanisms are thought to operate through the vascular system. Inflammatory cells generated from one site are ready to respond to an inflammatory stimulation elsewhere (Braunstahl et al 2001a, 2001b). Theoretically, improvement of upper airways inflammation should improve asthma symptoms and control. A limited number of studies indicate that this may occur (Krouse et al 2007).

Postnasal drip, and the aspiration of nasal secretions, has long been considered a factor in asthma. Although these symptoms are linked, the evidence indicates that nasal secretions are not aspirated into the lungs (Hurst 2009). However, in cystic fibrosis the bacteriology of the upper respiratory tract is replicated in the lower respiratory tract (Hare et al 2010). Anecdotally, many patients report that their asthma, chronic obstructive pulmonary disease and bronchiectasis improve when they have had surgery for chronic rhinosinusitis; high quality prospective studies are still non-existent.

Nasobronchial reflexes have also been implicated in the interactions between the upper and lower respiratory tracts. Mechanical or chemical stimulation of receptors in the nose, trachea and larynx might produce sneezing, coughing or bronchoconstriction in order to prevent deeper penetration of allergens or irritants into the airway (Sarin et al 2006). A neural reflex mechanism certainly contributes to the bronchoconstrictive effect and thus asthma aggravation after exposure to cold air. The association of nasobronchial reflexes with inflammatory exposure in the upper respiratory tract is less clear (Sarin et al 2006).

Airway inflammation, both allergic and infective, affects both the upper and lower respiratory tracts. Patients with lower respiratory tract diseases, such as asthma and chronic obstructive pulmonary disease, frequently have disordered breathing patterns. The evidence indicates that in these situations optimal management of disease processes in the upper respiratory tract may also benefit the lower respiratory tract (Krouse et al 2007).

NASAL HISTORY TAKING

The patient should be asked whether he/she is a nose/mouth breather. Mouth breathing is often linked to factors causing nasal obstruction and congestion. Generalized swelling of the nasal lining causing nasal obstruction is usually due to infection, allergy or nasal polyps. As well as nasal obstruction, these conditions are often associated with other additional symptoms. A septal deviation, or rarely benign or malignant neoplasms, may cause unilateral nasal obstruction; an S-shaped septal deviation can cause bilateral nasal obstruction. In children, adenoidal enlargement is a common cause of nasal obstruction and usually presents as persistent mouth breathing. A history of cosmetic rhinoplasty can be indicative of a weakened nasal valve area. In some patients their nasal obstruction can be linked to a previous episode of nasal trauma.

Snoring and obstructive sleep apnoea can be associated with nasal obstruction. Key questions include whether snoring occurs every night in every position, whether there are periods of apnoea, the quantity and quality of sleep and inappropriate daytime somnolence. The Epworth Sleepiness Scale is used to determine the level of daytime sleepiness (Table 2.3.1). Patients with a score of 12 or more need further medical assessment.

Table 2.3.1 Epworth sleepiness scale

Situation	Chance of dozing
Sitting and reading	
Watching television	
Sitting inactive in a public place (e.g. a cinema or meeting)	
As passenger in a car for > 1 hour	
Lying down to rest in the afternoon when circumstances permit	
Sitting and talking to a companion	
Sitting quietly after an alcohol-free lunch	
In a car, while stopped briefly in heavy traffic	
Total Epworth Sleepiness Score	

Use the following scale to choose the most appropriate number for each situation:
0 = would *never* doze or sleep
1 = *slight* chance of dozing or sleeping
2 = *moderate* chance of dozing or sleeping
3 = *high* chance of dozing or sleeping

Allergic symptoms of sneezing, itchy nose, itchy eyes and a clear nasal discharge indicate underlying allergy, which is frequently associated with asthma. Purulent secretions suggest acute/chronic rhinosinusitis. A nasal foreign body in a child usually causes a unilateral, offensive nasal discharge; in adults a unilateral bloodstained discharge may represent a neoplasm.

Facial pain, particularly over the sinuses, can be a multifaceted problem. Migraine, tension headache and temporomandibular pain can be associated with breathing pattern disorders (Bartley 2011). Chronic infective sinusitis rarely causes facial pain (Naranch et al 2002). Co-morbidities such as anxiety, depression, fibromyalgia, irritable bowel symptoms and low back pain often indicate that the 'sinus pain' is part of an overall central neural sensitization picture (Woolf 2011).

NASAL EXAMINATION

The external nose can be examined by observation and palpation. The nasal bones only occupy the superior one third of the external nose with the remaining portion being cartilaginous. A deformed exterior may often represent internal functional problems. Examination of the interior of the nose needs good lighting, appropriate instruments and occasionally the topical use of a vasoconstrictor to shrink the nasal mucosa. A headlight is necessary for a thorough examination and leaves both hands free for using instruments.

Cheap battery operated functional headlights can be obtained from many camping stores, but most therapists probably do not need to invest in one.

In children, where use of instruments is best avoided, simple upward pressure on the tip of the nose allows a surprisingly full examination of the vestibule and beyond. Similarly, in some adults, upward pressure on the nasal tip will demonstrate a dislocated and therefore disturbed septum. Using a handheld otoscope with a wide speculum can be helpful for illuminating the internal nose. If one holds a metal tongue depressor or a small mirror under the nostrils and asks the patient to breathe out through their nose, airway patency can be assessed. Both sides should fog over relatively equally (allowing for the nasal cycle), indicating normal nasal patency (Brescovici & Roithmann 2008). If there are concerns about nasal obstruction, a medical opinion is advisable.

TEACHING NASAL BREATHING

In clinical practice, nasal passage size and a patient's reported ability to breathe nasally often do not correlate. Through a number of mechanisms, defective breathing patterns can contribute to nasal congestion. For optimal airway hydration and mucus clearance, the mucosa needs exposure to the oscillatory stresses of breathing (Button et al 2008). Faulty breathing patterns also have the potential to cause nasal congestion. Nasal congestion is related to arterial pCO_2 levels. If arterial CO_2 levels are low due to hyperventilation, then the nose becomes congested (Bartley 2006). Slowing breathing depth and rate, and thus elevating arterial CO_2 levels to normal levels, can help relieve nasal congestion.

An initial problem is that some people, particularly those with a panic disorder, have an increased sensitivity to increasing arterial pCO_2 levels (Rassovsky et al 2006). Some patients feel as if they are suffocating when they slow their breathing. Clinically, many patients appear to overcome this sensation with specific breathing exercises (see also discussion of breath holding in chapters in Section 7 for retraining protocols).

It is also important for the therapist to encourage slow nasal diaphragmatic breathing; it is difficult to breathe rapidly diaphragmatically. Placing the tongue behind the top teeth on the hard palate is a useful manoeuvre, which can facilitate nasal breathing. Breathing in too quickly through the nose causes the lateral sidewalls of the external nose (nasal valves) to collapse inwards. Some patients have already discovered that pulling the soft tissues of the cheek away in a superolateral direction from the nasofacial groove tightens the sidewall of the nose, improving nasal breathing – Cottle's manoeuvre (Walsh & Kern 2006). Chronic mouth breathing may cause the muscles that open the sidewalls of the nose to weaken. After nasal breathing is initiated, it may take time before their muscle tone returns to normal. Similarly, the increased resistance associated with shifting from mouth breathing to nose breathing can also feel uncomfortable for many patients; however this increased resistance is important for optimal respiratory function.

NASAL SALINE IRRIGATION

Many patients find that nasal saline irrigation improves nasal congestion. Saline nasal irrigation may improve nasal mucosal function through several physiologic effects, including direct cleansing; removal of inflammatory mediators; and improved mucociliary function, as suggested by increased ciliary beat frequency (Rabago & Zgierska 2009). A recipe and instructions for nasal saline irrigation are included in Chapter 9.

A traditional yogic nose pipe (www.nosepipe.com) can be used. It is often possible to buy a nasal spray bottle with packaged salt (www.sinusrinse.com). Pulsed saline irrigation systems (www.ent-consult.com) are also available.

The practice of steam inhalation, used when a nasal infection is present, helps to not only cleanse and moisten the airways but research on essential oils suggests they may help kill unwanted bacteria. Xylitol is a five-carbon sugar alcohol that is generally believed to enhance the body's own innate bactericidal mechanisms. Increasing evidence indicates that a xylitol nasal spray may also help some patients suffering from chronic rhinosinusitis (Weissman et al 2011). In some countries, xylitol nasal spray is sold in health food shops (a xylitol nasal spray recipe is included in Chapter 9).

CONCLUSIONS

The upper and lower respiratory tracts interact with each other. Nasal dysfunction and disease frequently impact on the lower respiratory tract. Consideration of, and attention to the upper respiratory tract can benefit lower respiratory tract function.

REFERENCES

Ayoub, J., Cohendy, R., Dauzat, M., et al., 1997. Non-invasive quantification of diaphragm kinetics using m-mode sonography. Canadian Journal of Anaesthesia 44, 739–744.

Bartley, J., 2006. Nasal congestion and hyperventilation syndrome. American Journal of Rhinology 19, 607–611.

Bartley, J., 2011. Breathing and temporomandibular joint disease. Journal of Bodywork and Movement Therapies 15, 291–297.

Braunstahl, G.J., Overbeek, S.E., Kleinjan, A., et al., 2001a. Nasal allergen provocation induces adhesion molecule expression and tissue eosinophilia in upper and lower airways. Journal of Allergy and Clinical Immunology 107, 469–476.

Braunstahl, G.J., Overbeek, S.E., Fokkens, W.J., et al., 2001b. Segmental bronchoprovocation in allergic rhinitis patients affects mast cell and basophil numbers in nasal and bronchial mucosa. American Journal of Respiratory and Critical Care Medicine 164, 858–865.

Brescovici, S., Roithmann, R., 2008. Modified Glatzel mirror test reproducibility in the evaluation of nasal patency. Brazilian Journal of Otorhinolaryngology 74, 215–222.

Button, B., Boucher, R.C.; University of North Carolina Virtual Lung Group, 2008. Role of mechanical stress in regulating airway surface hydration and mucus clearance rates. Respiratory Physiology and Neurobiology 163, 189–201.

Cappo, BM., Holmes, D.S., 1984. The utility of prolonged respiratory exhalation for reducing physiological and psychological arousal in non-threatening and threatening situations. Journal of Psychosomatic Research 28, 265–273.

Cole, P., 2003. The four components of the nasal valve. American Journal of Rhinology 7, 107–110.

Eccles, R., 1996. A role for the nasal cycle in respiratory defence. European Respiratory Journal 9, 371–376

Elad, D., Wolf, M., Keck, T., 2008. Air-conditioning in the human nasal cavity. Respiratory Physiology and Neurobiology 163, 121–127.

Hare, K.M., Grimwood, K., Leach, A.J., et al., 2010. Respiratory bacterial pathogens in the nasopharynx and lower airways of Australian indigenous children with bronchiectasis. Journal of Pediatrics 157, 1001–1005.

Hurst, J.R., 2009. Upper airway. 3: Sinonasal involvement in chronic obstructive pulmonary disease. Thorax 65, 85–90.

Krouse, J., Brown, R., Fineman, S., et al., 2007. Asthma and the unified airway. Otolaryngology - Head and Neck Surgery 136, S75–S106.

Le Doux, J., 2003. The Emotional Brain. Phoenix, New York.

Morton, A.R., King, K., Papalia, S., et al., 1995. Comparison of maximal oxygen consumption with oral and nasal breathing. Australian Journal of Science and Medicine in Sport 27, 51–55.

Moss, M., Cook, J., Wesnes, K., et al., 2003. Aromas of rosemary and lavender essential oils differentially affect cognition and mood in healthy adults. International Journal of Neuroscience 113, 15–38.

Naranch, K., Park, Y., Repka-Ramirez, M., et al., 2002. A tender sinus does not always mean rhinosinusitis. Otolaryngology - Head and Neck Surgery 127, 387–397.

Plum, F., 1992. Breathing is controlled independently by voluntary, emotional and metabolically related pathways. Archives of Neurology 49, 441

Rabago, D., Zgierska, A., 2009. Saline nasal irrigation for upper respiratory conditions. American Family Physician 80, 1117–1119.

Rassovsky, Y., Abrams, K., Kushner MF 2006. Suffocation and respiratory responses to carbon dioxide and breath holding challenges in individuals with panic disorder. Journal of Psychosomatic Research 2006; 60, 291–298.

Rogan, M.P., Geraghty, P., Greene, C.M., et al., 2006. Antimicrobial proteins and polypeptides in pulmonary innate defence. Respiratory Research 7, 29.

Sahin-Yilmaz, A., Naclerio, R., 2011. Anatomy and physiology of the upper airway. Proceedings of the American Thoracic Society 8, 31–39.

Sarin, S., Undem, B., Sanico, A., et al., 2006. The role of the nervous system in rhinitis. Journal of Allergy and Clinical Immunology 118, 999–1016.

Selimoglu, E., 2005. Nitric oxide in health and disease from the point of view of the otorhinolaryngologist. Current Pharmaceutical Design 11, 3051–3060.

Setzer, W.N., 2009. Essential oils and anxiolytic aromatherapy. Natural Product Communications 4, 1305–1316.

Shannahoff-Khalsa, D., 1993. The ultradian rhythm of alternating cerebral hemispheric activity. International Journal of Neuroscience 70, 285–298.

Soudry, Y., Lemogne, C., Malinvaud, D., et al., 2011. Olfactory system and emotion: common substrates. European Annals of Otorhinolaryngology, Head and Neck Diseases 128, 18–23.

Swift, A., Campbell, I., McKown, T., 1988. Oronasal obstruction, lung volumes, and arterial oxygenation. Lancet 1, 73–75.

Tanaka, Y., Morikawa, T., Honda, Y., 1988. An assessment of nasal functions in control of breathing. Journal of Applied Physiology 65, 1520–1524.

Walsh, WE., Kern, RC., 2006. Sinonasal anatomy, function and evaluation. In: Bailey, B.J., Johnson, J.T. (Eds.), Head and Neck Surgery – Otolaryngology, fourth ed. Lippincott, Williams and Wilkins, Philadelphia, p. 312.

Weissman, J.D., Fernandez, F., Hwang, PH., 2011. Xylitol nasal irrigation in the management of chronic rhinosinusitis: a pilot study. Laryngoscope 121, 2468–2472.

Woolf, C.J., 2011. Central sensitization: implications for the diagnosis and treatment of pain. Pain 152, S2–S15.

Chapter 3

Patterns of breathing dysfunction in hyperventilation and breathing pattern disorders

Dinah Bradley

Introduction

Having been introduced to structural and functional influences on breathing (Chapters 2.1–2.3), as well as embryological and evolutionary, and nasal, influences, this chapter summarizes major features of both normal breathing patterns and what happens to individuals when breathing patterns become dysfunctional. The consequences of breathing pattern disorders (BPDs) – the umbrella term used to cover these conditions including chronic hyperventilation – are not only distressing to the patient but also expensive to our health care systems if they are not diagnosed and treated (once more serious pathologies have been ruled out). Greater detail of the multiple interacting relationships between biochemistry and psychology on BPDs – touched on in this chapter – are to be found in Chapters 4 and 5.

Too often, patients present to emergency rooms or to general practitioners with frightening symptoms which mimic serious disease (Lum 1987), though blood tests, heart checks such as electrocardiographs (ECGs), and thorough physical examinations reveal nothing out of the ordinary. Breathing pattern abnormalities and their sequelae (see below) are commonly missed by doctors and health care professionals, or else dismissed as 'over anxiousness', and no treatment options are offered.

Normal breathing

Optimal respiratory function offers a variety of benefits to the body:

- It allows an exchange of gases involving
  - the acquisition of oxygen (O_2)
  - the elimination of carbon dioxide (CO_2).

- The efficient exchange of these gases enhances cellular function and so facilitates normal performance of the brain, organs and tissues of the body.
- It permits normal speech.
- It is intimately involved in human non-verbal expression (sighing, crying).
- It assists in fluid movement (lymph, blood).
- It helps maintain spinal mobility through regular, mobilizing, thoracic cage movement.
- It enhances digestive function via rhythmic positive and negative pressure fluctuations, when diaphragmatic function is normal.

Any modification of breathing function from the optimal is capable of producing negative effects on these functions.

Rates and volumes

Normal resting breathing rates are between 10 and 14 breaths per minute, moving between 3 and 5 litres of air per minute through the airways of the chest. During the active inspiratory phase, air flows in through the nose, where it is warmed, filtered and humidified before being drawn into the lungs by the downward movement of the diaphragm and the outward movement of the abdominal wall and lower intercostal muscles. The upper chest and accessory breathing muscles remain relaxed. The expiratory phase is effortless as the abdominal wall and lower intercostals relax downward and the diaphragm ascends back to its original domed position aided by the elastic recoil of the lung. A relaxed pause at the end of exhalation releases the diaphragm briefly from the negative and positive pressures exerted across it during breathing. Under normal circumstances people are quite unaware of their breathing. Breathing rates and volumes increase or fluctuate in response to physical or emotional demands, but in normal subjects return to relaxed low-chest patterns after the stimuli cease.

Definition of HVS

Hyperventilation is a pattern of overbreathing, where the depth and rate are in excess of the metabolic needs of the body at that time. Breathlessness usually occurs at rest or with only mild exercise. Physical, environmental or psychological stimuli override the automatic activity of the respiratory centres, which are tuned to maintain arterial carbon dioxide ($PaCO_2$) levels within a narrow range. At that particular time, the body's CO_2 production is set at a certain level, and the exaggerated breathing depth and rate eliminates CO_2 at a faster pace resulting in a fall in $PaCO_2$, or arterial hypocapnia. This results in the arterial pH (acid/alkaline balance) moving into the alkaline region to induce respiratory alkalosis (Fig. 3.1).

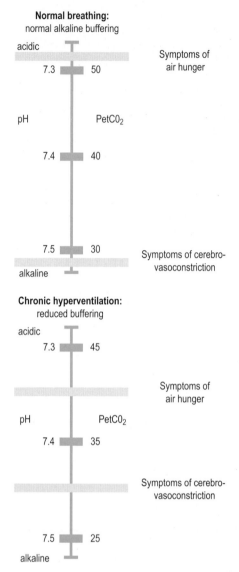

Figure 3.1 When hyperventilation continues for several hours or more, there is a drive to restore normal pH by excreting more alkaline buffer. This compensation permits CO_2 at a level of 5 mmHg to coexist with 7.4 pH. Such an individual becomes subject to reduced capacity to tolerate acidosis from any source, including breath-holding, and is also closer to the symptom line for reduced COP. *Reproduced from Gilbert 1999.*

Organic causes of increased breathing

It is important to exclude organic causes, where breathlessness is an appropriate respiratory response to a physical disease causing diminished arterial oxygen saturation (PaO_2) and elevated arterial carbon dioxide ($PaCO_2$) levels.

In true breathlessness, tachypnoea (rapid breathing) or hyperpnoea (increase in respiratory volume proportional to increase in metabolism), the respiratory centres are responding *automatically* to rising CO_2 production due to exercise or organic disease, and deeper and/or faster breathing response is appropriate.

Etiological breathing pattern disorder factors

Psychological factors

Anxiety
Social or work stress
Panic disorders
Personality traits, including perfectionism, high achiever, obsessive
Suppressed emotions, for example anger
Conditioning/learnt response
Action projection/anticipation
History of abuse
Mental tasks involving sustained concentration
Sustained boredom
Pain
Phobic avoidance
Misattribution of symptoms

Biochemical factors

Allergies
Diet
Exaggerated response to decreased CO_2
Drugs, including recreational drugs, caffeine, aspirin, alcohol, opiates
Hormonal, including progesterone
Exercise
Chronic low grade fever
Heat
Humidity
Altitude

Biomechanical factors

Postural maladaptations
Upper limb movement
Chronic mouth breathing
Cultural, for example, 'belly in, chest out', tight-waisted clothing
Congenital deformities
Overuse, misuse or abuse of musculoskeletal system
Abnormal movement patterns
Braced posture, for example, postoperative
Occupational, for example, divers, singers, swimmers, dancers, musicians

Other factors

Undiagnosed organic causes, including mild/asymptomatic asthma, interstitial lung disease, pulmonary hypertension, diabetic ketoacidosis, left ventricular failure.
Post-nasal drip, rhinitis.

The symptoms of hyperventilation are diverse. None is absolutely diagnostic. Consequently, clinicians rely on a suggestive group of symptoms. Each patient has a characteristic set of symptoms which can be amplified during an acute episode or when hyperventilation is exaggerated. The intermittent nature and variable intensity of the symptoms adds to the difficulty of diagnosis. In addition, many patients fail to mention some of their symptoms, either because they think they are unrelated or because they are ashamed to discuss them. Examples are hallucinations, phobias, sexual problems, fear of impending death or madness, and nightmares. Careful enquiries about the relationship of breathlessness to exercise usually reveals a variation in severity from day to day.

ACUTE HYPERVENTILATION

The diagnosis of an acute episode, either witnessed by the clinician or recalled by the patient, is relatively easy. The patient appears distressed and the pattern of respiration involves deep and rapid breaths using the accessory muscles visible in the neck and the upper chest. Wheezing may be heard as a result of bronchospasm triggered by hypocapnia. Oxygen saturations (measured by pulse oximetry (see Chapter 6.3), are within normal ranges (95–98%), and are commonly up to full saturations of 100%. A stressful precipitating event is usually reported.

Neurological signs

Hypocapnia reduces blood flow to the brain (2% decrease in flow per 1 mmHg reduction in arterial CO_2), causing frightening central nervous system symptoms. Poor concentration and memory lapses may result, with tunnel vision and onset in those susceptible of migraine-type headaches or tinnitus. Sympathetic dominance brings on tremors, sweating, clammy hands, palpitations, and autonomic instability of blood vessels causing labile blood pressures (Magarian 1982). Bilateral perioral and upper extremity paresthesiae and numbness may be reported. Unilateral tingling is most often confined to the left side. Dizziness, weakness, visual disturbances, tremor, and confusion – sometimes fainting or even seizures – are typical symptoms. Spinal reflexes become exaggerated through increased neuronal activity caused by loss of CO_2 ions from the neurons. Tetany and cramping may occur in severe bouts (Fried & Grimaldi 1993).

Metabolic disturbances

Two tests of nerve hyperexcitability produced by hypocapnia-induced *hypocalcemia* are Trousseau's sign and

Chvostek's sign. The Trousseau test consists of occluding the brachial artery into the arm by pumping the blood pressure cuff above the systolic pressure for 2.5 minutes. A positive sign is where paresthesia is felt severely within the period and the wrist and fingers arch in carpopedal spasm – termed 'main d'accoucheur' or obstetrician's hand. The Chvostek sign is when tapping the facial nerve at the point where it emerges through the parotid salivary gland elicits a contraction of the facial muscle that twitches the side of the mouth. This is also a test for *magnesium deficiency* (Werbach 2000). *Acute hypophosphatemia* also contributes to weakness and tingling.

Cardiac signs

Chest pain is another alarming symptom challenging the clinician to exclude heart disease. Epinephrine-induced ECG changes can occur in hyperventilation uncomplicated by coronary heart disease. One study suggests that up to 90% of non-cardiac chest pain is thought to be induced by HVS/BPD (De Guire et al 1992, 1996, Hamer et al 2006).

In older patients, established coronary artery disease can be exacerbated by vasoconstriction arising from hypocapnia, putting these patients at risk of coronary occlusion and myocardial damage. Alternatively, hyperventilation can trigger spasming of normal caliber coronary arteries. This type of variant angina (Prinzmetal's angina) occurs without provocation, usually at rest (Nakao et al 1997). This phenomenon is prevented by calcium channel blockers, which reduce calcium ion migration from the cells. To date, no specific studies of breathing retraining and outcome measurements for this type of angina have been done.

Syndrome X refers to those patients with a history of angina and a positive exercise test (chest pain within 6 minutes or less), yet who have normal angiography. Thought to be a functional abnormality of coronary microcirculation, it is much more common in women than in men (Kumar & Clark 2009).

Gastrointestinal signs

Rapid and/or mouth breathing instigates aerophagia from air gulping, causing bloating, burping and extreme epigastric discomfort. Irritable bowel syndrome (IBS) is listed as a common symptom of chronic overbreathing. Fear and anxiety may induce abdominal cramps and diarrhoea (Lum 1987). The median swallowing rate in healthy, non-dyspeptic controls is 3 or 4 per 15 minutes. In the absence of food, up to 5 ml of air accompanies saliva into the gastrointestinal tract with each swallow (Calloway & Fonagy 1985).

Some clinicians think aerophagia may exacerbate hiatus hernia (part of the stomach passes up through a weakened esophageal valve in the diaphragm into the chest cavity),

Case study 3.1 **Acute hyperventilation**

A 39-year-old man with profound deafness from past middle ear infections came into the emergency department with a severe headache, abdominal pain, and an inability to stand and walk. Numbness and pins and needles also affected his legs. He looked and felt distressed. Five doctors assessed him in the course of the 12 hours he spent in the department. The history obtained was fragmentary because a person skilled in sign language was not sought. The medical registrar called in the physician, who ordered a CT scan of the patient's head because of the headache, paresthesiae, and paraparesis. The CT scan was normal. They noted an increased respiratory rate but dismissed this finding, as both chest X-ray and ECG were normal and there were no abnormal cardiac signs. The surgical registrar and surgeon considered the abdominal pain warranted an ultrasound of the patient's abdomen and were relieved that this was normal. As the day wore on the symptoms improved, and the patient and the fifth doctor were reassured by the normal investigations. It was therefore decided to send him to the ward pending an investigation of a spinal cord lesion. Overnight, a sympathetic nurse found out that the man had just lost his 48-year-old partner. Her grown-up children had removed a lot of the patient's furniture from his house, believing it to be their mother's, and one of her sons had written off the patient's (uninsured) car in a crash. This set of misfortunes – bereavement, loss and depression – set up the acute hyperventilation, less apparent on admission, when the consequent symptoms were dominant. Eventually a signer was brought in and the symptoms and hyperventilation explained. The patient responded to this explanation and to counselling.

or may even be the cause in susceptible people. Case study 3.1 describes a patient with abdominal pain following acute hyperventilation.

CHRONIC HYPERVENTILATION

The diagnosis of chronic and intermittent hyperventilation is more difficult, as the patient will often only present when having an acute episode on top of chronic hyperventilation.

Often the patient will dwell on one symptom in a particular system and will be referred to a specialist, for example a cardiologist, gastroenterologist, neurologist, psychiatrist, or respiratory physician (Case study 3.2). Each will diagnose and investigate within the particular specialty, delaying the diagnosis for months, or even years. Some patients have such a thick folder of notes, including all their previous tests, that this in and of itself is considered diagnostic by some experienced physicians – the 'fat folder syndrome' (Lum 1975).

There are often attacks where there is no preceding stressful event. It is thought that in those with chronic hyperventilation the respiratory centre is reset to tolerate a lower than normal partial pressure of arterial carbon dioxide ($PaCO_2$) in the blood (Nixon 1989). In such patients a single sigh or one deep breath will reduce the $PaCO_2$ enough to bring on symptoms. See Chapter 5 for further discussion of unconscious and conditioned factors that may contribute towards hyperventilation.

Examination must exclude organic diseases of the brain and nervous system, diseases of the heart (particularly angina and heart failure), respiratory disease and gastrointestinal conditions, especially if there are suspicious symptoms in these systems.

Multidisciplinary assessment protocols, and questionnaire use, as described in later chapters, will help in development of diagnostic and assessment skills. (See Ch 5, and the chapters in Section 6.)

Case study 3.2 **An example of chronic HVS**

A 36-year-old woman was referred for an exercise ECG because of chest pain at rest and on exercise, though its relation to exercise was variable. The test was normal, but a detailed history was suspicious. She was a happily married woman with two children who were doing well. A senior bank officer, she had been promoted to a position for which she had had no past experience, nor was she given any orientation. She was meticulous in her work and it frustrated her that immediate mastery of the new job eluded her. This promotion and the move into a new house had coincided with the onset of the chest pain. The pain was left sub-mammary, coming on mainly during rest, but sometimes with light exercise. It was associated with breathlessness and some tingling of the left arm and around her mouth. She had previously enjoyed walking and keeping fit by going to the gym two days a week, but she had to give up these pastimes because of the chest pain and breathlessness. She looked anxious. Though her respiratory rate was normal, the two-hand test (HiLo test, see Fig. 6.2.1 in Ch. 6.2) revealed an upper-chest mouth-breathing pattern. Significant respiratory and cardiac disease was excluded by a normal PEF, chest X-ray, and normal resting and exercise ECGs. An HVPT was positive in producing chest pain and paresthesiae, and the ECG during the pain was normal. She was relieved by the normal tests and quickly saw the logic of the multiple stressors generating symptoms from hyperventilation. Over 6 weeks her attacks diminished and eventually stopped as she reduced her working hours and had breathing retraining with an experienced respiratory physiotherapist.

DIAGNOSIS

Clinical diagnosis of primary HVS would be made on the findings of specific or relevant tests and questionnaires, and after exclusion of organic disease.

When considering the myriad of balanced biochemical reactions which make up normal metabolism, and their dependence on the careful maintenance of an optimal pH, it is not surprising that respiratory alkalosis resulting from hyperventilation causes such widespread disturbances and symptoms (Fig. 3.2). Out of the mass of data some major threads emerge – changes in vasomotor tone, mainly reducing cerebral, coronary and cutaneous blood flow, diminished oxygen availability to tissues, and increased neuronal excitability of the peripheral nervous system:

- Buffering mechanisms protect the pH by renal excretion of bicarbonate (HCO_3). If this compensation is prolonged, chronic loss of buffer base reserves further stimulates respiration to avoid metabolic acidosis.
- Oxygen uptake is impaired by a leftshift of the oxyhaemaglobin dissociation curve (Bohr effect) leading to sensations of breathlessness (Fig. 3.3). As $PaCO_2$ is depleted, there is a linear reduction in cerebral blood flow (see above). The respiratory centre becomes reset to a lower CO_2 threshold. A chronic exhausting circle is established (Nixon 1993).
- Neuronal hyperexcitability is related again to falling CO_2 levels. These result in elevated sensory and motor nerve potentials and bursts of spontaneous discharges, giving rise to paresthesiae of the hands, trunk and around the mouth, as well as hypertonicity, cramps and carpopedal spasm of the muscles. The mechanism is uncertain. There is a dramatic lowering of serum phosphate which may influence calcium flux; calcium ions stabilize the nerve membrane potential. The same symptoms occur with hypocalcemia, but there is no evidence of reduced serum calcium levels in respiratory alkalosis (Magarian 1982).
- Hyperexcitability of cardiac muscle fibres and electrical conducting systems may cause atrial cardiac arrhythmias.
- As $PaCO_2$ falls there is a reduced coronary blood flow with myocardial hypoxia due to vasoconstriction, and sometimes spasming of coronary arteries. This may be one cause of anginal chest pain, which is of particular relevance to those with pre-existing coronary artery disease, with the risk of dislodging plaque and precipitating occlusion/infarction/death.

Chest pain in hyperventilation may also stem from:

- Sharp pains felt on inspiration from *pressure on the diaphragm* from aerophagia ('air gulping' from mouth breathing) (Evans & Lum 1981).

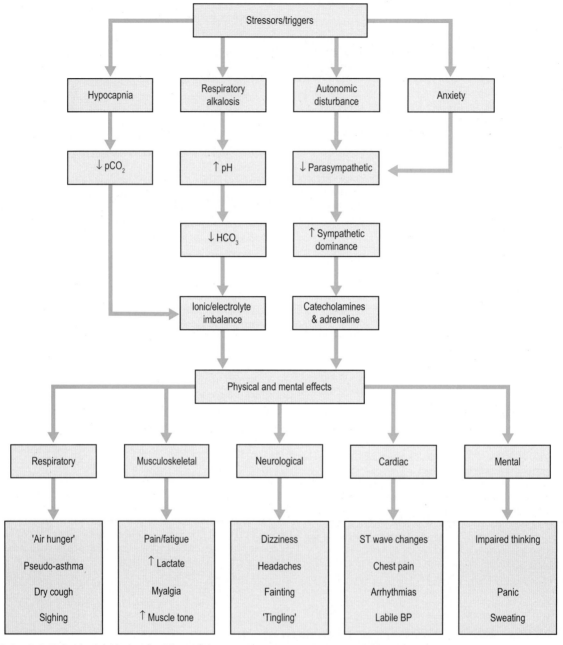

Figure 3.2 Pathophysiological explanations of the symptoms. *Adapted from Bradley 1994.*

- A typical dull and diffuse pain due to *intercostal muscle fatigue and spasm* (Evans & Lum 1981).
- Heavy retrosternal pain, sometimes radiating to the neck and arms, which mimics angina, lasts longer, and does not abate at rest nor become worse with continued activity as with classic angina; nor does it respond to nitrolingual sprays (anti-anginal medications) (Magarian 1982).
- Nasal congestion and headaches (Bartley 2005).
- Esophageal reflux is another source of central chest discomfort outside the respiratory system.

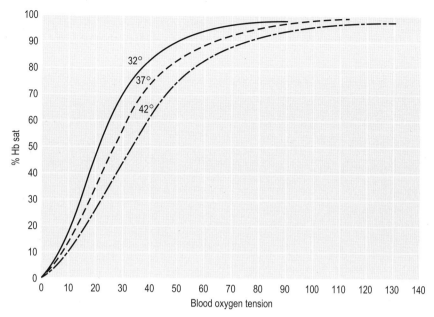

Figure 3.3 Oxygen dissociation curve of blood at a pH of 7.4 showing variations at three temperatures. For a given oxygen tension, the lower the blood temperature the more the haemoglobin holds onto its oxygen, maintaining higher saturation. *Reproduced from Wilkins et al 2000.*

Hyperventilation may initiate bronchoconstriction in non-asthmatic subjects. As hyperventilators are often mouth breathers, air entering the bronchi is dry and increases the airway fluid osmolarity, rendering it more sticky and tenacious. This stimulates nicotinic and muscarinic receptors, releasing prostanoids and leukotrienes, which cause bronchospasm and mucosal damage.

During hyperventilation there is an additional reduction in peripheral vascular resistance, with a drop in mean arterial blood pressure. This can result in fainting or extreme light-headedness. However, compensatory increases in heart rate and cardiac output may eventually supervene with blood pressure (BP) rising above baseline, causing elevated or fluctuating BP levels.

Breathing pattern disorders secondary to other health problems

Observation of changes to patients during primary hyperventilation and disordered breathing patterns also needs to extend to disorders in which hyperventilation prevails as a coexisting complication. The aim in what follows is to provide a broad overview of common conditions and alert clinicians to secondary breathing pattern dysfunc-

tions in patients, which may complicate the original disorder and/or add unwarranted stressors.

Obstructive disorders

Starting with the most common obstructive lung disorders (asthma, chronic obstructive pulmonary disease (COPD) and emphysema), airways obstruction may be due to:

* Reversible factors (as in asthma), e.g. inflammation, bronchospasm or mucus plugging
* Irreversible factors (as in emphysema and chronic bronchitis), e.g. damaged alveoli leading to loss of elastic recoil of adjacent lung tissue, or scarred airway walls (Hough 1996).

Restrictive disorders

Restrictive lung disorders, with reductions in both lung volumes and lung compliance, include:

* Acute inflammations such as pleurisy or pneumonia
* Chronic disorders, often under the collective term, interstitial lung disease (ILD), which covers over 200 variants. Examples of these are fibrosing alveolitis, sarcoidosis, asbestosis, bird fancier's lung, pneumoconiosis ('coal miner's lung').

Breathing patterns

Breathing patterns often provide clues as to the type of condition involved:

- Rapid shallow upper-chest breathing suggests loss of lung volume seen in restrictive diseases, where the work of breathing is increased to maintain ventilation
- Prolonged exhalation time as witnessed in someone having an asthma attack indicates acute intrathoracic obstruction
- Prolonged exhalation (perhaps 'pursed-lip' in severe cases) caused by chronic intrathoracic obstruction in patients with COPD
- Prolonged inspiratory time occurs in acute upper airway obstruction as in croup or globus (throat spasm) (Wilkins et al 2000).

In all the above, accessory muscle use would be clearly visible, and mouth breathing would probably be the chosen route to move air in and out of the lungs. Helping the patients to reduce the work of breathing and diffuse anxiety, with the use of rest positions and relaxation techniques, may be of benefit (See Section 7 and Ch. 9).

Patients who are recovering from acute chest infections or asthma attacks require 'debriefing' to ensure correct breathing patterns are restored. This is particularly important in those with asthma, as hyperventilation is a very common secondary problem which may trigger attacks. Lowered CO_2 levels from chronic hyperventilating encourage catecholamine and histamine release into the blood, which in turn stimulates mast cells in the lung parenchyma, promoting bronchoconstriction and hyperinflation. Inhaling cold air via the mouth has also been shown to trigger bronchoconstriction (Gardner 1996).

Those working in pulmonary rehabilitation programmes with COPD patients need to be aware of breathing retraining measures to help maximize respiratory function and encourage relaxed breathing. Mild to moderately affected patients benefit more than those with more severe disease, with diaphragm flattening and reduced respiratory competence. But breathing assessment and retraining where necessary make a valuable adjunct to pharmacological therapies and in many cases help patients safely to reduce anxiety levels and medications.

PRE- AND POST-SURGICAL BREATHING PROBLEMS

Patients waiting to undergo an operation may hyperventilate in response to fear and pain, which may persist after surgery. Those who have been in chronic pain for long periods (waiting for hip replacement, for instance) may be especially vulnerable to HVS/BPDs.

Coronary bypass patients facing open-chest surgery are often briefed beforehand on the importance of deep breathing exercises to expand and clear the lungs of mucus secretions in order to prevent chest infection. Some at-risk patients (perhaps with coexisting COPD from smoking) are given incentive inspirometers – handheld devices to breathe through which make the work of inhalation harder, encouraging air entry down to the lung bases.

Part of the debriefing before the patient leaves hospital (and as part of any coronary rehabilitation programme) should be the restoration of normal, relaxed nose/abdominal breathing. Collapse of coronary bypass grafts may be a consequence of vasoconstrictive or vasospastic influences of chronic hyperventilation (Nixon 1989). As noted in Chapter 1, overbreathing results in increased collagen synthesis due to increased alkalosis, possibly accounting in part for negative influence on grafts, described by Nixon (Falanga 2002, 2005, Jensen et al 2008).

Conclusion

Chronic HVSs are common problems affecting the health of 10% of the normal population (Newton 2012). All health care professionals need to be aware of the effects of depletion of the body's buffering systems in response to chronic hyperventilation. They can be alerted by clearly visible abnormal changes in breathing patterns and postural changes, and this should prompt a search for symptoms and signs. (The subsequent application of diagnostic tests and the establishment of diagnoses and treatments are discussed in later chapters.) Checking respiratory rates and breathing patterns should be an essential part of all health care investigations, with treatment options offered to those with this omnipresent debilitating disorder.

REFERENCES

Bartley, J., 2005. Nasal congestion and hyperventilation syndrome. Am J Rhinol. 19 (6), 607–611.

Bradley, D., 1994. Discussion Paper. Physiotherapy Conference, New Zealand.

Calloway, S.P., Fonagy, P., 1985. Aerophagia and irritable bowel syndrome. Lancet 14 December, pp. 168 [letter].

De Guire, S., Gervitz, R., Kawahara, Y., et al., 1992. Hyperventilation

syndrome and the assessment and treatment for functional cardiac symptoms. American Journal of Cardiology 70, 67–677.

DeGuire, S., Gevirtz, R., Hawkinson, D., et al., 1996. Breathing retraining: a three-year follow-up study of treatment for hyperventilation syndrome and associated functional cardiac symptoms. Biofeedback & Self Regulation 21 (2), 191–198.

Evans, D.W., Lum, L.C., 1981. Hyperventilation as a cause of chest pain mimicking angina. Practical Cardiology 7 (7), 11–19.

Fried, R., Grimaldi, J., 1993. The psychology and physiology of breathing. Plenum, New York, pp. 186–187.

Falanga, V., 2002. Wounding of bioengineered skin: cellular and molecular aspects after injury. J Invest Dermatol 119, 65–660.

Falanga, V., 2005. Wound healing and its impairment in the diabetic foot. Lancet 66, 176–174.

Gardner, W.N., 1996. The pathophysiology of hyperventilation disorders. Chest 109, 516–554.

Gilbert, C., 1999. Hyperventilation and the body. Accident and Emergency Nursing 7, 130–140.

Hamer, H.P., McCallin, A., 2006. Cardiac pain or panic disorder? Managing uncertainty in the emergency department. Nursing and Health Sciences 8, 224–220.

Hough, A., 1996. Physiotherapy in respiratory care, second ed. Ch. 3. Stanley Thornes, Cheltenham.

Jensen, D., Duffin, J., Lam, Y., 2008. Physiological mechanisms of hyperventilation during human pregnancy. Respiratory Physiology & Neurobiology 161 (1), 76–78.

Kumar, P., Clark, M., 2009. Clinical medicine, seventh ed. W B Saunders, Edinburgh.

Lum, L.C., 1975. Hyperventilation: the tip and the iceberg. Journal of Psychosomatic Research 19, 75–78.

Lum, L.C., 1987. Hyperventilation syndromes in medicine and psychiatry: a review. Journal of the Royal Society of Medicine 229–221.

Magarian, G.J., 1982. Hyperventilation syndromes: infrequently recognised common expressions of anxiety and stress. Medicine 62, 219–226.

Nakao, K., Ohgushi, M., Yoshimura, M., et al., 1997. Hyperventilation as a specific test for diagnosis of coronary artery spasm. Am J Cardiol. 1, 80 (5), 545–549.

Newton, E., 2012. Hyperventilation from the emergency department. http://bit.ly/In8sDf (Accessed June 2013).

Nixon, P.G.F., 1989. Hyperventilation and cardiac symptoms. Internal Medicine 10 (12), 67–84.

Nixon, P.G.F., 1993. The grey area of effort syndrome and hyperventilation: from Thomas Lewis to today. Journal of the Royal College of Physicians of London 27 (4), 77–78.

Werbach, M., 2000. Adult attention deficit disorder: a nutritional perspective. Journal of Bodywork and Movement Therapies 4 (3), 182–118.

Wilkins, R., Kreder, S., Sheldon, R., 2000. Clinical assessment in respiratory care, fourth ed. Mosby, St Louis.

Chapter | 4 |

Biochemical aspects of breathing

Chris Gilbert (notes on food sensitivities and nutrition: Leon Chaitow)

CHAPTER CONTENTS

This chapter presents aspects of the biochemistry of respiration relevant to breathing pattern disorders, including psychological, allergic and nutritional factors. The focus is on the processes of the delivery of oxygen (O_2) to the tissues and the removal of carbon dioxide, and the powerful function that carbon dioxide performs on its way out of the body. There are a number of texts that provide a comprehensive picture of the biochemistry of breathing, including Comroe 1974, West 2008, Nunn 1993, and general physiology textbooks.

THE BIOCHEMISTRY OF BREATHING

Breathing itself – the mechanical, muscle-powered part of respiration – is a major focus of this book. With its functioning grossly visible, many breathing variables can be assessed easily from moment to moment. However, it is important to outline what happens deeper within the system where the actual gas exchange takes place, since respiration is ultimately a chemical matter.

Simply put, the body extracts oxygen from the inhaled air and exhales carbon dioxide. That formulation suggests that all we need to remember is that oxygen is useful and carbon dioxide is not. But oxygen can also be corrosive and toxic, and a deficiency of the waste gas carbon dioxide (CO_2) can cause fainting, seizures, or even death, so the useful/useless distinction is true only within certain limits. Maintaining limits is a complex task for the body, even more so because the supply of each gas fluctuates with each breath. This tidal oscillation must be smoothed out so that the brain and bodily tissues receive a steady supply of O_2, and also so that CO_2 in the body remains at a stable level. With regard to these two gases, we live in a narrow zone of homeostasis bordered on both sides by physiological disaster. Much of what goes wrong with breathing involves attempts to prevent this disaster, and that sometimes-misguided regulation is the focus of this chapter.

In understanding the biochemistry underlying breathing, one must keep several factors in mind simultaneously, because they all interact. The scales of the various factors are vastly different, ranging from the atomic, the molecular, the cellular, the circulatory, and to the large muscle activity of the chest and abdomen. Moreover, these factors do not all change simultaneously, and some are slower to react than others. There are layers of security operating to ensure a steady supply of O_2 to the brain and the heart.

In considering aberrations in the breathing pattern, it is helpful to keep the following rough classification in mind:

1. Compensations for pathology elsewhere (e.g. acidosis from diabetes or kidney problems)
2. Responses to extrinsic factors (such as allergy or drugs)
3. Responses to intrinsic factors (such as progesterone)
4. Pathological disorders of the breathing system itself
5. Psychogenic or functional breathing problems.

All of these must be compared to the idealized 'normal' picture of breathing presented below. The following are the main factors involved in the biochemical regulation:

- Saturation of blood with oxygen – the amount it is carrying; and the chemical status of haemoglobin – the amount of oxygen it is able to carry
- Saturation of the blood with carbon dioxide, mostly dissolved as carbonic acid
- The amount of the alkaline buffer bicarbonate in the blood
- The pH of the blood, the cerebrospinal fluid, and the body in general
- The retention or disposal of acid and alkaline components by the kidneys
- The breathing 'drive' – determined by multiple competing inputs
- The amount of actual and expected metabolic demand, especially physical exertion
- The mechanical actions of breathing – rate per minute, depth, nose vs. mouth breathing.

pH

The story might best begin with pH, as this factor influences every organ of the body. To review:

- The pH scale runs from 1 to 14, with 1 being most acidic and 14 most alkaline. The neutral midpoint is at 7. The more acidic a solution, the higher its proportion of hydrogen ions, which are positively charged and ready to combine with other molecules ('pH' designates partial pressure of hydrogen).
- Acidity facilitates many metabolic exchanges and must be kept in careful balance. Since pH describes the proportion of hydrogen ions available for combination and the pH is on a log scale, a small change in pH, for example from 7.4 to 7.2, means doubling the number of hydrogen ions present. The binding of hydrogen to negatively charged sites helps to regulate enzymatic action, endocrine secretion, integrity of protein molecules, and cellular metabolism, including oxygen absorption and release. A steady pH of 7.2 would seriously compromise many physiological functions.
- The body will sacrifice many other things in order to keep pH between 7.35 and 7.45. Outside of those limits lie ill effects of many kinds.

Carbon dioxide

The acidity of the blood is determined mainly by percentage of carbon dioxide, and so now we come to breathing. CO_2 is the end product of aerobic metabolism, and comes primarily from the mitochondria (energy producers within the cytoplasm) inside cells. It is the biological equivalent of smoke and ash. It is odourless, heavier than air, and puts out fires, including ours; if breathed in its pure form, it will quickly cause suffocation. CO_2 is present in the atmosphere at a concentration of around $\frac{3}{100}$ of 1% – low enough to be innocuous to us, but sufficient to sustain plant life.

Of all our excretions, CO_2 is the most lethal. To transport this substance from the tissues into the blood and then into the lungs for exhalation, the body converts CO_2 to carbonic acid (H_2CO_3), of which we have a perpetual surplus. Breathing saves us from poisoning: the human lungs exhale around 12 000 mEq carbonic acid per day, compared to less than 100 mEq of fixed acids from the kidneys. An increase in bodily activity produces even more CO_2, which means the blood becomes more acidic unless more CO_2 is excreted.

Therefore, changes in breathing volume regulate the moment-to-moment concentration of pH in the bloodstream (longer-term regulation of pH is shared with the kidneys). There is a tight interaction between the breathing volume, the amount of CO_2 production, the partial pressure of CO_2 in the arterial blood (indicated as $PaCO_2$), and blood pH. Note that the concentration of CO_2 in the blood, not the amount of oxygen, is the major regulator of breathing drive. Higher CO_2 level *immediately* stimulates more breathing; an abundance of CO_2 in the lungs means that one is breathing oxygen-poor air, that breathing has stopped, or that something else is happening which could lead to suffocation.

During exercise more CO_2 is produced, but since more oxygen is needed also, the greater drive to breathe should keep pH constant. Conversely, reduced exertion reduces oxygen need, and also lowers CO_2 production, which lessens the drive to breathe:

$$\textit{High } CO_2 = \text{high acidity} = \text{low pH}$$
$$= \text{higher breathing drive}$$
$$\textit{Low } CO_2 = \text{low acidity} = \text{high pH}$$
$$= \text{lower breathing drive}$$

The effects of different pH values, from acidosis to alkalosis, are shown in Table 4.1. Under normal circumstances, $PaCO_2$ and pH are linked as shown in the table. Changes in breathing rate and volume adjust pH of the blood up or down. This relationship can be altered by metabolic acidosis or alkalosis and by renal compensation, offsetting one scale relative to the other.

With breath-holding, CO_2 rises because more is being dumped into the bloodstream every second, and then released into the lungs. To feel the urgency of this drive to resume breathing, we need only hold the breath to the breaking point. It is not really oxygen deficiency that we are feeling but the accumulation of CO_2; we are exquisitely sensitive to its build-up in the bloodstream. In underwater swimming, hyperventilating before the plunge will permit a longer stay beneath the surface before the urge to breathe becomes unbearable. The reason is that hyperventilation has depleted the alarm substance (CO_2). The danger here is of brain hypoxia and underwater blackout because of the suppressed breathing drive.

Why do we have this complicated system which gives a waste gas on its way out of the body such a prime role in regulating breathing drive? Sensitivity to oxygen itself would appear to be a more direct way to regulate the breathing. However, the body's safeguards to preserve oxygen supply dictate against this. For one thing, there is a large reserve of oxygen in the bloodstream, such that under normal conditions about 75% of the oxygen inhaled is exhaled again without being utilized. Even with maximal exercise, perhaps 25% of the inhaled oxygen is returned unused. This large reserve makes direct indexing of oxygen a poor candidate for regulating breathing drive. The pool of available oxygen does not change quickly. The PaO_2 must drop from 100 mmHg to about 50 before the brain's hypoxia detectors are moved to demand an increase in breathing.

Breathing is the major regulator of the body's acid-base balance because it regulates CO_2. The body can apparently tolerate fluctuations in CO_2 better than it can afford oxygen fluctuations. Fine adjustments of breathing rate and depth can alter CO_2 rapidly, and this serves to maintain both adequate oxygen and proper pH (Figs 4.1 and 4.2).

Metabolic alkalosis and acidosis

Changes in pH caused primarily by transient aberrations in breathing are called respiratory alkalosis or acidosis. Many physiological conditions associated with illness or dysregulation affect pH as well, and can cause an alkaline or acidic condition for which the body tries to compensate by adjusting rate and depth of breathing. Distinguishing metabolic alkalosis/acidosis from respiratory is best done by blood analysis and careful consideration of medical factors. For example:

- In the case of ketoacidosis (excess metabolism of fats combined with insufficient carbohydrates, as in some weight-loss diets or poorly controlled diabetes), the acidic state of the blood promotes deeper, faster breathing because the breathing centres are responding to the higher acidity. This hyperventilation is not the anxiety-based type, but

Table 4.1 Relationship between arterial pH and $PaCO_2$, with effects

	pH	$PaCO_2$	Effects
Acidosis			
	7.1	90–100+	Coma
	7.2	70	Hypercapnia symptoms (drowsiness, confusion)
	7.3	50	Breathing reflex stimulated
	7.4	**40**	**Normal**
	7.5	30	Mild hypocapnia symptoms (light-headedness, weakness), breathing reflex suppressed
	7.6	20	Moderate hypocapnia symptoms (paresthesias, confusion, twitches)
	7.7	10	Coma
	7.8+	0	Death
Alkalosis			

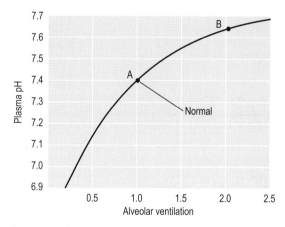

Figure 4.1 Change in plasma pH associated with relative alveolar ventilation. Normal alveolar ventilation = 1. Point A is normal pH and point B represents the change in pH associated with a two-fold increase in alveolar ventilation.

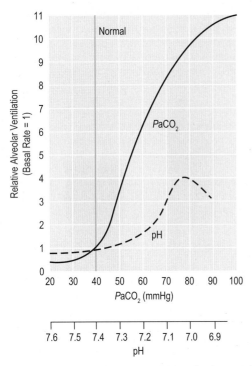

Figure 4.2 Stimulation of alveolar ventilation by decreased arterial pH or increased $PaCO_2$. *From Guyton 1971.*

kidneys detect excess acidity (a surplus of positively charged hydrogen ions) they will retain more bicarbonate to balance the acid, but the process is not fast; adjusting their filtration characteristics takes hours to days.

In the meantime, if bicarbonate buffering of excess acid is not sufficient or if the bicarbonate is depleted, a faster back-up buffering system is available – hyperventilation. Excessive breathing expels more CO_2 (acid), thereby moving pH closer to normal. In this case, one system's goals are subordinated to those of another system: the value of keeping $PaCO_2$ near 40 is sacrificed so that pH can remain around 7.4. This happens with acidosis, as in the above examples, and with alkalosis in the reverse.

Breathing more to compensate for metabolic acidosis has side effects which reflect both low CO_2 and high pH. In the short term these might include widespread vasoconstriction, interference with nerve function, cognitive and sensory disturbances, muscle weakness, and fatigue (see Ch. 3). Most of these will subside once the renal compensation sets in and the pH normalizes, but the CO_2 may remain low in order to maintain the proper pH, and so some consequence of low CO_2 cannot be avoided. Conditions which disrupt pH are not rare; since these conditions vary in duration and chronicity, the body must be able to adapt both quickly and in the long term to maintain homeostasis. Hyperventilation has many possible causes, which may be as varied as kidney failure and anxiety. Blood analysis of pH, bicarbonate, O_2 and CO_2 saturation all together will help distinguish the reason for any abnormalities. Medical determination of acid-base disorders is beyond the scope of this chapter, but if dire pathophysiology is ruled out, the distinction between compensated and non-compensated at least is important for a practitioner to know when working with hyperventilation:

- If the $PaCO_2$ is low, pH is high (alkaline) and bicarbonate level is normal, it is uncompensated, and the hyperventilation could be transitory, perhaps easily remedied.
- If the $PaCO_2$ is low but the pH is normal and the bicarbonate is low, this means that the kidneys have excreted more bicarbonate than usual to bring the pH down to normal. The person may then be in a chronic compensated state of hyperventilation, and it will be harder to get the breathing back to normal

represents the body's attempt to compensate for the blood imbalance by overbreathing in order to excrete CO_2 and bring the blood pH closer to normal.

- Diarrhoea results in loss of plasma bicarbonate ion, which is alkaline, and if the diarrhoea goes on too long acidosis develops. This stimulates corrective overbreathing in order to remove CO_2 (as carbonic acid) and normalize the pH. (See Ch. 3 for fuller coverage of metabolic acidosis as a source of hyperventilation.)
- Excessive vomiting, on the other hand, causes loss of hydrochloric acid, shifting the body chemistry toward alkalosis and depressing breathing (hypoventilation) enough to allow CO_2 to build up and restore pH.
- Use of steroids and diuretics can also bring on alkalosis.

Normal values are listed in Box 4.1.

Bicarbonate buffer (Fig. 4.3)

The bicarbonate ion (HCO_3^-) is derived from CO_2 during its ride in the bloodstream; CO_2 dissociates into hydrogen ions (H^+) and HCO_3^-. This bicarbonate reserve is adjustable as needed, up to a point, and constitutes a major alkaline buffer system that opposes rises in acidity. If the

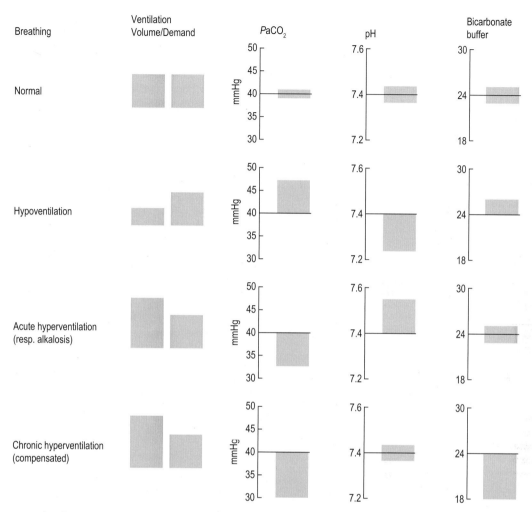

Figure 4.3 When breathing volume does not match what the body needs (demand) there are changes in Pa_{CO_2} which affect pH. The bars are meant to show directional shifts rather than exact values.

because without the buffering effect of normal amounts of bicarbonate, the blood becomes a little too acidic. Since the chemoreceptors regulating breathing are sensitive to pH as well as CO_2 itself, a rise in CO_2 – even if toward normal – will feel closer to suffocation. Learning to tolerate higher CO_2 by breathing less is therefore important in rehabilitating the breathing pattern.

People living at high altitudes need constant hyperventilation in order to compensate for the low oxygen pressure, but adaptation to low CO_2 blood level varies among individuals and is not always successful. According to West (2008):

Those born at high altitude have a diminished ventilatory response to hypoxia that is only slowly corrected by subsequent residence at sea level. Conversely, those born at sea level who move to high altitudes retain their hypoxic response intact for a long time. Apparently therefore ventilatory response is determined very early in life [p. 145].

OXYGEN TRANSPORT AND DELIVERY

The blood carries oxygen mainly in molecules of haemoglobin within red blood cells. Oxygen saturation refers to how close to maximal the haemoglobin is loaded with oxygen; near sea level, this is generally 97–98%, and above 95% considered normal.

An exquisite regulation of oxygen transport occurs inside the red blood cell. The readiness of haemoglobin to combine with oxygen (to form the compound oxyhaemoglobin) varies according to local pH as well as PaO_2. These changes ensure adequate oxygen supply. This variable affinity is important not only for absorbing oxygen in the lungs through the delicate walls of the alveoli, but also for releasing oxygen through the capillary walls, where oxygen diffuses into the tissues. Blood acidity promotes dissociation and release of oxygen from the haemoglobin, while alkalinity encourages retention of oxygen. The system adjusts to local conditions so that when pH is low and the blood more acidic, haemoglobin in that area is stimulated to release more oxygen. This is true of metabolically active tissues in general, but especially of muscles. An exercising muscle needs all the oxygen it can get, and this is facilitated by its chemical nature: 'an exercising muscle is acid, hypercarbic, and hot, and it benefits from increased unloading of O_2 from its capillaries' (West 2008, p. 81). Heat acts like acidity in reducing haemoglobin's affinity for oxygen.

In the lungs the need is to bind oxygen to haemoglobin, not to release it. Since the lungs maintain a more alkaline environment, the chemistry favours affinity between haemoglobin and O_2, and so oxygen is easily absorbed through the pulmonary capillary walls. This general effect of pH on oxyhaemoglobin dissociation is called the Bohr effect.

Regulating oxygen delivery through changes in pH may seem like a complicated mechanism, but it works well, and it is fast: a red blood cell coming from the heart is exposed to oxygen in the lung for about ¾ second. There are about 280 million molecules of haemoglobin in a single red blood cell, and each haemoglobin molecule can carry four molecules of oxygen. This is particularly relevant to hyperventilation: the resulting alkalinity causes the haemoglobin molecule to retain oxygen rather than release it. Under conditions of uncompensated hyperventilation, oxygen saturation (SaO_2), may reach 100%. This may sound good to a patient, but it really means less oxygen is available to the tissues. Increased breathing only makes the situation worse.

PSYCHOGENIC HYPERVENTILATION

Hyperventilation is a natural compensatory response to acidic blood, but hyperventilation may also be initiated and maintained by strictly mental stimuli, so that whatever factors drive anxiety may also drive the breathing. Strong emotions such as anxiety, apprehension, time urgency, resentment and anger manifest somatically in many people as increased breathing, as if preparing for action. If muscles contract, the increased CO_2 produced will balance the loss of CO_2 from heavier breathing. But in the absence of exertion, low CO_2 and respiratory alkalosis is the likely result. If this imbalance becomes chronic, the same renal compensation occurs as with metabolic alkalosis – dumping more bicarbonate into the urine. This adjustment constitutes a new equilibrium, as if the overbreathing is expected to continue. This adaptation most likely adds to the difficulty in restoring normal breathing habits.

Moreover, a biochemical feature of strong emotion is a rise in adrenaline and noradrenaline, and that has been shown (Heistad et al 1972) to boost the body's sensitivity to CO_2 by about 30%, which results in increased hyperventilation.

Cerebral blood flow

The effect of hyperventilation on the cerebral cortex is to reduce blood flow. This is partly through the vasoconstrictive effect of low CO_2 on smooth muscle, and partly through the effect of elevated pH. Cerebral blood flow has been found to be linearly related to arterial $PaCO_2$ (Hauge et al 1980), showing a 2% decline for each 1 mmHg drop in $PaCO_2$. A typical transient CO_2 drop in a person prone to hyperventilation might be 40 torr to 30 – a 25% reduction in fuel to the brain. The precise effects of such a change have not been studied, apart from findings such as a slowing in EEG frequency (Gotoh et al 1965). This reduction in blood flow is in the opposite direction from what is most efficient for alertness and effective thinking (Fig. 4.4).

The biochemistry of anxiety and activity

Anxiety is not merely a mental phenomenon; threat perception is supported by bodily changes designed to enhance readiness for action. Increased breathing is often one of those changes, and in the short term it is reasonable because it creates a mild state of alkalosis. This would help offset a possible surge of acid in the blood (not only carbonic acid but also lactic acid if muscle exertion is drastic enough, since lactic acid is given off by anaerobic metabolism). Long-distance runners, sprinters and horse trainers have experimented successfully with doses of sodium bicarbonate, which supplements the natural bicarbonate buffer and opposes the lactic acid load created by exercising muscles (Schott & Hinchcliff 1998, McNaughton et al 1999).

If action does not occur shortly after hyperventilation begins, homeostasis will be disrupted. This is common in cases of acute anxiety where no clear physical action is called for. If perception of threat continues, the physiological alarm condition continues also, sometimes even boosted by perception of the associated bodily changes. This body-mind tangle becomes an additional disturbance

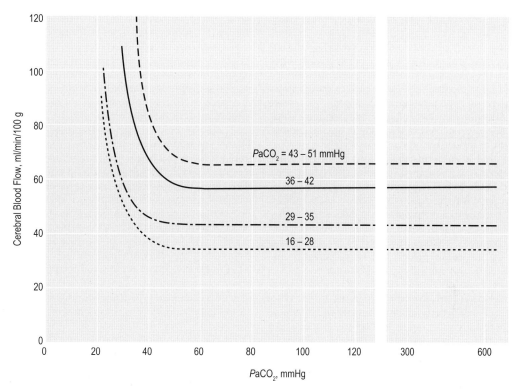

Figure 4.4 Changes in cerebral blood flow as a function of PaO_2 at different $PaCO_2$s. The solid line represents the normal $PaCO_2$ range. Note that both hypercapnia (higher $PaCO_2$) and hypoxaemia (lower PaO_2) increase blood flow, and that hypocapnia causes a sharp decrease.

to the person seeking safety by worrying and hypervigilance. A likely sequence of events in such cases, with changes in the chemical, behavioural and cognitive realms, is shown below:

- Initial threat perception (anxiety)
- Increased breathing
- Respiratory alkalosis and cerebral hypoxia
- Appearance of symptoms in several body systems
- Impairment of thought processes and disrupted mental stability
- Hyper-emotionality, sustained anxiety, faulty reality orientation and limited ability to cope with the anxiety trigger.

Some people are more susceptible than others to this sequence, and this variability may reflect constitutional factors which predispose some people to greater vasoconstriction for a given degree of hypocapnia. Using Doppler ultrasound to monitor changes in the size of the basilar artery in panic patients, Gibbs (1992) found a wide variance in arterial diameter in response to the same degree of hyperventilation. Those with the strongest artery constriction (as much as 50%) were those with the greatest panic symptoms (confirmed by Ball & Shekhar (1997) and Nardi et al (2001)).

Few sufferers of hyperventilation and panic are aware of the 'vicious circle' effect in which the unbalanced physiological state itself stimulates further anxiety. Several mental mechanisms can sustain this cycle:

1. Misinterpretation of physical symptoms as medical problems (worry about heart attack, brain tumour and lung cancer are common)
2. Cognitive impairment leading to a feeling of 'losing one's mind' – fear of insanity
3. The general feeling of being out of control – such effects as disequilibrium, accelerated heart rate, sweating, muscle weakness and paresthesias are alarming when they have no obvious source.

Unstable breathing

L. C. Lum (1976, 1981) proposed that the most drastic neurological consequences of hyperventilation result not from a low level of CO_2 but from sudden drops or fluctuations. Irregular breathing has been shown to accompany anxiety states (Han et al 1997). The increased variability from breath to breath may appear in rate, volume, or CO_2 level; the exact effects on the stability of cortical functions have not been studied systematically, but given the close relationship between the mechanical and chemical variables of breathing, one could postulate a loose, ragged coupling in which pH, haemoglobin oxygen-retention, respiratory drive and $PaCO_2$ struggle to adjust to each other because of the fluctuating anxiety affecting the system.

Patel (1991) described a common pattern during stress and anxiety of hyperventilation alternating with brief apnoea. Attention to sensory input, sudden memory intrusion or indecision is likely to suspend the breath, and the restoration of regular breathing (such as sighing) may, if excessive, lead to more instability. By focusing on what might happen next, the apprehensive individual brings the imagined future into the present and the body is stimulated to react. When the conscious mind invokes a 'manual override' because of anticipated threat, the body is forced into a mismatch between actual and anticipated metabolic needs. Physiology follows the play of thoughts and feelings – if the mental process is chaotic and jerky with abrupt changes, then so will be the breathing.

Neuronal excitability increases with CO_2 reduction, at least in the short term (Macefield & Burke 1991). With varying degrees of hyperventilation, sensory and muscular evoked potentials were found to rise even though the stimulus remained the same, and paresthesias and muscle twitches occurred if CO_2 dropped far enough. Low CO_2 also facilitates rapid muscle response (Bishop et al 2004).

Neural regulation of breathing

Acute shifts in CO_2 seem to challenge homeostasis. Breathing is largely regulated by two types of chemoreceptors: central, in the medulla, and peripheral, in the carotid and aortic bodies. Both are sensitive to CO_2 concentration, but there is evidence that the peripheral receptors fine-tune and modulate the output of the central receptors (Forster & Smith 2010).

Having two separate sources of control may provide safeguards, but it also opens the way for discoordination, in the same way that two musicians playing together create the chance for discord that would not occur with one alone. The unevenness of breathing and CO_2 level in anxious individuals, particularly those with panic disorder, may reflect difficulty in coordination between neural control centres. The sub-threshold (sub-symptom) effects in response to sudden shifts in breathing may contribute to the pervasive uneasiness and restlessness common in chronic hyperventilators, and could feed back into the mental state to compound the anxiety. Add to this the restricted cortical circulation, and critical thinking and discrimination are further compromised.

Persistence of hyperventilation

Hyperventilation tends to persist in many people, and once a pattern of overbreathing is established it can be maintained by only a 10% increase in minute volume, which could be achieved by a combination of deeper breaths, faster breathing, or an occasional sigh (Saltzman et al 1963). Such subtle differences are difficult to detect without instrumentation. A clear marker of chronic hyperventilation is a delayed return to baseline after hyperventilation provocation (Hardonk & Beumer 1979).

Persistence of emotion may explain the persistence of hyperventilation, but there may also be a physiological factor. In one study, 90 patients diagnosed with hyperventilation syndrome were asked to hyperventilate for a few minutes, focus on a negative emotional memory, and then resume normal breathing and indicate when they thought their breathing was actually back to normal. More than half of them signalled 'normal' when their CO_2 was less than 80% of their baseline, or resting level, while only 4% of the control subjects did so (King 1990).

This study, by including the negative emotional focus, confounded the effect of emotional persistence with the effect of hyperventilation itself, but it still offers valuable observations about a possible trait in hyperventilators. It may be that enough experience with this hypocapnic state creates habituation to this compromised chemical condition and changes the threshold for normality. Gardner (1996) found chronic hyperventilation to be a very persistent, stubborn pattern, subsiding only during the later stages of sleep. If such individuals routinely perceive their breathing as normal when it is not, this misperception would work against improvement. Similar in principle is acceptance of poor posture or chronic muscle tension, not really noticing the problem yet still constrained by it in some way. Breathing rehabilitation therefore should include help in recognizing optimal breathing as well as learning to create and sustain it without constant attention.

Panic attacks during relaxation

Panic attacks which happen suddenly, without apparent reason, are a frequent experience for those with panic disorder. Sitting quietly watching television or driving long distances are often associated with a sudden onset of breathlessness. Nocturnal panic attacks which awaken the individual from deep sleep may seem to challenge any psychological explanation, unless one postulates possible dream content, but such speculation is hard to confirm objectively.

Ley (1988a, 1988b) has offered a plausible explanation for this phenomenon based on the body's adaptation to chronic hyperventilation. The long-term reduction in bicarbonate buffer concentration, offsetting lowered $PaCO_2$, returns pH to normal, but the equilibrium is an uneasy one, dependent on the hyperventilation continuing. This situation makes the individual more susceptible than ever to a rise in CO_2 (more acidity) because the alkaline buffer has been reduced. Consequently a change in breathing toward normal, away from hyperventilation, would feel closer to suffocation than if the person possessed normal bicarbonate buffering capacity.

Ley proposed that during certain deep sleep stages (not paradoxical sleep) and during sedentary states, the breathing is most likely to slow, and since the system has been set to expect a certain amount of hyperventilation, it is caught by surprise by the more normal breathing. Core temperature drops between 0.8 and 1.1°C. Lowered metabolism reduces the production of CO_2, adding to the already low level created by hyperventilation. Timing is important; if the breathing volume does not keep pace exactly with shifting metabolic requirements, there will be a period of mismatch. In Ley's words:

> The chronic hyperventilator…is vulnerable to the effects of decreases in metabolism because a decrease in CO_2 may lower an already abnormally low resting level of $PaCO_2$ beyond the threshold of severe respiratory alkalosis and thereby produce those sensations of hypocapnia (e.g. dyspnea) that mark the panic attack. Thus, the chronic hyperventilator teeters on the brink of calamity. If the metabolic production of CO_2 drops suddenly, as when one sits down or lies down to relax, while minute volume remains constant, the sensations of hypocapnia will increase in intensity and thereby lead to the familiar symptoms which mark the panic attack.
>
> Ley 1988b, p. 255

Citing a study by Bass & Gardner (1985), Leznoff (1997) has observed that:

> patients who chronically hyperventilate for reasons of anxiety do not achieve adequate renal compensation by excretion of bicarbonate because they do not hyperventilate during sleep. Thus they experience the physiologic and somatic consequences of uncompensated hypocarbia.

GENERAL SUMMARY

High body priorities are to maintain pH around 7.4 and ensure adequate oxygen supply and delivery. Excess breathing excretes more CO_2 than is being produced, so pH moves higher, toward the alkaline end (low $PaCO_2$ promotes alkalosis). Insufficient breathing retains more CO_2 than is being produced, so pH drops toward the acidic end. The pH in the short term is adjusted by increases or decreases in breathing volume.

Bicarbonate is an alkaline buffer which cushions abrupt rises in acidity. With the continued respiratory alkalosis created by chronic hyperventilation, the kidneys attempt

to return pH to normal, excreting bicarbonate. This creates a new false equilibrium which works against resuming normal ventilation, which now creates sensations of breathlessness as $PaCO_2$ rises, less buffered by bicarbonate.

Muscle contraction, or any increase in metabolism, produces more CO_2, but normally the breathing increases also, resulting in more exhalation of CO_2. When respiration is matched to metabolic need, the level of $PaCO_2$ and pH stays stable. However, anticipated metabolic production (set off by apprehension, anxiety, preparation for exertion, discomfort, or chronic pain) will raise breathing volume. If the exertion does not occur, $PaCO_2$ will drop because the anticipatory increased breathing is not followed by increased muscle activity.

With higher $PaCO_2$ (lower pH), haemoglobin is stimulated to release more oxygen to the tissues. But a deficit of CO_2 promotes oxygen retention by the haemoglobin molecule. Thus, at a time when vasoconstriction is being promoted by alkalosis and high pH, release of oxygen is further inhibited by the Bohr effect. The system does not seem to have a mechanism for handling anticipatory anxiety unaccompanied by exertion, and this may constitute a functional, chemical loophole suffered by sentient beings able to project into the future.

ALLERGIC, DIETARY AND NUTRITIONAL FACTORS

Food allergy is an immunological event, involving immunoglobulin E (IgE), whereas food intolerance involves adverse physiological reactions of unknown origin, without immune mediation. Food intolerance may involve food toxicity or idiosyncratic reactions to foods, sometimes related to enzyme deficiency or pharmacological responses (Hodge et al 2009).

Lum (1996) has observed that food intolerance, with bloating after meals, 'splints the diaphragm', requiring expert dietary management, and that pseudo-allergy is common, with many patients inaccurately attributing symptoms to an 'allergy' to particular foods:

> In two-thirds of such cases of pseudo-allergy, the symptoms have been shown to be due to a conditioned reflex of hyperventilation on exposure, with a similar mechanism common in allergy to perfumes, and industrial gases.

Gray & Chan (2003) note that there are numerous complex mechanisms underlying food intolerances, and that these are incompletely understood. They assert that 'far fewer reactions are due to true allergy [i.e. involving the immune system] than is commonly believed.'

Many experts hold to the opinion that the symptoms that are associated with food and environmental intolerances are more likely a response to anxiety rather than true chemical reactions (Leznoff 1997, Simon et al 1993). As Ley (1988c) presciently pointed out – the fact that a panic attack follows exposure to a substance does not discriminate between two possibilities: that the individual reacted to the substance, leading to hyperventilation and a panic attack, that the 'the experience of panic attacks is the cause of the heightened sensitivity.'

It would certainly be helpful to be able to make a clear distinction between frank food allergy (hypersensitivity) reactions and food intolerance responses; however, these terms remain a source of much confusion and little certainty.

MECHANISMS

Foodstuff in the gut is usually reduced enzymatically to molecular size (short chain fatty acids, peptides, and disaccharides) for absorption or elimination; however, it has been noted for some years that food antigens and immune complexes also find their way across the mucosal barrier to enter the bloodstream. The rate of entry seems to relate directly to the load of antigenic material in the gut lumen (Bischoff 2011, Mitchell 1988). Mitchell states:

The presence of specialised membranous epithelial cells…appears to allow active transport of antigen across the mucosa even when concentrations of antigen are low.

Box 4.2 lists the factors which can damage the gut wall. Permeability is retarded by defensive mechanisms, including enzyme and acid degradation, mucus secretion and gut movement and barriers, which reduce absorption and adherence.

Gut wall irritation resulting from bacterial or yeast overgrowth (Guarner et al 2006), or from higher levels of toxic load (dysbiosis), can increase the rate of transportation of undesirable molecules into the bloodstream – the so-called 'leaky-gut syndrome'. A variety of immunological defensive strategies occur to counter the entry of toxins and antigens into the system; however, a degree of adaptive tolerance seems to be a common outcome. Mitchell states that animal studies suggest strongly that the liver, along with the age of first exposure, the degree of the antigenic load, and the form in which the antigen is presented, all play roles in regulation of the antigen-specific tolerance (hyporesponsiveness) which emerges from this process (Mitchell 1988, Roland 1993). Early feeding patterns seem to be a critical factor in determining subsequent antibody responses to foods, with eggs, milk, fish and nuts rating as among the greatest culprits (Mitchell 1988, Brandtzaeg

---

Box 4.2 What damages the gut wall?
(Dinan & Cryan 2012, Deitch 1990, Iocono 1995, Jenkins 1991, O'Dwyer 1988, Isolauri 1989, Hollander 1985, Bjarnason 1984)

- Drugs (antibiotics, steroids, alcohol, NSAIDs)
- Age
- Allergies (specific genetically acquired intolerances)
- Infections of the intestine – bacterial, yeast, protozoal, etc.
- Chemicals ingested with food (pesticides, additives, etc.)
- Maldigestion, constipation (leading to gut fermentation, dysbiosis, etc.)
- Emotional stress which alters the gut pH, negatively influencing normal flora
- Major trauma such as burns (possibly due to loss of blood supply to traumatized area)
- Toxins which are not excreted or deactivated may end up in the body's fat stores

---

2010). Apparently most people show the presence of serum antibody responses to food antigens, involving all classes of immunoglobulins. It is assumed that antibodies assist in elimination of food antigens via the formation of immune complexes which are subsequently phagocytosed. Failure to remove these complexes may result in tissue deposition and subsequent inflammation (Brandtzaeg 2010). Sometimes the immune response to food antigens involves IgE, and sometimes not. The true food allergy exists, as do other responses which fall short of the criteria which would attract this label, and these are the food intolerances. An approach to the food-intolerant patient is shown in Figure 4.5.

Mast cells

Mast cells in the lung, intestines, and elsewhere are critical to the allergic response, occurring as mucosal and connective tissue variants. Mast cells have surface receptors with a high affinity to IgE but, critically, also to non-immunological stimuli including food antigens. How violent an allergic reaction is, involving the interaction of mast cells with IgE or other stimuli, depends on the presence of a variety of mediators such as histamine and arachidonic acid (and its derivatives such as leukotrienes) which augment inflammatory processes (Wardlaw 1986, Holgate 1983).

Histamine is secreted by mast cells during exposure to allergens, and the level of circulating histamine rises during prolonged hyperventilation (Kontos et al 1972). Histamine causes local inflammation and oedema as well as bronchiole constriction. This last effect is especially

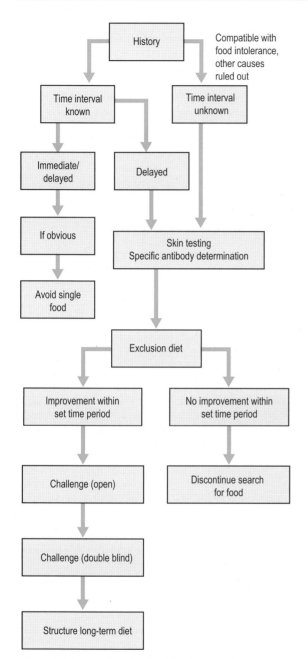

Figure 4.5 Approach to the food-intolerant patient.

A summary of the evidence relating food sensitivity to asthma and other bronchial conditions is given below:

- Avoidance by lactating mothers of milk, eggs, fish and nuts – and avoidance by the infant (up to 12 months) of the same foods plus soy, wheat and oranges – reduced allergic disease (including asthma) in 58 cases compared with 62 controls (Spector 1991).
- In adults who have asthma the prevalence of food allergy in one double-blind, placebo-controlled study was 2%, and in children 6.8%. Where asthma is poorly controlled, food allergy should be suspected. The main culprits identified are egg, milk, peanuts, soy, fish, shellfish and wheat (Onorato 1986, James 1997).
- Another study showed that up to 10% of asthma may involve food allergy. This is more likely if the patient has a history of atopic dermatitis (egg, peanuts and milk were identified as the main foods to cause a reaction). If asthma is refractory to standard medication, food allergy should always be considered (Plaut 1997).
- Food intolerance is identified in various studies to be a trigger in up to 50% of asthma patients (Warner 1995, Metcalf 1989, Wilson 1988, Bahna 1991).

a reaction to food (Box 4.3). Wilson and colleagues demonstrated (1982) that even in the absence of an immediate episode of bronchospasm, a reaction to foods (cola drinks were being tested) can modify the function of the bronchial wall, although the mediating pathways are unclear (see Fig. 4.6).

Testing for intolerances and even frank allergies is not straightforward. Various factors may cause confusion, including the following (Roberson 1997):

- Demonstration of IgE antibodies in serum may be confounded because of the presence of other antibody classes
- Cytotoxic blood tests commonly produce false positive results
- Skin testing is an effective means of demonstrating the presence of inhaled allergens; however, this is not the case for food allergens (Rowntree et al 1985)
- Early in life the skin test response to food may be lost even though IgE antibodies are present in serum.
- Skin testing is inefficient in assessing delayed sensitivities and fails to accurately evaluate metabolic intolerances to foods (Hamilton 1997).

It is suggested that, following positive skin tests and/or radio-allergo-sorbant (RAST) tests, an *elimination diet* should be introduced to assess for food intolerances (James 1997) (see also Fig. 4.5).

relevant to asthmatics, but can affect anyone to some degree, adding to breathing difficulty.

At times a rapid response is noted to ingested and absorbed antigens; however, hours or days may elapse before a reaction manifests (Mitchell 1988). In the context of this text the relation between food intolerance and respiratory symptoms is of particular relevance. Both allergic rhinitis and bronchial asthma may result from

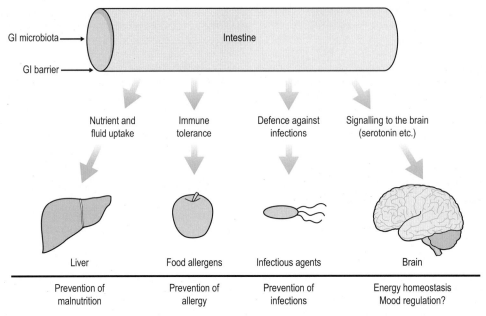

Figure 4.6 The intestines' impact on health. The gastrointestinal tract contributes to health by ensuring digestion and absorption of nutrients, minerals and fluids; by induction of mucosal and systemic tolerance; by defence of the host against infectious and other pathogens; and by signalling from the periphery to the brain.

An elimination diet involves a food or food family being excluded for a period – commonly 3 weeks – during which time symptoms are assessed. If there is an improvement, a challenge is initiated as the food is reintroduced. If there is benefit when the food is excluded, and symptoms emerge when it is reintroduced, the food is then excluded for not less than 6 months. This process offers the simplest, safest, and most accurate method of assessing a food intolerance, but only when it is applied strictly.

Strategies

Oligoallergenic diets, elimination diets, challenge studies and rotation diets are variations which attempt to identify and then minimize the exposure of an individual to foods which provoke symptoms. A variety of elimination diets, challenge studies and rotation diets are variations which attempt to identify and then minimize the exposure of an individual to foods which provoke symptoms. Evidence of the value of such approaches is listed in Box 4.4.

Summary

Breathing disorders as severe as asthma, and as mild but irritating as chronic rhinitis, may be aggravated, or at times triggered, by food intolerances which are not frank allergies. Reduction or avoidance of factors in the diet which load the defensive mechanisms of the body is a choice

---

Box 4.4 **Dietary strategies and asthma**

- 74% of 50 patients with asthma experienced significant improvement without medication following an elimination diet. 62% were shown to have attacks provoked by food alone and 32% by a combination of food and skin contact (Borok 1990).
- When 113 individuals with irritable bowel syndrome were treated by an elimination diet, marked symptomatic improvement was noted. 79% of the patients who also displayed atopic symptoms, including hay fever, sinusitis, asthma, eczema and urticaria, showed significant improvements in these symptoms as well (Borok 1994).
- A moderate to high intake of oily fish has been shown to be associated with reduced risk of asthma, presumably due to high levels of eicosapentaenoic acid (EPA) which inhibits inflammatory processes (Hodge 1996, Thien 1996).
- A vegan diet which eliminated all dairy products, eggs, meat and fish as well as coffee, tea, sugar and grains (apart from buckwheat, millet and lentils) was applied to 35 asthmatics, of whom 24 completed the 1-year study. There was a 71% improvement in symptoms within 4 months and 92% after 1 year (Lindahl 1985).

patients may make if the evidence is presented to them in a coherent way, and strategies are offered which allow them to possibly enhance their quality of life. Clinical experience suggests that after a period of exclusion (6 months at least), cautious reintroduction of previously poorly tolerated foods may no longer provoke symptoms, especially if the foods are rotated (i.e. not eaten on a daily basis). Other strategies include desensitization, using homeopathic injection or orally administered dilutions of the food(s) in question (Reilly 1994, Kahn 1995).

DIETARY LINKS TO ANXIETY, PANIC ATTACKS AND PHOBIC BEHAVIOUR

Ley (Timmons & Ley 1994) states that emotional arousal gives rise to conditionable changes in ventilation, and it appears that the connection between the emotions and breathing is a reciprocative relationship, in which changes in one lead to corresponding changes in the other (p. 80; see Ch. 5 for further coverage of conditioning). This suggests that feelings of anxiety may predispose to hyperventilation, which behaviour then reinforces the feelings of anxiety, forming a potentially destructive cycle. Ley's statement, of course, also suggests that hyperventilation predisposes towards feelings of apprehension and anxiety. Opinions differ as to the relative hierarchy of importance between these two factors, i.e. which comes first, anxiety or hyperventilation, making this a very practical chicken and egg conundrum. And although Gardner (in Timmons & Ley 1994, p. 102) expresses the view that there is ample evidence that 'chronic hyperventilation can occur in the absence of manifest anxiety' – which suggests the possibility of eggs without chickens, or vice versa – the fact remains that anxiety is established as a common instigator of hyperventilation.

Anxiety as an emotional state usually attracts psychosocial therapeutic attention. If, however, it could be shown that there exist common dietary factors which encourage anxiety, these triggers could be seen to be precursors to the breathing pattern changes which follow. This would offer the opportunity, in such individuals, for relatively simple dietary interventions (exclusions) that could potentially reduce or eliminate the anxiety state which may represent the main precursor to hyperventilation. A variety of such dietary triggers have been identified (Werbach 1991) and some of the key features of this phenomenon are summarized below:

- Buist (1985) has demonstrated a direct connection between clinical anxiety and elevated blood lactate levels, as well as an *increased lactate: pyruvate ratio.* This ratio is increased by alcohol, caffeine and sugar. Experimentally infused lactate is likely to provoke panic attacks, including hyperventilation, in people prone to panic, but not in those who are not prone to panic. The lactate leads to peripheral alkalosis by being converted to bicarbonate. This lactate effect is paralleled by that of breathing 5% CO_2 for a short time: panickers are more likely to panic, but not those who are not panickers. The hypothesis proposed by some researchers is that sensitivity to lactate and CO_2 comes from the fact that both are precursors of suffocation; panickers are more sensitive to build-up of these chemicals for reasons that may be either chemical or psychological. Wemmie (2011) reports that both CO_2 and lactate alter pH balance, influencing neuronal function via pH-sensitive receptors, provoking hyperventilation and panic. Esquivel et al (2010) propose that 'the shared characteristics of $CO_{(2)}$/H(+) sensing neurons overlap to a point where threatening disturbances in brain pH homeostasis, such as those produced by $CO_{(2)}$ inhalations, elicit a primal emotion that can range from breathlessness to panic.'

- *Alcohol* inhibits gluconeogenesis from blood lactate, which directly raises the lactate: pyruvate ratio (Alberti & Natrass 1977). In an experimental placebo-controlled study involving 90 healthy male volunteers, an increase was shown in state anxiety following administration of ethanol as compared with placebo (Monteiro 1990). In this study separate infusions were made of either ethanol or diazepam. The Spielberger State Anxiety Inventory was applied, demonstrating significant increases in state anxiety following ethanol infusion, as compared to significant reductions in feelings of tension which were reported after the placebo administration. The implication is that in dealing with anxiety-prone people, alcohol intake should be moderated or eliminated, if at all possible. Duke (2011) reports that acute alcohol intake may lead to hyperventilation because of disinhibition of central respiratory regulation centres, along with increases in dead-space ventilation. On the other hand in chronic alcohol users there is a generalized decrease in all lung capacities (vital, functional residual and inspiratory capacity).

- *Caffeine* was shown to have anxiogenic effects on patients with anxiety, particularly those suffering from panic disorders. In an experimental controlled study (Charney 1985) 21 agoraphobic patients with panic attacks or panic disorder and 17 controls ingested caffeine 10 mg/kg of body weight. Caffeine was found to produce significantly greater increases in subject-rated anxiety, nervousness, fear, nausea, palpitations, restlessness and tremors in the patients compared with the controls. 71% of the patients reported that the behavioural effects were similar to those experienced during panic attacks. Similar results have been reported by Nardi et al (2007) who noted an association between hyperventilation and hyperreactivity to caffeine. The implication is that in dealing with anxiety-prone people, caffeine intake should be moderated or eliminated, if at all possible.

The blood-glucose–hyperventilation connection

Diet has another effect on breathing disorders, namely that the level of glucose in the blood moderates the effect of low CO_2. These two factors are independent: that is, an individual may be in a hypoglycaemic state and may or may not be hypocapnic also. The combination amplifies the negative effects of each on the brain by diminishing cerebral circulation and therefore interfering with neural metabolism. The brain requires both glucose and oxygen to function, and the cortex is more sensitive to fuel interruptions than any other area. The brain uses approximately 20% of the glucose available in the blood at any one time.

Lum (1996) has noted that when the blood glucose is below the middle of the normal range (i.e. below 4.4 mmol/l) the effects of overbreathing are progressively exaggerated, and that this can trigger hyperventilation and associated symptoms such as panic attacks. Dietary modification, to help maintain blood glucose in the upper half of the normal range, is therefore important, involving a high protein/low carbohydrate pattern of eating.

This means that if episodes of hyperventilation are reported to occur in late morning or late afternoon, or any time relatively far-removed from a previous meal, the coincidence of hypoglycaemia and hyperventilation should be considered. A partial remedy would consist of prescribing a hypoglycaemic diet (high protein, frequent meals).

In addition, an individual's response to a hyperventilation challenge test will vary according to the blood sugar level. To maximize the chance of obtaining a positive test (duplicating the conditions under which the symptoms are more likely to appear during voluntary hyperventilation), fasting should be requested for at least 4 hours before the challenge is carried out. Depending on the efficiency of a person's insulin regulation, fasting may make little difference for the effects of hyperventilation, or it may make a very large difference.

The progesterone–hyperventilation connection

During the latter half of the menstrual cycle, progesterone begins to rise and peaks around the 22nd day, or a week after ovulation. Apart from promoting thickening of the uterine wall, progesterone also stimulates respiration. Some research suggests that it first stimulates acidosis, which in turn increases breathing to compensate. Other research supports progesterone's direct stimulation of breathing. Either way, hyperventilation is the result. Apart from increasing minute volume, progesterone also increases the sensitivity of CO_2 receptors in the respiratory centres of the brain (increased sensitivity implies that an urge to breathe would develop sooner).

$PaCO_2$ level is systematically related to the menstrual cycle, reaching its highest point before ovulation and its lowest point when progesterone and oestradiol levels have peaked (Slatkovska et al 2006). The average drop during the luteal phase is around 20–25%. $PaCO_2$ remains depressed for many days, with all the potentially symptom-generating effects on vasoconstriction, nerve conduction, muscle tension, anxiety, etc. Hyperventilation may contribute to severity of other premenstrual symptoms; there is much individual variability (Damas-Mora et al 1980). When a woman's breathing pattern is essentially normal, the premenstrual drop may not be enough to cause disruption because it is still in the low–normal range. But if a woman already has a tendency toward hyperventilation, a safety reserve is absent and the $PaCO_2$ may drop into the zone which can cause symptoms (Fried 1993).

Ott et al (2006) observe that:

> *In women with PMS the sensitivity of the respiratory center to CO_2 is increased more than normal by progesterone, or some other secretory product of the corpus luteum, resulting in pronounced hyperventilation with the associated clinical signs and symptoms.*

Dunnett et al (2007) found that several participants in a study of fibromyalgia (FMS) patients 'changed' their diagnosis during the course of a menstrual cycle, fulfilling the diagnostic criteria post-ovulation, when hyperventilation patterns were more evident – indicating lower pain thresholds – but never during the follicular phase when pain thresholds were higher, and breathing more normal.

Progesterone helps to maintain pregnancy and so also remains high throughout pregnancy, continuing to stimulate breathing. Some degree of hyperventilation is common, if not universal, during pregnancy, and this chronically depressed CO_2 may, if added to an already existing pattern, aggravate anxiety and other symptoms. Jensen et al (2005) report that sensitivity to CO_2 increases during pregnancy, probably due to the effects of gestational hormones. Altered levels of progesterone during menopause may disrupt stability further by its effect on breathing.

Women are at higher risk for anxiety disorders, and there may be a contribution to this liability by their periodic hormonal shift which disrupts their breathing pattern and thus their biochemistry. The progesterone effect is independent of other factors; in one study in which men were given either progesterone or a control substance, only the progesterone produced a higher basal temperature and decreased $PaCO_2$.

Exercise and biochemistry

Another peril of chronic hyperventilation is poor tolerance of exercise. The increased activity creates more carbonic acid (with aerobic exercise) and lactic acid once the anaerobic threshold is reached. But hyperventilators have a smaller buffer zone as a result of loss of bicarbonate, so blood acidity of any sort is relatively unopposed. This increases the chance of premature fatigue, feelings of breathlessness, dyspnoea and muscle pain. In addition, the large exercise-induced swings in metabolism create lag times and increase the chance of mismatches between metabolic demand and breathing volume.

REFERENCES

Alberti, K., Natrass, M., 1977. Lactic acidosis. Lancet 2, 25–29.

Bahna, S., 1991. Asthma in the food sensitive patient. Journal of Allergy and Clinical Immunology 87 (1), part 11, 174, abstract 144.

Ball, S., Shekhar, A., 1997. Basilar artery response to hyperventilation in panic disorder. American Journal of Psychiatry 154 (11), 1603–1604.

Bass, C., Gardner, W.N., 1985. Respiratory and psychiatric abnormalities in chronic symptomatic hyperventilation. Br Med J 290, 1387–1390.

Bischoff, S., 2011. Gut health: a new objective in medicine? BMC Medicine 9, 24.

Bishop, D., Edge, J., Davis, C., et al., 2004. Induced metabolic alkalosis affects muscle metabolism and repeated-sprint ability. Med Sci Sports Exerc 36, 807–813.

Bjarnason, I., 1984. The leaky gut of alcoholism – possible route for entry of toxic compounds. Lancet i, 79–182.

Borok, G., 1990. Childhood asthma – foods that trigger? South African Medical Journal 77, 269.

Borok, G., 1994. IBS and diet. Gastroenterology Forum (April), 29.

Brandtzaeg, P., 2010. Food allergy: separating the science from the mythology. Nat. Rev. Gastroenterol. Hepatol. 7, 389–400.

Buist, R., 1985. Anxiety neurosis: the lactate connection. International Clinical Nutrition Review 5 (1), 1–4.

Charney, D., 1985. Increased anxiogenic effects of caffeine in panic disorders. Archives of General Psychiatry 42, 233–243.

Comroe, J.H., 1974. Physiology of respiration, second ed. Year Book Medical Publishers, Chicago.

Damas-Mora, J., Davies, L., Taylor, W., et al., 1980. Menstrual respiratory changes and symptoms. British Journal of Psychiatry 136, 492–497.

Deitch, E., 1990. Intestinal permeability increased in burn patients shortly after injury. Surgery 107, 411–416.

Dinan, T., Cryan, J., 2012. Regulation of the stress response by the gut microbiota. Psychoneuroendocrinology 37 (9), 1369–1378.

Duke, J., 2011. Alcohol and substance abuse. In: Anesthesia Secrets, fourth ed. pp. 336–342.

Dunnett, A., et al., 2007. The diagnosis of fibromyalgia in women may be influenced by menstrual cycle phase. Journal of Bodywork and Movement Therapies 11, 99–105.

Esquivel, G., Schruers, K.R., Maddock, R.J., et al., 2010. Acids in the brain: a factor in panic? J Psychopharmacol. 24 (5), 639–647.

Forster, H.V., Smith, C.A., 2010. Contributions of central and peripheral chemoreceptors to the ventilatory response to CO_2/H^+. J Appl Physiol. 108 (4), 989–994.

Fried, R., 1993. The psychology and physiology of breathing. Plenum, New York, pp. 174–176.

Gardner, W.N., 1996. The pathophysiology of hyperventilation disorders. Chest 109, 516–534.

Gibbs, D.M., 1992. Hyperventilation-induced cerebral ischemia in panic disorder and effects of nimodipine. American Journal of Psychiatry 149, 1589–1591.

Gotoh, F., Meyer, J.S., Takagi, Y., 1965. Cerebral effects of hyperventilation in man. Archives of Neurology 12, 410–423.

Gray, J., Chan, W., 2003. Encyclopedia of food sciences and nutrition, second ed. Academic Press, London, pp. 2621–2626.

Guarner, F., Bourdet-Sicard, R., Brandtzaeg, P., et al., 2006. Mechanisms of disease: the hygiene hypothesis revisited. Nat Clin Pract Gastroenterol Hepatol 3, 275–284.

Guyton, A.C., 1971. Textbook of medical physiology, fourth ed. W B Saunders, Philadelphia.

Hamilton, K., 1997. Allergy/hypersensitivity/intolerance. In: Roberson, K. (Ed.), Asthma: clinical pearls in nutrition and complementary medicine. I T Services, Sacramento, California.

Han, J.N., Stegen, K., Simkens, K., et al., 1997. Unsteadiness of breathing in patients with hyperventilation syndrome and anxiety disorders. European Respiratory Journal 10, 167–176.

Hardonk, J., Beumer, H., 1979. Hyperventilation syndrome. In: Vinken, P., Bruyn, G. (Eds.), Handbook of clinical neurology. North Holland, Amsterdam, pp. 309–360.

Hauge, A., Thoresen, M., Walloe, L., 1980. Changes in cerebral blood flow during hyperventilation, and CO_2 rebreathing in humans by a bidirectional, pulsed, ultrasound Doppler blood velocity meter. Acta Physiologia Scandinavia 110, 167–173.

Heistad, D., Wheeler, R., Mark, A., et al., 1972. Effects of adrenergic stimulation in man. Journal of Clinical Investigation 51, 1469–1475.

Hodge, L., 1996. Consumption of oily fish and childhood allergy risk. Medical Journal of Australia 164, 136–140.

Hodge, L., Swain, A., Faulkner-Hogg, K., 2009. Food allergy and intolerance. Australian Family Physician 38 (9), 706–707.

Holgate, S., 1983. Mast cells and their mediators. In: Holborrow, E., Reeves, W. (Eds.), Immunology in

Medicine, second ed. Academic Press, London.

Hollander, D., 1985. Aging-associated increase in intestinal absorption of macro-molecules. Gerontology 31, 133–137.

Iocono, G., 1995. Chronic constipation as a symptom of cow's milk allergy. Journal of Pediatrics 126, 34–39.

Isolauri, E., 1989. Intestinal permeability changes in acute gastroenteritis. Journal of Pediatric Gastroenterology and Nutrition 8, 466–473.

James, J., 1997. Food allergy – what link to respiratory symptoms? Journal of Respiratory Diseases 18 (4), 379–390.

Jenkins, A., 1991. Do NSAIDs increase colonic permeability? Gut 32, 66–69.

Jensen, D., Wolfe, L.A., Slatkovska, L., et al., 2005. Effects of human pregnancy on the ventilatory chemoreflex response to carbon dioxide. American Journal of Physiology – Regulatory Integrative and Comparative Physiology 288 (5), 57–65.

Kahn, J., 1995. Homeopathic remedy relieves allergic asthma. Medical Tribune, 5 Jan, pp. 11.

King, J., 1990. Failure of perception of hypocapnia: physiological and clinical implications. Journal of the Royal Society of Medicine 83 (Dec), 765–767.

Kontos, H., Richardson, D., Raper, A., 1972. Mechanism of action of hypocapnic alkalosis on limb blood vessels in man and dog. American Journal of Physiology 223, 1296–1307.

Ley, R., 1988a. Panic attacks during relaxation and relaxation-induced anxiety: a hyperventilation interpretation. Journal of Behavior Therapy and Experimental Psychiatry 19, 253–259.

Ley, R., 1988b. Panic attacks during sleep: a hyperventilation-probability model. Journal of Behavior Therapy and Experimental Psychiatry 19, 181–192.

Ley, R., 1988c. Hyperventilation and lactate infusion in the production of panic attacks. Clinical Psychology Review 8, 1–18.

Leznoff, A., 1997. Provocative challenges in patients with multiple chemical sensitivity. J Allergy Clin Immunol 99, 438–442.

Lindahl, O., 1985. Vegan regimen with reduced medication in treatment of bronchial asthma. Journal of Asthma 22 (1), 44–55.

Lum, L.C., 1976. The syndrome of chronic habitual hyperventilation. In: Hill, O.W. (Ed.), Modern trends in psychosomatic medicine. Butterworth, London.

Lum, L.C., 1981. Hyperventilation and anxiety state. Journal of the Royal Society of Medicine 74, 1–4.

Lum, C., 1996. Treatment difficulties and failures: causes and clinical management. Biological Psychology 43 (3), 243.

Macefield, G., Burke, D., 1991. Paraesthesiae and tetany induced by voluntary hyperventilation: increased excitability of human cutaneous and motor axons. Brain 114, 527–540.

McNaughton, L., Dalton, B., Palmer, G., 1999. Sodium bicarbonate can be used as an ergogenic aid in high-intensity, competitive cycle ergometry of 1 h duration. European Journal of Applied Physiology 80 (1), 64–69.

Metcalf, D., 1989. Diseases of food hypersensitivity. New England Journal of Medicine 321 (4), 255–257.

Mitchell, E.B., 1988. Food intolerance. In: Dickerson, W., Lee, H. (Eds.), Nutrition in the clinical management of disease. Edward Arnold, London.

Monteiro, M., 1990. Subjective feelings of anxiety in young men after ethanol and diazepam infusions. Journal of Clinical Psychiatry 51 (1), 12–16.

Nardi, A., Valença, A., Lopes, F., et al., 2007. Caffeine and 35% carbon dioxide challenge tests in panic disorder. Hum. Psychopharmacol. 22 (4), 231–240.

Nardi, A., Valença, A., Nascimento, I., 2001. Hyperventilation challenge test in panic disorder and depression with panic attacks. Psychiatry Research 105 (1), 57–65.

Nunn, J.F., 1993. Applied respiratory physiology. Butterworth-Heinemann Medical, Oxford.

O'Dwyer, S., 1988. A single dose of endotoxin increases intestinal permeability in healthy humans. Archives of Surgery 123, 1459–1464.

Onorato, J., 1986. Placebo-controlled double-blind food challenge in asthma. Journal of Allergy and Clinical Immunology 878, 1139–1146.

Ott, H.W., Mattle, V., Zimmermann, U.S., et al., 2006. Symptoms of premenstrual syndrome may be caused by hyperventilation. Fertility and Sterility 86 (4), 1001e17–1001e19.

Patel, C., 1991. The complete guide to stress management. MacDonald Optima, London; Plenum Press, New York.

Plaut, M., 1997. New directions in food allergy research. Journal of Allergy and Clinical Immunology April 1997, 7–10.

Reilly, D., 1994. Is evidence for homeopathy reproducible? Lancet 344, 1601–1606.

Roberson, K. (Ed.), 1997. Asthma: Clinical pearls in nutrition and complementary medicine. I T Services, Sacramento, California.

Roland, N., 1993. Interactions between the intestinal flora and xenobiotic metabolizing enzymes and their health consequences. World Review of Nutrition and Diet 74, 123–148.

Rowntree, S., Cogswell, J., Platts-Mills, T., et al., 1985. Development of IgE and IgG antibodies to food and inhalant allergens in children. Archives of Diseases in Children 60, 727–735.

Saltzman, H.A., Heyman, A., Sieker, H.O., 1963. Correlation of clinical and physiologic manifestations of sustained hyperventilation. New England Journal of Medicine 268, 1431–1436.

Schott, H.C., Hinchcliff, K.W., 1998. Treatments affecting fluid and electrolyte status during exercise. Veterinary Clinics of North America Equine Practice 14 (1), 175–204.

Simon, G., Daniell, W., Stockbridge, H., et al., 1993. Immunologic, psychological, and neuropsychological factors in multiple chemical sensitivity. a controlled study. Annals of Internal Medicine 119 (2), 97–103.

Slatkovska, L., Jensen, D., Davies, G., et al., 2006. Phasic menstrual cycle effects on the control of breathing in healthy women. Respiratory Physiology & Neurobiology 154 (3), 379–388.

Spector, S., 1991. Common triggers of asthma. Postgraduate Medicine 90 (3), 50–58.

Thien, F., 1996. Oily fish and asthma. Medical Journal of Australia 164, 135–136.

Timmons, B.H., Ley, R., 1994. Behavioral and psychological approaches to breathing disorders. Plenum Press, New York.

Wardlaw, A., 1986. Morphological and secretory properties of bronchoalveolar mast cells in respiratory diseases. Clinical Allergy 16, 163–173.

Warner, J., 1995. Food intolerance and asthma. Clinical and Experimental Allergy 25 (suppl. 1), 29–30.

Wemmie, J.A., 2011. Neurobiology of panic and pH chemosensation in the brain. Dialogues Clin Neurosci. 13 (4), 475–483.

Werbach, M., 1991. Nutritional influences on mental illness. Third Line Press, Tarzana, CA.

West, J., 2008. Respiratory physiology: the essentials. Lippincott, Williams and Wilkins, Philadelphia.

Wilson, N., 1988. Bronchial hyperreactivity in food and drink intolerance. Annals of Allergy 61, 75–79.

Wilson, N., Vickers, H., Taylor, G., et al., 1982. Objective test for food sensitivity in asthmatic children: increased bronchial reactivity after cola drinks. British Medical Journal 284, 1226–1228.

Chapter 5

Interaction of psychological and emotional variables with breathing dysfunction

Chris Gilbert

Breathing problems, from whatever source, cause stress in many systems. This stress includes an attempt to restore normal functioning, seeking a return to homeostasis. If a problem (body or mind) is forcing the patient to adapt in some way, then a therapist can be helpful in many ways, depending on discipline: physical manipulation, suggesting exercises, providing hope, reducing overbreathing, treating trigger points, improving dietary habits, or improving mental outlook. Such measures can be seen as helping homeostasis along. The general payoff for an increased ability to adapt is less sense of threat, and this becomes a psychological matter. Regardless of the presence or absence of disease, acute vs. chronic, functional or organic, there is a person experiencing it all, and a person in distress can disrupt his breathing so much that other interventions are thwarted.

This chapter presents information about interactions between mind and body, which essentially means the person communicating with different aspects of self. Because of the close coupling of breathing with consciousness, many things can go wrong which have nothing to do with organic pathology. This resonating interface can also be used for improving the situation, if only by reducing the negative mental input which disrupts smooth functioning of the respiratory system.

THE DIAPHRAGM AND THE PHRENIC NERVE

The diaphragm is the muscular equivalent of an umbilical cord linking us to the environment; it keeps us alive by pulling fresh air into the lungs and returning used air back out into the world. This process is not a mindless one, but is very responsive to our thinking. The word 'diaphragm' is related to the Greek word for *mind:* the diaphragm muscle is controlled by the phrenic nerve, and its Greek root, *phren*, designates the mind as well as the muscle. The Random House College Dictionary (Merriam-Webster 1991) definition of the word 'phrenic' is the following: '1. Of or relating to the diaphragm. 2. Of or relating to the mind.'

Considering such an odd dual meaning, one might conclude that the Greeks were confused, but the confusion is rather in the modern thinking which attempts to separate mind and body into separate compartments. Ancient physicians had only their native senses for observing the action of breathing in themselves and others. This provided what no modern mechanical breathing monitor can offer – simultaneous registration of mental and breathing processes. With this opportunity for observation, parallels and correlations could be drawn between moments of emotion and changes in breathing rate, depth, regularity and body displacement. Interruption of attention, style of focusing, state of calmness or distress, degree of mental effort – such 'mental' variables can be observed in oneself and to a degree in others. These variables all interact with the breathing pattern via the phrenic nerve.

EMOTIONAL DISRUPTION OF OPTIMAL BREATHING

'Optimal breathing' can be defined first as a match between the rate of air exchange and the body's immediate needs. This applies not only to oxygen intake but also to carbon dioxide release. The metabolic demand for oxygen changes according to factors such as level of arousal, digestion, need for body heat and exercise. The need for excretion of carbon dioxide also changes according to exercise, digestion and general metabolism as well as disease states that alter the pH of the blood, such as acidosis due to kidney disease.

Keeping the blood gases and pH closely balanced is very important physiologically. As expressed by Jennett (1994, p. 73):

When there are not other overriding drives affecting breathing, the neural control system acts to maintain a constant arterial PCO$_2$. This must mean that the volume of CO$_2$ expired continually balances the volume produced by tissue metabolism. Measurements show that alveolar and arterial concentrations of CO$_2$ stay constant, which means that the volume of gas breathed out from the functional (alveolar) volume of the lungs must vary precisely with the rate of metabolic CO$_2$ production. In rest and activity, when the system is left to itself, it is so efficient that the matching occurs virtually breath-by-breath, even when metabolic activity is continually changing.

Optimal breathing, therefore, is what the body continuously seeks, using its various sensing systems to quickly adjust breathing depth and rate. This homeostatic stability is obviously important, yet it must sometimes yield to other priorities. Some, such as vocalizing, yawning, coughing and breath-holding, are transient and easily terminated, but other conditions can affect this stability in more drastic and long-term ways.

Of particular interest in this chapter are psychological factors which alter breathing. In texts about respiratory therapy, especially in descriptions of hyperventilation, statements such as 'Emotional stress can also affect breathing' or 'Psychogenic sources of hyperventilation should be considered' are routinely offered, but details are usually lacking. This chapter presents some of these details, together with speculation as to why breathing is so sensitive to emotions.

Memory, associations and the ability to imagine and anticipate all complicate the picture of breathing regulation. What may be optimal for the organism at a given moment, at a certain level of exercise and arousal, may not be so optimal in the next few moments if action is demanded. Action requires muscle contraction, which in turn calls for more oxygen. Prolonging the time during which the muscles can function well provides a survival advantage. Therefore, anticipating this need for action and preparing for it by increased breathing is a natural process in humans and animals. Other things happen also, such as muscle tensing, larger cardiac stroke volume and adrenaline surge, but breathing affects the basic fuel supply, without which nothing will work.

Bloch et al (1991) studied how breathing patterns vary when associated with different emotional states. Cross-cultural research has yet to be done, but in a population of French subjects, anger, erotic love and tenderness varied consistently in duration of post-expiratory pause, breathing amplitude and breathing rate. For sadness, joy and fear, the time ratio of inhalation to exhalation differentiated the emotions most clearly. The original article includes sample breathing traces for each emotion and also general stereotypes of the breathing pattern associated with each major emotion, showing that they are clearly differentiated.

Anticipation of action may be very certain, as when falling out of a tree, or it may be a prediction based on odds. This 'betting' is often unconscious, the result of fear conditioning creating a negatively charged image which is somehow coded as to intensity. If a person once fell out of a tree, this fact is remembered at many levels, and being in a tree again will activate those memories and their associated physical adaptations. Conscious recall is not necessary for these anticipatory preparations to occur. The system ends up adjusting the breathing and other survival-related variables because of a recognized sensory cue.

This mechanism predates the development of higher consciousness, and it triggers preparation faster than conscious awareness can decipher the meaning of a cue. This speed is of course an advantage; the disadvantage is that the conscious mind is removed from the decision circuit, in the same way that a nation's military, in an emergency, may act without consulting the chief executive (see LeDoux (2003), for description of direct routes from amygdala to effector systems, bypassing conscious decision-making).

Some specific ways in which breathing adjusts to differing conditions are described below.

Depth and rate of breathing

Both depth and frequency of breathing are adjustable depending on the body's need (or expected need) for air. These two are adjustable independently; in the case of pregnancy, for example, or a broken rib, depth of breathing will be reduced, but breathing faster will compensate for it. Some combination of depth and rate is calculated by the brain to increase or decrease air exchange.

Compared to increasing frequency, increasing the depth of respiration is more effective for boosting alveolar ventilation, but only up to a point. Increasing the depth of a breath is opposed by the elastic forces which bring about exhalation; breathing faster is opposed by the friction of moving air in and out of the airways. The relative importance of these two adjustments in the case of preparatory breathing is not known. Rapid breathing is common during anticipatory anxiety, as are increased sighing and deep breaths. Complicating this picture is the role of emotion-based vocalization: crying, screaming or shouting. Either deeper or faster breathing could help prepare for vocalizing activity.

Breathing faster does not necessarily indicate hyperventilation, which depends on the amount of air being exchanged rather than the rate of breathing; if more air passes through the system than the body needs, this qualifies as hyperventilation, which can be maintained with even three or four deep breaths per minute. Breathing faster than normal, or panting, may happen in a variety of situations: for example in a person who is anxious, overheated (panting helps dissipate heat), or who has restricted abdominal and thoracic expansion. Fresh air not exposed to the alveoli enters and leaves the body unchanged. A column of air can be moved up and down within the dead space of the system (mouth, trachea and airways above the alveoli) by panting, with little actual air exchange.

Finally, rapid breathing increases airway turbulence. This aids the sense of smell, but smooth laminar airflow is compromised; this becomes more important in obstructive lung disease, including asthma, when the airways are narrowed.

The regularity, or stability, of the breathing cycle may reflect changes in appraisal of external demands as well as inner distractions and associations. Susceptibility to panic attacks is one factor clearly affecting breathing stability;

Burkhardt et al (2010) studied panic disorder patients for breathing stability during 15 minutes of sitting quietly. There were several indications of less stable breathing, with higher variability for minute volume and end-tidal CO_2.

Breath-holding

Some life situations call for vigilant silence, a concealment response which may inhibit or suspend breathing altogether. Uncertainty about what action to take next, or waiting a moment for more information, will be reflected in the breathing as the mind switches between action preparation, focused attention and concealment. Each of these primary states calls for a particular modulation of breathing: focused attention on the environment benefits from smooth, steady breathing which stabilizes the 'sensory platform'. To focus sensory attention precisely or when attempting to remain undetectable, the breathing may be suspended for a few moments.

If breathing is reduced or paused, oxygen reserve slowly falls and CO_2 rises, which stimulates more breathing (often a sigh) which pushes CO_2 down – and the cycle starts over again (see Chapter 3 for details).

The human capacity for imagination allows us to create any scenario at any time, often in enough detail for our bodies to respond as though the scene were real. Therefore, the mere act of thinking about situations that would require action, concealment, vigilance or emotional expression is likely to cause corresponding changes in the breathing.

Location of breathing

Chest vs. abdomen

Optimal breathing when we are awake primarily makes use of the diaphragm, resulting in moderate abdominal expansion, with some involvement of intercostal muscles so that the lower rib cage expands. By contrast, chest breathing makes more use of the pectoral, scalenes, trapezius, sternocleidomastoid and upper intercostal muscles. All but the scalenes are collectively termed accessory breathing muscles because they are recruited either when diaphragmatic breathing is difficult or for extra-deep breathing. Scalenes are more primary breathing muscles, although they are more active in chest breathing. These two styles of breathing are end points on a continuum rather than discrete categories – one can breathe with any combination of chest and abdominal breathing.

Reasons for chest breathing

When asked either to take a deep breath or to breathe rapidly, nearly everyone breathes into the chest, unless they actually intend to breathe abdominally (a trained singer, for instance). They also frequently take this voluntary breath through the mouth rather than the nostrils. Chest, or thoracic, breathing seems to be the preferred route for consciously mediated intentional breathing, while abdominal breathing is the main route for relaxed, automatic breathing.

Why should this be? Inquiring into this matter involves speculating about the differences between the types of breathing, what functions they may play, and what conditions might initiate each type.

ACTION PROJECTION

One major reason for an organism to override the automatic regulation of breathing is to prepare for action. The word 'prepare' implies projecting oneself into and predicting the future. Ordinarily, breathing rate and volume closely follow immediate metabolic needs, with breathing changing at the moment when increased muscle activity demands more oxygen. But fuller breathing in advance of action confers a physiological advantage, not only by boosting oxygen saturation to the maximum, but also by lowering CO_2, which would help to balance the surge of CO_2 and acidity produced by sudden exercise. A familiar example is breathing deeply before lifting a heavy weight. This preparation is in the same category as postural adjustments; conscious mediation, if time allows, fine-tunes the preparation to the size of the expected effort.

Exercise physiologists have established that there is an instantaneous jump in ventilation at the onset of exercise (Taylor et al 1989, Levitzky 2007). It is thought to be mediated by something other than simple metabolic demand, because the rise outstrips any current oxygen deficit. In Taylor's words:

> Phase I appears to be neurally mediated by a learned response related to an anticipation of exercise and/or an increased proprioceptor input from muscles and joints at the onset of exercise. Phase I is load independent and accompanied by increases in heart rate and sympathetic activity [p. 214, emphasis added].

This Phase I shift in breathing seems to be triggered by conscious anticipation of exercise, and represents a well-established route from the mind to the breathing muscles. This route would be the logical means by which more subtle action projection from emotional sources might influence the breathing.

Preparation for emergency action can be complex; if a cerebral cortex is good for anything, it would be when a decision is required whether to freeze, attack or flee, and when, and how. This moment-to-moment anticipatory planning in a perceived crisis depends on cognitive and perceptual processes, combining observation, prediction and experience. Just as posture and balance will shift according to changes in anticipated movement, the breathing pattern will also be modulated by what exactly is being predicted. Thus the breath-holding typical of watchful observation increases the stability of the sense organs, and also reduces breathing movement and sound which might interfere with concealment. This suppression of breathing is then normally balanced by a deep breath just before leaping into action.

Both respiratory suspension and overbreathing in preparation for action are unbalanced, in the sense that the individual is not living entirely in the present. The projection into the future creates a discrepancy between actual and anticipated metabolic needs. Consider a sprinter in an awkward starting position, waiting for the pistol, or a baseball pitcher just before delivering a pitch, one leg raised high. Such positions are not meant to be held for long. If the expected action is carried out as planned, the awkward position turns out to facilitate performance. But if the starting pistol does not fire or the baseball pitch is delayed, the posture becomes untenable.

This prolonged action projection can explain much about human breathing pattern problems: with their ability to predict, project, extrapolate and imagine, people are well equipped to anticipate threats which might require action. When this occurs, the body obligingly prepares for such action with increased breathing or else erratic alternation between breath-holding and overbreathing. The trouble arises when the threat is non-physical and not imminent; for instance, anxiety about planning a wedding 3 months hence, or anger over being insulted by something written in a letter. Situations like these do not logically require an immediate increase in breathing, but when the mind is thinking about a threat the body seems to take no chances; it prepares for action as if the event were just around the corner and involves a physical challenge. If such feelings become habitual, then the preparation will become chronic.

Action projection and accessory breathing muscles

There are several possible reasons why this preparation for action would be linked with overuse of the accessory breathing muscles:

1. The diaphragm is the main mechanism of automatic breathing, and does not need input from the conscious mind to operate well. Normal breathing at rest is primarily abdominal and lower thoracic, reflecting diaphragm action with little or no activity of accessory breathing muscles. Thoracic breathing, on the other hand, is on call as a back-up system, especially for breathing preparatory to action. A good alternate term for the accessory breathing

muscles might be discretionary breathing muscles, since they are the primary route for voluntary or emotional input.

An example of voluntary input to breath control is preparing to blow up a balloon with an extra-deep breath; an example of emotional input is perceiving an approaching person as hostile and threatening. In the first case the person consciously decides to take a deep breath in order to inflate the balloon. In the second case the person probably does not consciously decide to increase breathing, but it happens anyway because of the emotion of fear or anger. In either case, the possibility of a need for fast action is translated into activation of accessory breathing muscles. This route seems responsive to any emotion which might lead to rapid action. Expanding thoracic volume can function either as a supplement to diaphragmatic breathing or as a substitute for it, depending on the circumstances.

2. Another reason for thoracic breathing is simply protective: during physical confrontation the abdomen is vulnerable to attack, and protection of this vital region would improve odds of survival. Tensing the abdominal muscles offers protection, but since such tensing flattens the abdomen and restricts expansion, it will interfere with diaphragmatic breathing. Switching to thoracic breathing solves this problem.

3. Thoracic breathing increases cardiac output and heart rate, just the opposite of abdominal breathing. This would furnish an advantage during emergency action. It may be that some people like the feeling of enhanced readiness, and if so, this thoracic breathing becomes reinforced. The common military posture of tensed abdomen and expanded chest boosts activity of the cardiac system, working against relaxed economical breathing but maximizing preparation for action.

4. Rapid action also requires stabilizing the spine and trunk. Leaping into action, whether fleeing or attacking, involves close motor coordination of the trunk and the pelvis. This calls on the abdominal muscles such as rectus and transversus abdominis and external and internal obliques, which during abdominal breathing are normally relaxed (Richardson et al 1999). When these muscles are recruited for action preparation, the auxiliary breathing mechanism must be brought into play. Many muscles have a dual involvement in postural control and breathing movements. Even the diaphragm, specialized as it is for breathing, contributes to spinal and pelvic stabilization, in part by assisting with pressurization and displacement of the abdominal contents, allowing the transversus abdominis to increase tension in the thoracolumbar fascia or to generate intra-abdominal pressure.

Any gross body movement might interfere with abdominal breathing, leaving accessory muscle breathing as the back-up. Complex interactions take place whenever the need for core stability occurs. The involvement of the diaphragm in postural stabilization suggests that situations might easily occur where contradictory demands are evident – for example, where postural stabilizing control is required at the same time that respiratory functions create demands for movement.

5. Finally, there is a common association of mouth breathing with chest breathing (see below). Airway resistance to mouth breathing is far less than to nasal breathing (Barelli 1994), making it easier to draw air in through the mouth. Also, the air passage into the chest and upper lungs is shorter than to the abdomen and the base of the lungs. Together, these facts give an advantage to the mouth/chest route for rapid air intake as preparation for action, including shouting or other vocalization.

Thus it makes sense that reliance on the accessory breathing muscles and the mouth intake route would be more closely linked with voluntary breathing. The greater efficiency of using the diaphragm and relaxing the external abdominal muscles requires a context of safety and relative inactivity. At moments of urgency, greater respiratory efficiency may be sacrificed in favour of the mixed demands that the action orientation may take.

Nose breathing vs. mouth breathing

We can breathe through the mouth, the nose, or a combination of the two, and psychology enters even here: from Barelli, 1994, p. 52:

> Nasal breathing is **involuntary. Mouth, or voluntary,** breathing occurs when there is difficulty breathing through the nose, such as in exertion, under stress, and – in particular – when cardiac, pulmonary, or other illness hampers the supply of oxygen to the tissues.

Significant anxiety triggers preparatory breathing, and the lungs may be filled with less effort, and more quickly, by mouth breathing. A state of surprise or startle will cause the jaw to drop open, perhaps for this reason.

The nasal route adds at least 50% more resistance to air flow, so one might think that lowered resistance by bypassing the nostrils is a good thing. But the pressure rise in the lungs during exhalation makes the air denser, simulating a lower altitude where the air is richer in oxygen per unit volume, and this improves perfusion into the alveoli. Also, the increased resistance introduced into the system by nasal inhalation increases the vacuum in the lungs, resulting in a 10–20% increase in oxygen transported (Cottle

1987). Finally, diaphragmatic movement improves venous return to the heart, reducing its workload.

Maurice Cottle, a renowned rhinologist, includes among the functions of nasal breathing:

> ... *slowing down the expiratory phase of respiration and ventilation, and the interposing of resistance to both inspiration and expiration which in turn helps to maintain the normal elasticity of the lungs, thus assuring optimal conditions for providing oxygen and good heart function. Breathing through the mouth usually affords too little obstruction and could lead to areas of atelectasis and poor ventilation of the low spaces in the lung [p. 146].*

If a momentary state of alarm and action preparation becomes more chronic or habitual, then the physiological factors cited above become important factors in altering the default breathing pattern. Mouth breathing can also develop during chronic nasal obstruction, such as sinus problems or injury to the nose. Once established, the habit may not subside even after the obstruction is cleared.

CONDITIONED BREATHING RESPONSES

The preceding describes most of the breathing adaptations to stress of various sorts. They could be called generic in the sense that they are standard responses to common stimuli such as a loud noise, obvious physical threat, or a clear requirement to prepare for physical exertion. The breathing pattern of any individual will also be altered by such experiences as hearing of the death of a loved one or being physically threatened by someone, but these are relatively rare events for most people while breathing disruptions are relatively common. Many stimuli capable of eliciting these breathing changes are unique to the individual as a result of personal experience; it is in this category that careful inquiry may be repaid by better understanding of what triggers this action preparation style of breathing.

Here the concept of psychophysiological time travel – memory and anticipation – may be useful. As discussed elsewhere (Gilbert 1998), an individual's significant emotional incidents become liable to time-shifting from the past to the present. The concept of memory is familiar enough, but when a reactivated memory triggers body responses similar to the original experience, or has flashbacks with a somatic accompaniment, then there is confusion in the system between past and present reality.

Traumatic conditioning (also known as fear conditioning) has been extensively studied in both man and animals. The general principles derive from studies of conditioning dating back to Pavlov's work with salivating dogs, but the difference between that situation and a modern office worker hearing the approaching footsteps of a dreaded supervisor is conceptually very small. Classical conditioning is a ubiquitous and protective learning mechanism which does not require conscious thought.

To understand how conditioning relates to breathing disorders in humans requires knowledge of several intermediate steps:

1. An autonomic response such as salivation can be elicited by an appropriate stimulus (e.g. food on the tongue). If a neutral stimulus such as a bell precedes the food by just a moment, the salivation will begin to occur in response to the bell, because it gives more advance warning of the food. In time the salivation will occur to the bell alone, *without the food*, apparently because the bell has merged in some way with the food stimulus.

2. A foot shock will produce an alarm/defence reaction, the unconditioned response to the shock. This includes a rise in heart rate and blood pressure, limb withdrawal, a spike in adrenaline, and disrupted breathing. This happens on the first trial, with no learning required. But if a bell, a change in lighting, a floor vibration, or any other neutral stimulus precedes the shock, the alarm response will soon be triggered by the neutral stimulus *whether or not the shock is delivered*. The neutral stimulus becomes a *conditioned* stimulus (synonyms are 'conditioning' or 'conditional'). This is how fear conditioning works – a formerly neutral stimulus acquires the power to set off the alarm response on its own.

3. Learning that involves fear is more rapid than learning involving things such as food and salivation because there is a potential threat to survival. The connection is established sometimes after a single trial; there is obviously an advantage to learning certain connections quickly because Nature often does not provide a second chance. Imagine, for instance, that a hawk swoops down on a rabbit and grabs it with sharp talons. Suppose the rabbit gets away with only a wound, and remembers the sound of the approaching hawk's wings. It would be very useful for the rabbit to associate the sound with remembered pain and terror. The faster the rabbit's response to this warning stimulus the next time, the more likely it is that the rabbit will take effective evasive action.

   The concept of evasive action introduces the variable of intention, which presupposes a kind of consciousness. The initial simple defence or escape response may be automatically conditioned, but the subsequent actions (such as jumping into a narrow crevice where the hawk cannot follow) may call for more than the default blind leap or freezing response. In other words, the introduction of conscious control of the next move adds to the animal's advantage.

4. Many conditioning experiments are arranged so that the foot shock is terminated by the animal withdrawing its foot. A neutral stimulus such as a bell still precedes the shock, thus providing a warning. In this case foot withdrawal becomes conditioned by the neutral stimulus alone, and the experimenter can turn off the shock apparatus with confidence that the withdrawal response will not soon be extinguished. The bell alone will set off a leg muscle contraction. Since the shock can be avoided completely by the quick foot withdrawal, the subject may not even realize that the shock threat has gone. (This is now termed 'operant conditioning' rather than 'classic,' because the animal is operating on the environment rather than reacting passively, as with autonomic responses.)

5. Since leg withdrawal is in the realm of voluntary muscle control rather than strictly autonomic, the response is brought into the domain of choice: thinking about what to do next. This allows the use of memory in a less automatic way, and involves judgment. For instance, in the hawk–rabbit example, the automatic response may be to jump without regard to direction, on the chance that the swooping hawk will miss its target. But suppose the rabbit hole is a few inches away but in a particular direction. A simple jumping reflex would not be that specific; aiming toward the hole requires memory and judgment. Thus a reflex blends with directed action.

6. In human beings, breathing control moves in a broad zone between automatic and voluntary. The mode of breathing seems to be selected automatically depending on what is anticipated in the next few seconds: breath-holding may accompany indecision or freezing; a deep gasp might prepare for major exertion or crying out; a sharp exhale might accompany anger, frustration, or aggression.

Behavioural research on man and animals has clarified the links by which breathing can be altered in the absence of an appropriate stimulus. The brain is doing its best to prepare for something based on projection from past experience, and consciousness is not necessarily part of this process. Since animals as low as snails have been successfully conditioned, the conditioning mechanism must have evolved before the development of a large cortex which allows a wide choice among possible actions. This means that certain breathing changes, difficult to explain otherwise, could represent conditioned responses to stimuli that either carry the signal of threat directly, or were associated with a threat signal.

One advantage of bypassing consciousness is that of speed. The extra milliseconds resulting from more synaptic connections could be critical in avoiding danger. The term 'head start' refers to an advantage obtained in a race, but it can also refer to the advantage of anticipation by 'using the head' – whether through conscious anticipation or with an unconscious conditioned response. The disadvantage of being guided by conditioned responses is that the interpretation and response are not guided by consciousness, so a slammed door might, for example, be mistaken for a gunshot by a combat veteran, and his reaction occurs before he can realize it's only a slammed door.

Experimental conditioning of breathing changes

There is clear evidence that respiratory responses can be conditioned. Ley (Ley et al 1996, Ley 1999) confirmed this by monitoring end-tidal CO_2 in college students while they coped with brief mental stressors such as doing calculations in their heads or counting backwards by sevens from 200. This was sufficient to increase their skin conductance, heart rate and breathing rate, and also to shift CO_2 in the direction of hyperventilation. In this situation there was no clear threat which would justify activating the bodily stress response, so either a psychosocial threat (a blow to the ego) was present from the risk of failing the test, or else the effort involved in the mental tasks activated the body changes.

Ley presented a specific sound to the subjects along with the 'start' instructions, linking the tone with the demand to perform. Eventually, sounding the tone became sufficient to set off the same stress responses even when no task performance was required. Hyperventilation was now conditioned to the neutral tone.

It might be objected that this is a consciously mediated common-sense association, and that the subject simply looks for clues and responds to them. But this conscious process seems to be secondary or peripheral, not necessary for the conditioned responses to occur. Conditioning of this nature can be demonstrated in very primitive organisms such as earthworms, snails and fruit flies. So it seems reasonable to conclude that disruption of breathing can occur because of associations to environmental stimuli, independent of conscious awareness.

Other conditioning experiments with breathing were carried out by Van den Bergh and colleagues (1997), and the findings may be relevant for understanding the origins of certain breathing disorders. Subjects were exposed to low concentrations of particular smells along with either normal room air or a 7% concentration of CO_2. (This procedure is often used in panic studies to test for sensitivity to excess CO_2, since the gas quickly stimulates increased breathing.)

After a few pairings of a particular odour with the high-CO_2 air, the odour by itself, in ordinary room air, would stimulate both an increase in breathing and complaints of breathlessness, chest tightness and other respiratory-related sensations. Females tended to respond by breathing faster, and males by breathing more deeply. But either way, the fact that stimuli paired with 'bad air' (high CO_2 content) could later provoke an increase in breathing volume using normal air suggests a mechanism whereby dyspnoea, uneasy breathing and hyperventilation could seem to appear out of nowhere. Ley's findings with conditioned sounds show that the effect is not due only to the sense of smell, but also spans other senses. See also Pappens et al (2012) for a study of interoceptive fear conditioning using occlusion of breathing and a conditioned stimulus.

In Van den Bergh et al's words (1997):

Patients with hyperventilation may be excessively attentive to typical respiratory complaints. Attentional direction may therefore prime both reporting more complaints of that type during acquisition and subsequently facilitate their conditioning …
Occurrences of hyperventilation may be considered learning episodes in which subjects increasingly learn to attend to and anxiously interpret 'normal' somatic variations, which may produce complaints and cause altered breathing as well. Eventually, the relationship between hyperventilation and somatic complaints may become reversed over time within an individual.

In light of these findings the authors also discuss the phenomenon of multiple chemical sensitivity, since many of the symptoms overlap with hyperventilation. It is possible that panic-like reactions to particular airborne chemical compounds, particularly irritant gases and strong odours, are in part classically conditioned responses rather than 'mechanical' immune responses. If so, reduction of the response strength through graduated exposure (desensitization) might offer an alternative to rigid control of the environment.

FEAR CONDITIONING AND THE AMYGDALA

For humans at least, a feeling of non-specific alarm sometimes occurs before any conscious awareness of the relevant stimulus. Irrational avoidance, along with rapid pulse, sweating, dread, a freeze reaction and sudden disruption of breathing are well-known components of post-traumatic stress disorder: re-experiencing some aspect of a traumatic experience. A person undergoing such an episode may feel temporarily out of control for no clear reason.

The mechanism which probably explains such moments actually involves a bi-level memory system. Neuroscientist Joseph LeDoux (1996, 2003) has been prominent in this area, and his book *The Emotional Brain* presents classic research on the distinction between explicit and implicit memory. This difference corresponds to two somewhat independent memory systems based on the hippocampus and amygdala, respectively. These two structures, part of the limbic system deep within the temporal lobes of the cerebrum, are essential for memory storage. Memory is not a unitary phenomenon; our conscious, or 'explicit,' memories depend on the hippocampus, while our protective, survival-oriented memories are maintained by the amygdala. This second type of memory does not require conscious knowledge, and so this can explain the previous observations about conditioned responses which may defy logic, yet are faster than our voluntary responses.

The amygdala has abundant chemical and neural outputs to effector systems involved in emergency action. On its command, blood pressure rises, muscles tense and heart rate increases. Breathing may stop and then become more rapid as the brain attempts to prepare for an ambiguous threat not necessarily perceived by the person's conscious mind. Nerve pathways lead directly from the thalamus to the amygdala, bypassing the cortex and the conscious mind and allowing sensory information to be fed directly to a brain site responsible for initiating emergency action. This is comparable to a military system being authorized to mount an emergency response before consulting the government. When such a system works well, its power is usually limited to creating an initial state of readiness, with further actions requiring instructions from higher decision centres. Interrupting current activity, including irrelevant distracting thoughts, would be the first step, followed by locking full attention onto the threatening stimulus, and then taking action to avoid a risky situation. Nearing the edge of a cliff, for example, would activate memory of any previous falls, and the sensitized amygdala might initiate/withdrawal startle response quickly, without significant cortical input.

The hippocampus-based explicit memory system is elaborate, extensive and can access the rest of the cortex for fine-tuning decisions. But amygdala-based memories seem linked to any event which has caused a fear reaction. If these memory traces match new sensory input, commands may go out to attack, hide, run, brace for action, or something more specific than a simple freeze or avoidance reaction. When conscious judgment and experience is bypassed, this can of course be a problem. Mistakes can be made which imperil the organism from without (such as attacking, when running away would be better) or from within (such as issuing a reflex command for a rise in blood flow and pressure which the system cannot handle).

Thus the amygdala reigns over the body like an ever-vigilant watchdog, its permanent archive of danger-related stimuli linked with its primitive repertoire of emergency actions. The conscious mind, like the watchdog's owner, gets the news more slowly; its compensating advantage is (supposedly) superior judgment and broader access to experience, both personal and secondhand, and its ability to foresee consequences. Planning and carrying out a shifting, adaptive coping strategy requires the highest levels of the brain/mind, but the more information is integrated, the more neural activity is needed, and this takes time. Ideally, the differences between the two systems are smoothly coordinated as might occur between the military and legislative branches of a government, so that the strengths of each contribute to the final outcome.

Incidental learning

Incidental learning involves conditioning to the entire context of a traumatic incident. Suppose a woman is assaulted in an elevator in which a particular song is playing. The resulting fear conditioning would probably make her uneasy about elevators in general, especially because they possess the biologically prepared factor of confinement. The assault would also boost her fear of strangers. If she later hears the same music that was playing in the elevator, she may feel an unaccountable dread. Her breathing quickens, muscles tense, her heart starts to pound, and she sweats, yet she may not know why. This is the result of the brain's fear conditioning system trying to warn her. The amygdala has stored a multisensory 'snapshot' of the context of the elevator assault, and it is now activating the fear response, leaving the woman's conscious self bewildered as to why she is so uneasy. She may identify the music as the trigger, but she does not have to consciously remember that the same music was playing in the elevator. Her amygdala memory system has already done that.

In this case the brain's protection system has gone woefully wrong. The woman may avoid the new context in which the song is heard, or she may develop fear about what seems to be a surge of 'out of the blue' anxiety. Yet if she were the rabbit instead, as in the previous example, with a hawk swooping down to grab her and the sound of the hawk's wings substituted for the elevator music, then the stimulus would be very relevant indeed, and reacting to it might save her life. It is probably beyond the capacity of the amygdala's memory system to designate certain details of a context as relevant and others as irrelevant. Indeed, there may be a biased rule built into the system: making the error of over-reacting to a harmless stimulus means a brief flurry of anxiety and avoidance, a recoverable expenditure of energy. On the other hand, making the error of ignoring a stimulus which actually signals the familiar danger returning could be fatal.

Another discovery from this area of study is that there are many more neural connections from the amygdala to higher cortical areas than there are in the opposite direction. The system seems to be set up to deliver danger-relevant information to higher cortical areas so that the initial responses can be refined or controlled by judgment and experience. This inhibitory downward control is weaker, as by both the neural connections and the fact that phobias are more easily acquired than eradicated. Anxiety shifts priority to survival issues; at these times, loops of neurons in the amygdala perpetuate the connections between memory, perception and alarm, and the cortex must struggle to oppose this process.

Worse yet, these conditioned fears may not be entirely erasable. In LeDoux's words:

> *Unconscious fear memories established through the amygdala appear to be indelibly burned into the brain. They are probably with us for life. This is often useful, especially in a stable, unchanging world, since we don't want to have to learn about the same kinds of dangers over and over again. The downside is that sometimes the things that are imprinted in the amygdala's circuits are maladaptive. In these instances, we pay dearly for the incredible efficiencies of the fear system.*
>
> LeDoux 1996, p. 252

HYPNOTIC INVESTIGATIONS

Hyperventilation as a chronic syndrome or behavioural tendency is squarely in the category of disorders often called 'functional,' 'psychophysiological' or 'psychosomatic.' But it is not always so clearly delineated; disruption of the optimal breathing pattern can happen in subtle ways. Increased variability from breath to breath is known to correlate with anxiety states (Han et al 1997, Beck et al 2000). Low $PaCO_2$ and increased frequency of sighing are typical of those with panic disorder, even when not panicking (Wilhelm et al 2001a). These generalizations miss individuals who do not have a chronic breathing pattern disorder, but who do experience disrupted breathing under particular conditions. The conditions can provoke either an amygdala 'alarm' discharge or some specific, learned breathing response, as well as occasional panic.

Conway, and Freeman and colleagues (Conway et al 1988, Freeman et al 1986) have used hypnosis to investigate the sources of these hyperventilation episodes in a number of patients. Based on this research, they suggest that 'hyperventilators' is not a uniform category but consists of at least two groups: the chronic and the episodic. Many people are subject to hyperventilation episodes but breathe normally most of the time. They are susceptible to particular stimuli associated with some original event of intense emotion, and when reminded of this event are likely to breathe in a way that lowers CO_2 quickly, setting off many symptoms of hyperventilation, and sometimes including panic:

> *It has been considered that emotional events, particularly involving loss, separation and impotent anger, are the precipitating factors that may initiate a trend to hyperventilation...On some occasions the important initiating event, psychological strain or life event was evident from the history, but in others questioning under hypnosis revealed psychological triggers, not elucidated previously, which provoked marked falls in $PetCO_2$. Since it is a feature of many psychosomatic illnesses that the initiating factors are repressed and only the somatic symptoms remain, this technique may be of considerable help in some patients in whom therapy may not be progressing as well as might have been expected.*

Freeman et al 1986, p. 80

One marker for panic disorder consists of delayed return of end-tidal CO_2 to a normal range following voluntary hyperventilation (Wilhelm et al 2001b). A delayed return to baseline after another 3 minutes is also a positive diagnostic sign for hyperventilation syndrome, as based on symptom reports. Conway and colleagues (1988) found that those who showed slow return to baseline tended to be habitual overbreathers, and were usually most bothered by the physiological distress accompanying hyperventilation. This group would probably score higher on the Anxiety Sensitivity Index (see Ch. 6.4), meaning they were hypersensitive to the sensations of anxiety. But another group of subjects were most sensitive instead to specific emotional triggers such as bereavement, anger, separation, loss and grief. The onset of their hyperventilation episodes tended to come and go more quickly and did not turn into a habit.

This suggests that the emotion-triggered group may have more trouble dealing with such recalled experience, or perhaps that their respiratory systems are more closely tied to certain intense emotions. They did not appear to have the 'bad breathing habit' that Lum (1975) suggested is typical of hyperventilators; instead, their predisposition for plummeting CO_2 lay waiting to be triggered. These moments may seem to be unpredictable and the trigger unknown. However, hypnosis proved invaluable in uncovering triggers for hyperventilation attacks which were not easily apparent from either personal histories or the subjects' own awareness and recollection of events (Conway et al 1988, p. 303). These were not necessarily repressed memories; the hyperventilation was simply linked to the memory of certain experiences.

In another study (Freeman et al 1986), patients diagnosed as having hyperventilation syndrome were studied during hypnotic recall of emotionally disturbing experiences, particularly those associated with the reported symptoms. Drops in $PetCO_2$ were measured and compared to a control group without symptoms of hyperventilation, during similar hypnotic recall of emotionally disturbing experiences. The average drop in 27 patients was 18.2 mmHg, while in 10 controls the mean drop was 5 mmHg. The range was also much larger in the patients, and overall the difference between the two groups was highly significant.

This study showed at least that individuals who reported several symptoms indicating hyperventilation (including chest pain and palpitations, dizziness, etc. – not exclusively respiratory symptoms) displayed rather strong hyperventilation in response to recalling emotionally disturbing events, whereas the control subjects did not. Bereavement, loss of control, grief and anger were common topics associated with the symptoms.

Hypnosis is not essential for eliciting such symptoms, but the researchers chose it for its value in focusing attention on the memories. There is no guarantee with hypnosis that the recalled information is true, because hypnosis can blur the subject's distinction between real and imaginary. This has led to controversy regarding whether recovered memories of childhood abuse are authentic or are products of inadvertent hypnotic suggestion. It is possible that hypnosis can provide a way of digging deeper into the memory systems, perhaps accessing impressions in the amygdala or overcoming inhibition within the hippocampal–cortical memory system.

Donald Dudley and colleagues investigated the effect of emotional states on variables of breathing. The model was similar to that used by Conway: obtain a baseline, engage the subject in discussion of emotionally meaningful and disturbing topics, and observe how breathing changes. This was done sometimes with and sometimes without hypnosis, so the effect of hypnosis was probably to facilitate or enhance the emotional intensity rather than create a distinct new experimental situation.

In his book, Dudley (1969) presents many instructive case studies as well as statistical summaries. Action orientation was seen as related to increased breathing, while inaction (such states as withdrawal, apathy, and depression) was related to decreased breathing. In general, other arousal-related variables such as pulse rate, skin temperature, and catecholamine secretion were not well correlated with the breathing changes. This suggests that adjustments to breathing signify a sensitive fine-tuning of oxygen delivery, directed by shifts in emotion and cognition.

Dudley's conclusions from study of a number of patients with asthma or other breathing-related disorders are listed below:

1. In a pneumographic study of 22 subjects, respiratory patterns were found to vary closely with the emotional state.

2. Increased rate or depth or both and sighing were found chiefly with anxiety but sometimes during anger and resentment. Decreased rate or depth or both were found when the subjects felt tense and on guard with feelings of anxiety or anger and when feeling sad or dejected.

3. Irregularity of respiration was commonly associated with anger, particularly when the feeling was suppressed. It was also associated with feelings of guilt and occurred during weeping.

4. A prolongation of expiration during periods of emotional disturbance was found in a higher proportion of subjects with asthma than in those with anxiety. In three asthmatic subjects this change was associated with wheezing and dyspnoea, and in one with dyspnoea alone.

5. Discussions of attitudes and conflicts known to be associated with respiratory symptoms (dyspnoea and chest discomfort) evoked such symptoms in more than half of the subjects, and the symptoms were related to changes in the respiratory pattern.

6. It is concluded that respiratory symptoms associated with emotional disturbances may arise from altered respiratory function in response to symbolic stimuli to action and often are related to conflict concerning such action (Dudley 1969, pp. 98–99).

Dissociation

A 'resurrected' emotional memory can drastically disrupt breathing, either with or without conscious awareness. Breathing is not the only body reaction triggered; any organ system can be so conditioned. The phenomenon is consistent with LeDoux's observations about implicit memory, contextual or incidental conditioning, and what is known about dissociation and repression. In victims of traumatic stress, evidence of dissociation at the time of the original trauma is considered a significant predictor for developing post-traumatic stress disorder (Van der Kolk et al 1996, p. 314). 'Dissociation' refers to compartmentalizing of experience, such that a traumatic experience is not properly integrated into a unitary sense of self. It is as if the person retreats either from the experience as it occurs or from the subsequent memory of the experience. This process may manifest as disorientation, altered body image, tunnel vision, a sense of unreality, altered time sense, unusual detachment, and out-of-body experiences. Pierre Janet, at the end of the 19th century, proposed the concept of 'memory phobia' to explain instances of dissociation, and Sigmund Freud used Janet's ideas as a springboard for his own.

Dissociation seems to be an emergency manoeuvre for coping with something unbearable and still remaining conscious by achieving some psychological distance; it is the mental equivalent of running away. Though it may help endure what is happening at the moment, dissociation interferes with memory storage and creates a fragmentation of experience, so that later reminders of the incident may stimulate only isolated aspects of the memory. This explains the flashbacks of the traumatized combat veteran and the victim of rape. Hyperventilation triggered by reminders of bereavement or grief may fit in this same category.

HYPERVENTILATION-RELATED COGNITIVE AND PERFORMANCE DEFICITS

Many authors have observed and collected data on transient mental deficits resulting from hyperventilation. Low CO_2 is known to cause cerebral vasoconstriction, which in turn causes brain hypoxia of variable degree. The EEG is generally slowed by this hypoxia. A surge of research occurred in the 1940s and 1950s, stimulated by study of Second World War combat pilots experiencing dangerous problems in performance (Hinshaw et al 1943, Balke & Lillehei 1956). $PaCO_2$ in student pilots during training flights was found to be as low as 15 mmHg (Wayne 1958). Various studies have found loss of concentration, memory, motor coordination, reaction time, judgment and general intellectual functioning. Wyke (1963) summarized most of this early literature, which at times had poor experimental controls for such factors as possible distraction by other symptoms, and also impaired motor coordination interfering with manual test responses.

Van Diest et al (2000) used a demanding test of visual attention and discrimination to measure the cognitive and performance effects of overbreathing. Trials were run under conditions of both normal and deep breathing and $PaCO_2$ was allowed to fall naturally during one trial of hyperventilation, while in another trial the $PaCO_2$ was unobtrusively replaced in order to maintain normal $PaCO_2$ in the subject. Subjects were 42 'normal' women (those with signs of hyperventilation or panic were excluded). The task was presented in the 3 minutes during recovery from the hyperventilation. With these controls applied, there was a clear deficit in performance, both in slower reaction times and in more errors, in a subset of subjects during the 'true hyperventilation' trials in which $PaCO_2$ was actually lowered. Subjects whose performance suffered generally had brief apnoeas during the 3-minute recovery stage. The resulting performance deficits were tentatively explained as due to 'prolonged central hypoxia'. The authors describe other data showing that while $PaCO_2$ recovered faster in subjects with apnoeas, oxygen saturation stayed lower.

Breathing pauses during the recovery stage are common because the breathing drive is reduced by the lower $PaCO_2$ level. Recovery from brief hyperventilation poses a conflict for the brain's regulatory centres: CO_2 returns to normal in the blood more quickly after hyperventilation if there are apnoeas during recovery, but at those moments of suspended breathing there is no oxygen taken in, and because of the persisting vasoconstriction the brain is in a more vulnerable state.

The most focused research on this matter was by Han et al (1997) with data gathered from 399 patients with either hyperventilation syndrome or anxiety disorders, as compared with 347 normal controls. The observations were brief, consisting of a 5-minute quiet breathing baseline period, then 3 minutes of hyperventilation followed by another 5 minutes of quiet breathing. The authors found that recovery to baseline $PaCO_2$ was slower in the patient group than in the control group. The incidence of pauses during recovery was clearly higher in the control subjects than in the patients, and this difference was especially obvious in younger subjects. Control subjects seemed to terminate the hyperventilation more definitively, whereas the patient group in effect kept on hyperventilating to some degree, at least by not pausing. If the conclusions of Van Diest's study described above can be generalized from the smaller number of subjects, it means that the slow-recovering hyperventilators *without* apnoeas are less prone to errors of performance and perception. The authors speculate that the resistance to pausing may indicate a higher level of vigilance.

Ley & Yelich (1998) reviewed several studies which found lower $PaCO_2$ in naturally occurring stressful situations. Young adolescent students were differentiated into high and low test-anxious by a standard questionnaire; during a task performance, end-tidal CO_2 was lower in the first group than the second (36.6 mmHg vs. 38.3 mmHg) with breath rate also faster in the first group, which also reported significantly more symptoms on the Nijmegen Questionnaire (assessing hyperventilation). The authors concluded:

the propensity to hyperventilate may exist as a trait which requires stressful conditions for its expression as a negative emotional state. This suggests the possibility that hyperventilatory complaints may, to some extent, be state-dependent and thus contingent on the context in which hyperventilation appears.

Music performance anxiety ('stage fright') has been studied with attention to breathing patterns. Studer et al (2011, 2012), focusing on university classical music students, used the Nijmegen Questionnaire and self-reports about anxiety before performance. End-tidal CO_2 level was also measured in the 2012 study, and was found to correlate with performance anxiety. In general, reports of hyperventilation-related symptoms increased as the reported anxiety increased, although no measure was taken of objective performance quality.

CONCLUSIONS

Aside from medical problems, there are still many factors in the psychological and behavioural realms competing for control of breathing (Fig. 5.1). Successful regulation must take all factors into account, with special consideration for priorities of survival. The human brain adds a layer of complication with its power to imagine, project and recall, often stimulating breathing reflexes without apparent reason. Chapter 7.4 presents some psychological techniques which engage the conscious mind to improve self-regulation, but all therapeutic approaches to disturbed breathing patterns must deal with the influence of perception, emotion and consciousness.

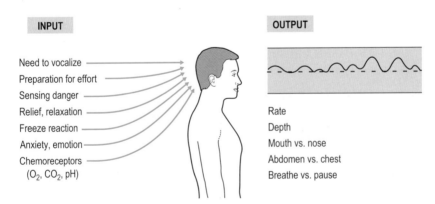

Figure 5.1 Final modulation of the breathing act includes input from many possible sources: the need for vocalization (a cry for help, a shouted warning, perhaps a growl), preparation for exertion, the need to freeze and become perhaps less noticeable, the need to maximize sensory acuity by stilling the body, the need to either remain calm or return to a baseline state of calmness. These inputs too often conflict with each other, but if there is the hint of a threat to survival, that seems to have priority over all other considerations.

REFERENCES

Balke, B., Lillehei, J., 1956. Effects of hyperventilation on performance. Journal of Applied Physiology 9, 371–374.

Barelli, P., 1994. Nasopulmonary physiology. In: Timmons, B.H., Ley, R. (Eds.), Behavioral and psychological approaches to breathing disorders. Plenum, New York.

Beck, J.G., Shipherd, J.C., Ohtake, P., 2000. Do panic symptom profiles influence response to a hypoxic challenge in patients with panic disorder? A preliminary report. Psychosomatic Medicine 62, 678–683.

Bloch, S., Lemeignan, M., Aguilera, N., 1991. Specific respiratory patterns distinguish among human basic emotions. International Journal of Psychophysiology 11 (2), 141–154.

Burkhardt, S.C., Wilhelm, F.H., Meuret, A.E., et al., 2010. Temporal stability and coherence of anxiety, dyspnea, and physiological variables in panic disorder. Biological Psychology 85 (2), 226–232.

Conway, A.V., Freeman, L.J., Nixon, P.G.F., 1988. Hypnotic examination of trigger factors in the hyperventilation syndrome. American Journal of Clinical Hypnosis 30, 296–304.

Cottle, M.H., 1987. The work, ways, positions and patterns of nasal breathing (relevance in heart and lung illness). Reprinted in: Barelli, P., Loch, W.E.E., Kern, E.R., Steiner, A. (Eds.), Rhinology. The collected writings of Maurice H. Cottle, MD. American Rhinologic Society, Kansas City, Missouri.

Dudley, D.L., 1969. Psychophysiology of respiration in health and disease. Appleton-Century-Crofts, New York.

Freeman, L.J., Conway, A., Nixon, P.G.F., 1986. Physiological responses to psychological challenge under hypnosis in patients considered to have the hyperventilation syndrome: implications for diagnosis and therapy. Journal of the Royal Society of Medicine 79 (Feb), 76–83.

Gilbert, C., 1998. Emotional sources of dysfunctional breathing. Journal of Bodywork & Movement Therapies 2, 224–230.

Han, J.N., Stegen, K., Simkens, K., et al., 1997. Unsteadiness of breathing in patients with hyperventilation syndrome and anxiety disorders. European Respiratory Journal 10, 167–176.

Hinshaw, H.C., Rushmer, R.F., Boothby, W.M., 1943. The hyperventilation syndrome and its importance in aviation medicine. Journal of Aviation Medicine 14, 100–114.

Jennett, S., 1994. Control of breathing and its disorders. In: Timmons, B.H., Ley, R. (Eds.), Behavioral and psychological approaches to breathing disorders. Plenum, New York.

LeDoux, J.E., 1996. The Emotional Brain. Simon & Schuster, New York.

LeDoux, J., 2003. Synaptic Self: How Our Brains Become Who We Are. Penguin Books, New York, pp. 122.

Levitzky, M.G., 2007. The Control of Breathing. In: Levitzky, M.G. (Ed.), Pulmonary Physiology, seventh ed. McGraw-Hill, New York (Chapter 9).

Ley, R., 1999. The modification of breathing behavior: Pavlovian and operant control in emotion and cognition. Behavior Modification 23, 441–479.

Ley, R., Ley, J., Bassett, C., et al., 1996. End-tidal CO_2 as a conditioned response in a Pavlovian conditioning paradigm. Paper presented at the Annual Meeting of the International Society for the Advancement of Respiratory Psychophysiology, Nijmegen, The Netherlands.

Ley, R., Yelich, G., 1998. Fractional end-tidal CO_2 as an index of the effects of stress on math performance and verbal memory of test-anxious adolescents. Biological Psychology 49 (1–2), 83–94.

Lum, L.C., 1975. Hyperventilation: the tip and the iceberg. Journal of Psychosomatic Research 19, 375–383.

Merriam-Webster, 1991. Random House Webster's college dictionary. Random House, New York.

Pappens, M., Smets, E., Vansteenwegen, D., et al., 2012. Learning to fear suffocation: A new paradigm for interoceptive fear conditioning. Psychophysiology 49 (6), 821–828.

Richardson, C., Jull, G., Hodges, P., et al., 1999. Therapeutic exercise for spinal segmental stabilisation in low back pain. Churchill Livingstone, Edinburgh.

Studer, R.K., Danuser, B., Hildebrandt, H., et al., 2011. Hyperventilation complaints in music performance anxiety among classical music students. Journal of Psychosomatic Research 70 (6), 557–564.

Studer, R.K., Danuser, B., Hildebrandt, H., et al., 2012. Hyperventilation in anticipatory music performance anxiety. Psychosomatic Medicine, 2012, epub.

Taylor, A., Rehder, K., Hyatt, R., et al., 1989. Clinical respiratory physiology. W B Saunders, Philadelphia.

Van den Bergh, O., Stegen, K., Van de Woestijne, K.P., 1997. Learning to have psychosomatic complaints: conditioning of respiratory behavior and somatic complaints in psychosomatic patients. Psychosomatic Medicine 59, 13–23.

Van der Kolk, B., Van der Hart, O., Marmar, C.R., 1996. Dissociation and information processing in posttraumatic stress disorder. In: Van der Kolk, B., McFarlane, A., Weisaeth, L. (Eds.), Traumatic stress. Guilford Press, New York.

Van Diest, I., Stegen, K., Van de Woestijne, K.P., et al., 2000. Hyperventilation and attention: effects of hypocapnia on performance in a Stroop task. Biological Psychology 53, 233–252.

Wayne, H.H., 1958. Clinical differentiation between hypoxia and hyperventilation. Journal of Aviation Medicine 29, 307.

Wilhelm, F.H., Trabert, W., Roth, W.T., 2001a. Characteristics of sighing in panic disorder. Biological Psychiatry 49, 606–614.

Wilhelm, F.H., Gerlach, A.L., Roth, W.T., 2001b. Slow recovery from voluntary hyperventilation in panic disorder. Psychosomatic Medicine 63 (4), 638–649.

Wyke, B., 1963. Brain function and metabolic disorders: the neurological effects of hydrogen-ion concentration. Butterworth, London.

Chapter | **6.1** |

Dynamic Neuromuscular Stabilization: assessment methods

Pavel Kolar, Alena Kobesova, Petra Valouchova, Petr Bitnar

The assessment of a breathing pattern is a significant and 'insightful' entranceway into the assessment of postural functions. It allows for an assessment of the respiratory-stabilization function of the diaphragm and its collaboration with other muscles of the trunk (Kolar 2006). The examination can be performed in various positions, such as supine, sitting or standing. Further, we can describe from the clinical assessment the quality of the respiratory-stabilization pattern based on observation and palpation. Dynamic Neuromuscular Stabilization (DNS) is an approach based on developmental kinesiology. See Chapter 2.1 for more detail of developmental kinesiology.

An infant does not need to be taught to breathe or stabilize the spine correctly because genetically determined programmes occur automatically as a result of maturation of the central nervous system (CNS). Starting at 5 months of age, any healthy infant demonstrates an ideal pattern of dual respiratory-stabilization function. In any position (supine, prone, sitting, quadruped or standing), ideal postural and movement stereotypes occur (Kolar & Kobesova 2010). In DNS, we compare a patient's breathing, posture and movement patterns with those of a healthy 5-month-old or older infant. The assessment and treatment procedures described below can be utilized in patients suffering from various painful syndromes of the locomotor system as well as in patients with primary breathing problems. Postural-respiratory function is indivisible in that the muscles of the torso play a simultaneous role in stabilization and breathing (Kolar et al 2012, McGill et al 1995). An impaired breathing pattern goes hand in hand with impaired postural stabilization (Kolar et al 2012, Smith et al 2006). Therefore, the treatment addresses both functions simultaneously. Without a normal breathing pattern, no other movement pattern can be normal. An altered respiratory-postural pattern is a matter of intra- and inter-muscular coordination controlled by the CNS, which is hardly measurable. If indicated, the clinical assessment (observation and palpation) is combined with pulmonary function tests, instrumental balance assessment, electromyography, dynamic MRI imaging or other tests to support the diagnosis and to objectivize treatment results.

DNS: CLINICAL EXAMINATION OF DUAL RESPIRATORY-POSTURAL FUNCTION

Standing posture assessment

First, the patient's primary stance should be observed. The initial alignment of the chest and the pelvis is critical for both the quality of the breathing pattern and the postural-stabilization function. As previously mentioned (see

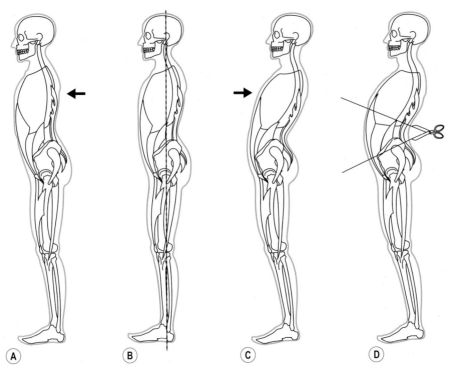

Figure 6.1.1 Chest-spine-pelvis alignment. **A** Forward-drawn chest position. Chest is positioned in front of the pelvis. **B** Optimal alignment, chest positioned above the pelvis, normal spinal curvatures, optimal balance between the anterior and posterior musculature. **C** Thorax positioned behind the lumbosacral junction. **D** 'Open scissors' syndrome: 'inspiratory' (cranial) chest position and an anterior pelvic tilt. Abnormal chest–pelvis relationship results in **A,C,D** situations in patients with abnormal spinal curvatures in the sagittal plane and hyperactivity of the paraspinal muscles.

Fig. 2.1.3, Ch. 2.1), the thorax should be positioned so that the anterior-posterior axis between the insertion of the diaphragm's pars sternalis and the posterior costophrenic angle is almost horizontal. The axis of the lower thoracic aperture and the pelvic axis are parallel to the chest, which is 'positioned' above the pelvis (Fig. 6.1.1B). Only such an alignment allows for ideal respiratory-postural coordination between the diaphragm, pelvic floor and the abdominal muscles. In healthy individuals, the parallel cranio-caudal movement of the diaphragm and the pelvic floor and the synchronous changes in the diameter of the abdominal wall occur during breathing. Therefore, posture may affect the recruitment of these muscles (Talasz et al 2011). Based on an ideal (physiological) standing posture derived from developmental kinesiology, the above-described alignment between the thorax and pelvis and the coordinated muscle activity can be observed in a 14- to 16-month-old healthy infant (Fig. 6.1.2).

An inspiratory position of the thorax known as the 'inspiratory alignment of the thorax' is usually accompanied by an anterior pelvic tilt. Clinically, this abnormal posture is known as 'open scissors' syndrome (Fig. 6.1.1D). A forward shift of the thorax presents another common

deficit (Fig. 6.1.1A), as well as a thorax positioned behind the lumbosacral junction, which is the result of an incorrect spinal curvature in the sagittal plane (Fig. 6.1.1C). This malalignment is often observed in individuals with spinal stenosis or ankylosing spondylitis and it is typically accompanied by a kyphotic or semi-flexed posture.

The increased activity of the upper portion of the abdominal musculature together with a drawing-in of the abdominal wall are considered typical deficits. This is referred to as an 'hour-glass syndrome' (Fig. 6.1.3). Constant isometric activation of the upper sections of the abdominal wall and the inability to relax the abdominals prevents the diaphragm from sufficient caudal descent during inspiration and during postural strain. Abdominal movement closely correlates with diaphragmatic movement, in other words, abdominal movement increases diaphragmatic excursions (Wang et al 2009). Shoulder alignment should also be noted. Their protraction often suggests dominance and shortening of the pectoral muscles. The rib cage elevates when shoulder retraction is attempted and there is a muscle imbalance between the upper and lower trunk stabilizers (the pectoral and abdominal muscles).

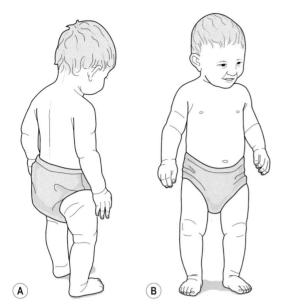

Figure 6.1.2 Physiological stabilization of the spine, chest and pelvis, i.e. optimal, genetically determined posture. Neutral position of the thorax and the scapulae; upper chest and shoulder blade fixators are relaxed and in balance with lower fixators; optimal balance between the anterior and posterior core musculature; upright spine and a neutral position of the pelvis. Such muscle coordination and optimal alignment between the chest and the pelvis and proper spinal stabilization are maintained during all the movements and in any posture – supine, prone, quadruped, sitting, etc. Neutral chest position is maintained through the entire respiratory cycle, during inspiration and expiration.

The shape of the thorax is also important for the physiological stabilization of the spine. Common deviations in the shape of the thorax are especially associated with rib tilting. A long (asthenic) thorax is flat in the anterior-posterior direction and the ribs are markedly hanging with narrow intercostal spaces. An asthenic thorax demonstrates a significant difference in the size of the perimeter of the thorax during inspiration and expiration or with significant breathing excursions and results in quite good ventilation ability. A barrel-chest is the opposite of an asthenic thorax, in which the ribs run horizontally and the intercostal spaces are wide. The anteroposterior diameter of the thorax is increased, the chest is in a permanent inspiratory alignment and has a low ventilation capacity (van Schayck et al 1995). The barrel chest configuration is typical but not specific to chronic obstructive pulmonary disease and it is often associated with an abnormal postural development. A newborn's chest is barrel-shaped and the rib cage geometry changes during early childhood development (Openshaw et al 1984). An abnormal postural development can result in anatomical changes,

including the thoracic area (Park et al 2006). A barrel-shaped chest is anatomically disadvantageous for stabilization function. As far as shape deviations, the position of the posterior angles of the lower ribs in relation to the spine is the most significant. If aligned too far ventrally (in front of the spine), the function between the spinal extensors and the intra-abdominal pressure cannot be balanced. In this situation, paravertebral muscle overactivity is observed leading to a greater tendency toward spinal problems in these individuals. Non-physiological postural development usually leads to this deviation in shape. We often observe a barrel-shaped chest in patients with chronic back pain and after failed back surgery syndromes. In many of these patients, an abnormal postural development is considered to be the primary etiology of their chronic pain syndromes. Also, a barrel-shaped chest is a mere consequence of the ageing effect (Maitre at al 1995). Ageing is related to changes in the CNS, including neuronal loss, reduction in the components of myelin and intracellular enzymes, decreased receptor concentration, etc. At the same time, changes in the peripheral nervous system occur (Wickremaratchi & Llewelyn 2006) and one can assume that such processes have an influence on sensory-motor postural control, as well as having an anatomical consequence. The ageing process can be viewed as a reverse process of postural-locomotion development. In many aspects, the posture of ageing individuals resembles a newborn's posture (spinal kyphosis, barrel-shaped chest, decrease range of motion, semi-flexed posture).

However, a distinction has to be made between a developmental thoracic deformity and congenital thoracic malformations. Pes excavatus presents as a depression of the sternum with an anterior protrusion of the ribs. Pes carinatum is a reverse deformity with the sternum protruding anteriorly (Maitre at al 1995). Usually, such deformities result in rather esthetic issues (Jaroszewski et al 2010, Kelly et al 2008), however, sometimes they may influence ventilatory parameters (Jaroszewski et al 2010) and they do not automatically result in abnormal postural stabilization (Schoenmakers et al 2000) or an abnormal respiratory pattern. This type of chest malformation may be inconvenient with respect to stabilization and respiratory stereotype, especially when associated with scoliosis (Schoenmakers et al 2000) or with a connective tissue disorder (Kelly et al 2005). It is our experience that, unlike developmental chest deformities, physical therapy and other rehabilitation interventions do not usually result in changes of the anatomical parameters in congenital types of malformations. Only a few studies show benefits of conservative treatment on chest wall geometry (Haecker 2011, Moreno et al 2011). If necessary, the deformity needs to be surgically corrected (Jaroszewski et al 2010). All clinicians should be aware that chest pain, dyspnoea, decreased endurance, decreased exercise tolerance and increased fatigue may occur in patients with a severe form of pectus excavatum (Jaroszewski et al 2010).

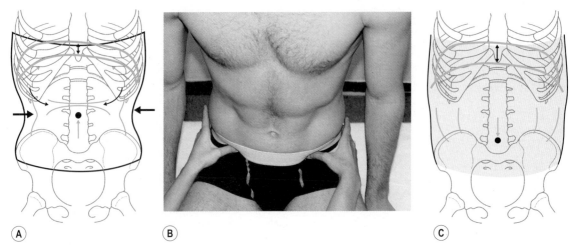

Figure 6.1.3 'Hour-glass syndrome'. **A** Constant concentric activation of the abdominal wall, especially in its upper section, with the umbilicus in a cranial and a 'drawn-in' position. Such muscle coordination results in a cranial position of the diaphragm and limits diaphragmatic descent during postural tasks, thus altering postural stabilization. During postural activity, the diaphragmatic excursion is small and the direction of activation is toward the centrum tendineum (blue arrows) because the diaphragmatic attachments on the lower ribs are not stabilized via an eccentric abdominal contraction. **B** Clinical picture of an 'hour-glass syndrome'. The activity of the upper abdominal wall predominates; the patient cannot eccentrically activate the lower section of the abdominal wall (pushing clinician's thumbs outwards and caudally). **C** Correct model of stabilization. Balanced function of all the abdominal wall sections, the diaphragm descends during postural tasks and its costal attachments are stabilized. Note opposite direction of the blue arrows and greater diaphragmatic excursion when compared to **A**. The umbilicus moves caudally as a result of increased intra-abdominal pressure and diaphragmatic descent. The abdominal wall expands proportionally in all the directions.

Assessment of the breathing pattern and the diaphragm's respiratory function

Movement of the ribs (thorax) and the abdominal cavity are observed. During diaphragmatic breathing, the diaphragm descends caudally, flattens and compresses the internal organs caudally. With inspiration, for example, the kidney shifts several centimetres caudally while during expiration it migrates cranially (Xi et al 2009). The thoracic and abdominal cavities symmetrically expand. It is important that during physiological diaphragmatic breathing, the lower aperture of the thorax also expands in addition to the abdominal cavity. The sternum moves ventrally. During rib palpation, it is observed that the intercostal spaces expand and the lower thorax expands proportionately in the lateral, ventral and dorsal directions (Fig. 6.1.4B). Simultaneously, both thumbs then palpate the dorsolateral aspect of the abdominal wall below the 12th rib and observe whether the palpated area expands during inspiration. The inhalation wave reaches as far as the lower abdominal wall, i.e. the patient can also breathe into the abdominal wall just above the groin (Fig. 6.1.4A). The sternum does not change its position in the transverse plane. The accessory breathing muscles (scalenes, pectorales, upper trapezius, etc.) are physiologically relaxed during resting breathing.

In a pathological scenario, the sternum moves craniocaudally and the thorax expands only minimally while the intercostal spaces do not expand. The accessory muscles are activated during inspiration. A patient's inability to perform diaphragmatic breathing suggests an insufficient or impaired synchronization between the diaphragm and the abdominal muscles. This is often caused by an inability to relax the abdominal wall (especially the upper portion). The nature of the breathing pattern and its control usually correlate with the results of clinical tests focused on the stabilizing function of the spine.

If the upper chest stabilizers (pectoralis, upper trapezius, scalenes, SCM) dominate and pull the thorax into an 'inspiratory position', the thoracic position is commonly accompanied by impaired costovertebral joint mobility. This dysfunction is compensated for by movement in the thoracolumbar junction even during breathing (see Fig. 6.1.1D). The spine moves into extension during inspiration while during expiration it moves into flexion. With thoracic spine straightening, the entire thorax moves cranially; however, physiologically, it should remain in a neutral position during inspiration and expiration (see Fig. 6.1.2).

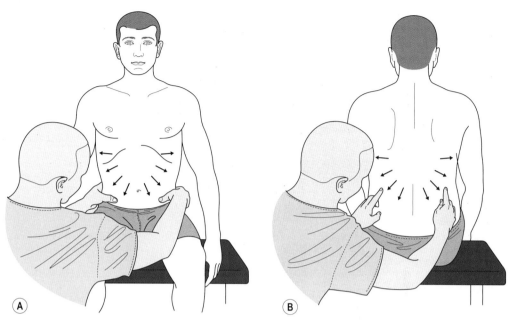

Figure 6.1.4 Assessment of the respiratory–postural function of the diaphragm. With inspiration, the individual should be able to expand all sections of the abdominal wall while maintaining an upright sitting position and relaxed shoulders. The clinician palpates the area above the groin from the front (**A**); and between and below the lower ribs from behind (**B**). To assess solely the postural diaphragmatic function, the client is asked to exhale and push actively against the clinician's fingers. The expansion should be relatively strong, symmetrical and without any pathological synkineses (i.e. the chest, pelvis and spine position remain neutral). The same position can be used for training. The clinician guides the patient manually and verbally.

When assessing the breathing pattern as described above, the patient's natural pattern is examined, i.e. without any specific instruction or corrections. The area between and below the lower ribs is observed and palpated. Most of the patients, including individuals with dysfunction as well as healthy individuals, do not demonstrate an ideal pattern as their default movement stereotype. However, it is the ability to modify the stereotype that matters. The second step of the assessment consists of patient instruction. The patient is instructed to relax the upper chest stabilizers, sit upright and breathe into the lower chest cavity and into the latero-dorsal aspects of the abdominal wall as well as into the lower abdominal wall above the groin. The examiner guides the patient verbally and manually. Most of the patients are 'locked' in their insufficient stereotype. They cannot follow the instruction and cannot modify their respiratory-postural stereotype. The overactivity of certain muscles or muscle sections (constantly substituting for the insufficient ones), overloading of certain spinal or joint segments and finally, pain syndromes are all results of the constant uniformity. From our experience, the ability to better modify the breathing and/or movement patterns and the ability to better follow the clinician's instructions indicate better prognosis – the treatment will be shorter and simpler and the results will last longer.

Assessment of the diaphragm's postural function

During the assessment, the patient sits at the edge of a treatment table, feet unsupported, arms relaxed along the trunk. The same rule as described above is utilized. First, the patient's natural pattern is observed and then, if necessary, the patient is instructed in how to correct it. The upper extremities are freely positioned without the patient leaning on them. Laterodorsal portions of the abdominal wall are palpated below the lower ribs from behind (see Fig. 6.1.4B) and the groin area is palpated from the front medially to the anterior superior iliac spines above the femoral heads (see Fig. 6.1.4A). The patient, while holding their breath, is asked to expand the laterodorsal sections of the abdominal wall posteriorly and laterally or to push their abdominal wall caudally and ventrolaterally against the pressure of the examiner's thumbs. In this test, the abdominal wall is assessed during increased abdominal pressure.

A symmetrical pressure of the abdominal wall against the examiner's thumbs is considered to be the correct pattern. Through activation of the diaphragm, an eccentric bowing out of the abdominal wall in all its sections occurs first. This is followed by an isometric contraction of the abdominal muscles. This principle is clearly apparent in a weightlifter when lifting a heavy load (see Fig. 2.1.7, Ch. 2.1).

The test is positive if the patient is not able to freely activate the palpated abdominal wall or if the pressure against the resistance from the examiner's thumbs is asymmetrical or bilaterally weak and the upper portion of the rectus abdominis and the external obliques dominate. The abdominal wall is drawn in at its upper half and the umbilicus migrates cranially (see Fig. 6.1.3A,B). The patient also substitutes the activation of the lower abdominal wall with a posterior pelvic tilt. Activation of muscles in the palpated area without symmetrical bowing out of the lower abdomen is also considered incorrect.

Additional assessment approaches are described in Chapters 6.2, osteopathy; 6.3, physiotherapy; 6.4, psychology; 6.5, questionnaires and manual methods and 6.6, capnography.

Treatment and rehabilitation methods, based on DNS methodology, are summarized in Chapter 7.1b.

REFERENCES

Haecker, F.M., 2011. The vacuum bell for conservative treatment of pectus excavatum: the Basle experience. Pediatr Surg Int. 27 (6), 623–627.

Jaroszewski, D., Notrica, D., McMahon, L., et al., 2010. Current management of pectus excavatum: a review and update of therapy and treatment recommendations. J Am Board Fam Med. 23 (2), 230–239.

Kelly, R.E., Jr., Cash, T.F., Shamberger, R.C., 2008. Surgical repair of pectus excavatum markedly improves body image and perceived ability for physical activity: multicenter study. Pediatrics. 122 (6), 1218–1222.

Kelly, R.E., Jr., Lawson, M.L., Paidas, C.N., et al., 2005. Pectus excavatum in a 112-year autopsy series: anatomic findings and the effect on survival. J Pediatr Surg. 40 (8), 1275–1278.

Kolar, P., 2006. Facilitation of agonist-antagonist co-activation by reflex stimulation methods. In: Liebenson, C. (Ed.), Rehabilitation of the spine – a practitioner's manual, second ed. Lippincott Williams & Wilkins, Philadelphia, pp. 531–565.

Kolar, P., Kobesova, A., 2010. Postural – locomotion function in the diagnosis and treatment of movement disorders. Clinical Chiropractic. 13 (1), 58–68.

Kolar, P., Sulc, J., Kyncl, M., et al., 2012. Postural function of the diaphragm in persons with and without chronic low back pain. J Orthop Sports Phys Ther. 42 (4), 352–362.

Maitre, B., Similowski, T., Derenne, J.P., 1995. Physical examination of the adult patient with respiratory diseases: inspection and palpation. Eur Respir J. 8 (9), 1584–1593.

McGill, S.M., Sharratt, M.T., Seguin, J.P., 1995. Loads on spinal tissues during simultaneous lifting and ventilatory challenge. Ergonomics. 38 (9), 1772–1792.

Moreno, C., Delgado, M.D., Martí, E., et al., 2011. Conservative treatment of the pectus carinatum. Cir Pediatr. 24 (2), 71–74.

Openshaw, P., Edwards, S., Helms, P., 1984. Changes in rib cage geometry during childhood. Thorax. 39 (8), 624–627.

Park, E.S., Park, J.H., Rha, D.W., et al., 2006. Comparison of the ratio of upper to lower chest wall in children with spastic quadriplegic cerebral palsy and normally developed children. Yonsei Med J. 47 (2), 237–242.

Schoenmakers, M.A., Gulmans, V.A., Bax, N.M., et al., 2000. Physiotherapy as an adjuvant to the surgical treatment of anterior chest wall deformities: a necessity? A prospective descriptive study in 21 patients. J Pediatr Surg. 35 (10), 1440–1443.

Smith, M.D., Russell, A., Hodges, P.W., 2006. Disorders of breathing and continence have a stronger association with back pain than obesity and physical activity. Aust J Physiother. 52 (1), 11–16.

Talasz, H., Kremser, C., Kofler, M., et al., 2011. Phase-locked parallel movement of diaphragm and pelvic floor during breathing and coughing – a dynamic MRI investigation in healthy females. Int Urogynecol J. 22 (1), 61–68.

van Schayck, C.P., Dompeling, E., Putters, R., et al., 1995. Asthma and chronic bronchitis. Can family physicians predict rates of progression? Can Fam Physician. 41, 1868–1876.

Wang, H.K., Lu, T.W., Liing, R.J., et al., 2009. Relationship between chest wall motion and diaphragmatic excursion in healthy adults in supine position. J Formos Med Assoc. 108 (7), 577–586.

Wickremaratchi, M.M., Llewelyn, J.G., 2006. Effects of ageing on touch. Postgrad Med J. 82 (967), 301–304.

Xi, M., Liu, M.Z., Li, Q.Q., et al., 2009. Analysis of abdominal organ motion using four-dimensional CT. Ai Zheng. 28 (9), 989–993.

Osteopathic assessment of structural changes related to BPD

Leon Chaitow

The information in this chapter is designed to assist all professionally trained manual practitioners or therapists. There is no suggestion that the descriptions in this chapter should be used as a basis for application of the treatment, unless competency has been achieved in anatomy, physiology, soft tissue and osseous manipulation methods, by individuals who are appropriately licensed to perform the methods involved.

Many (but not all) of the methods described in this chapter have their roots in osteopathy, however, the title of the chapter should be taken to refer to the author's (LC) professional background and philosophical bias, rather than being seen as a claim that everything mentioned in the chapter is 'osteopathic' in origin.

STRUCTURE–FUNCTION

Chapter 2.2 highlighted the interdependence of structure and function. Clinical experience – and common sense – suggest that rehabilitation of BPD is likely to be more effectively achieved following identification and appropriate normalization of associated articular and soft tissue changes.

The treatment of respiratory dysfunction by means of osteopathic manipulative therapy (OMT) dates back to the beginning of the 20th century (Smith 1920). It is logical that a therapeutic system which had normalization of the musculoskeletal system as a primary therapeutic goal should see breathing dysfunction as an appropriate focus for its work (Riley 2000, Knott et al 2005, Hruby & Hoffman 2007).

There is ample scope for biomechanical dysfunction to appear in the 'machinery' of breathing, involving as it does the thoracic cage acting as a pump, coordinated by complicated central controls. This involves integrated muscular contractions and relaxations, together with a network of fascial accommodations, all modulated by neural activity – inducing movement in almost every joint in the body, but particularly involving the thoracic cage with its multiple pivoting and rotating articulations.

Functional symmetry

Ward et al (2002) have described important osteopathic objectives involving 'restoration of three-dimensionally patterned functional symmetry', when attempting to manage dysfunction (local or global, for example in relation to respiratory function), potentially involving:

1. Identification of patterns of ease/bind, loose/tight, short/weak, etc. in a given body area, achieved by sequential palpation and assessment of soft tissue shortness and/or articular restrictions (Cleland et al 2006, Heiderscheit & Boissonnault 2008), followed by:
2. Release of areas identified as tight, restricted, tethered, possibly involving myofascial release (MFR), muscle energy techniques (MET), neuromuscular technique (NMT), positional release technique (PRT), joint mobilization (or if indicated, manipulation), (some of these methods will be discussed further in Ch. 7.2) (Flynn et al 2001).
3. Identification and appropriate deactivation of myofascial trigger points contained within these structures (see below for assessment methods, and Ch. 7.2 for treatment) (Dommerholt et al 2006).
4. Facilitation in tone of inhibited (weak) musculature, ideally involving self-care, home exercises (Lewit 2009).

5. Use of high velocity thrust (HVT) methods should only be applied if appropriate to the status (age, structural integrity, inflammatory status, pain levels, etc.) of the individual, and should be reserved for joints that fail to respond adequately to soft tissue mobilization. Ross et al (2004) have made the useful observation following research, that manual therapy interventions (including HVLA) tend to affect regions of the spine, rather than specific, 'targeted', segments.
6. Re-education and rehabilitation (including home work involving prescribed exercises). This should involve work on posture, breathing and patterns of use in order to restore functional integrity and prevent recurrence, as far as is possible. Exercise (home work) needs to be focused, time-efficient, and within the patient's easy comprehension and capabilities, if compliance is to be achieved (Vance 2003). See also Chapter 9 for home care options, as well as self-applied methods described throughout different chapters in the book.

FUNCTIONAL ASSESSMENT APPROACHES

See Chapter 6.1 and Chapter 6.3, for additional manual assessment methods.

Janda (1996), Janda et al (2006) and Lewit (2009) suggest that altered movement patterns should be tested as part of a screening examination for locomotor dysfunction. Prior to palpation and/or manual assessment methods, observation of posture and movement is suggested, accompanied, or followed, by light palpation to confirm the accuracy of what is observed.

Postural patterns such as those described and illustrated in Chapter 2.2 (crossed syndromes for example) offer immediate information regarding tissues that are probably shortened, lengthened and/or restricted: in particular see Figs 2.2.1, 2.2.3, 2.2.4, 2.2.5 (Hruska 1997, Pryor & Prasad 2002).

Any tendency for the head to be carried forward of the body should be considered in relation to accompanying breathing pattern changes. Courtney (2009) points out that forward head posture 'is a well-known response to obstructed breathing and is common in children with chronic nasal allergy and mouth breathing because this head position opens the upper airways.' For more on this topic see notes later in this chapter under the subheading: *Assessment of shortness in accessory (and obligatory) breathing muscles.*

The functional assessments described below are followed in this chapter by descriptions of specific tests for shortness of muscles associated with respiratory function as well as identification of myofascial trigger points in these muscles. In addition, rib assessment methods are detailed. It is important to emphasize that individually none of the assessments is diagnostic – only indicative. It requires a cluster of supportive test results, combined with information relating to the individual's history and current symptom status, to change an indication, a suggestion, into something more definitive – and even then this should be a tentative diagnosis.

NOTE: All assessment and palpation results should be charted.

OSTEOPATHIC ASSESSMENT

An osteopathic approach to the evaluation of respiratory function includes taking account of the following elements relating to the act of breathing (Chila 1997):

- *Category*: does breathing involve the diaphragm? the lower rib cage? both? The pattern should be charted. The ideal would be both.
- *Locus of abdominal motion*: does abdominal movement occur as far as the umbilicus? as far as the pubic bone? The locus should be charted. A full breath should be palpable anteriorly to the pubis, as well as involving lateral rib expansion.
- *Rate*: rapid? slow? The breathing rate should be recorded before and after treatment, with an ideal in the range of 10 to 14 cycles per minute (see Ch. 7.1a).
- *Duration of cycle*: are inhalation and exhalation phases equal? or is one longer than the other? This ratio between these should be noted. Ideally exhalation to take longer than inhalation.

Additionally, a series of observations and palpation methods can usefully be combined into a sequence such as that outlined below.

The patient's breathing function should be evaluated by palpation and observation, seated, supine, side-lying and prone, following on from a standard evaluation of posture in which head position, shoulder rounding, crossed syndromes (see Ch. 2.2) are noted and charted.

A. Seated: the HiLo or 'two-hand' test (Fig. 6.2.1)

The patient is asked to place a hand on the upper abdomen and another on the upper chest (Fig. 6.2.1). The hands are observed as the individual inhales several times. If the upper hand (chest) moves first, and especially if it also moves superiorly rather than slightly antero-superiorly, and moves significantly more than the hand on the

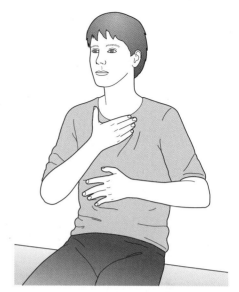

Figure 6.2.1 Hand positions for breathing function assessment using HiLo or two-hand test. *Reproduced with kind permission from Chaitow & DeLany 2010. Adapted from Bradley D 1998.*

abdomen, this should be noted as suggesting a dysfunctional – upper chest – pattern of breathing.

B. Palpation for symmetry of motion on inhalation

The practitioner stands behind the seated patient and places, and rests, his hands gently over the upper trapezius area. The patient is asked to inhale while the practitioner notes whether his hands move significantly toward the ceiling, bilaterally or unilaterally. If so, the upper fixators of the shoulder/accessory breathing muscles, and the scalenes, are overworking, and, as most of these are postural muscles (see discussion on muscle types in Chapter 2.2), are likely to be shortened. Specific muscles should subsequently be assessed individually as outlined later in this chapter.

C. 1st rib palpation test (Fig. 6.2.2)

A number of alternative tests are listed. None is necessarily more sensitive than another. As with many manual tests confirmation of a result by using a different method enhances the validity of the findings.

The patient is seated and the practitioner stands behind and places his hands so that the fingers can draw posteriorly the upper trapezius fibres lying superior to the 1st rib.

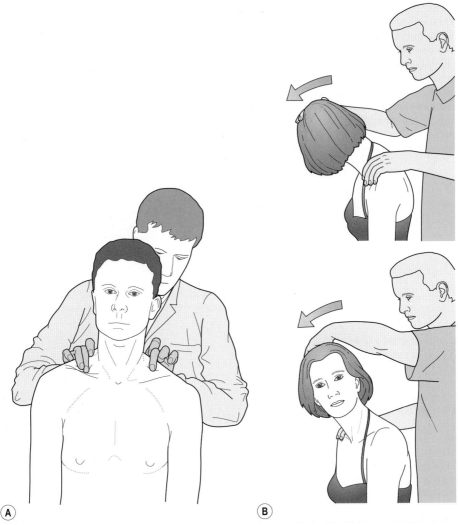

Figure 6.2.2 A 1st rib palpation test. *From Greenman 1996.* **B** Cervical rotation, lateral flexion test for 1st rib restriction. *Lindgren et al. 1989, Lindgren 1997.*

The tips of the practitioner's middle and index, or middle and ring fingers can then most easily be placed on the superior surface of the posterior shaft of the 1st rib. Caution: This is frequently an extremely sensitive area and pressure should be modulated accordingly. Symmetry is evaluated as the patient inhales.

Alternatively:

The patient exhales and shrugs his shoulders and the palpated 1st ribs are assessed to evaluate whether the first ribs behave asymmetrically or asymmetrically, i.e. whether one moves superiorly more than the other. If there is asymmetry, the rib that moves superiorly more than its pair, is probably elevated.

Alternatively:

The patient exhales fully and the palpated 1st ribs are assessed to evaluate whether they behave symmetrically or asymmetrically, i.e. whether one moves inferiorly more than the other. If there is asymmetry, the rib that fails to move inferiorly as far as its pair is probably elevated.

NOTE: Clinical experience suggests that both first ribs may be elevated in someone who chronically uses an upper chest pattern of breathing, and that the tests described above may identify the more dysfunctional of the two, even though both may require normalizing, possibly using methods described in Chapter 7.2.

Alternatively:

The cervical rotation lateral flexion test, as advocated by Lindgren et al 1989, Lindgren 1997, is used to screen for elevation of the first rib. The patient is seated with the practitioner standing behind. The practitioner passively rotates the neck away from the side of the 1st rib being tested. The cervical spine is then passively, and gently, side-flexed in the sagittal plane. If an obvious reduction in side-bending mobility is noted, this suggests an elevated first rib on the side opposite that from which the cervical spine has been rotated. Lindgren et al (1989) report this test to be reliable, with good agreement with imaging evidence. See Figure 6.2.2b.

Subsequent to the most obvious rib being treated, re-assessment may reveal that the other rib is also elevated, requiring attention.

The commonest restriction of the 1st rib is into elevation ('locked in inhalation') and the likeliest soft tissue involvement is of anterior and medial scalenes (Kuchera & Goodridge 1997). The superior aspect of this rib will palpate as being more prominent, and even light touch might be reported as uncomfortable (Greenman 1996).

1st rib elevation suggests probable involvement of scalene and sternomastoid, as well as upper trapezius muscles. These should be individually assessed for shortness, hypertonicity and/or trigger point presence (see below).

D. Seated assessment of lateral expansion (Fig. 6.2.3)

The practitioner is behind the patient and places his hands on the patient's lower ribs, laterally, with thumbs either side of the spinous processes of approximately T9/10. On inhalation the degree of lateral excursion (the hands pushed apart), and the degree of symmetry is noted. There should be a degree of lateral expansion and it should be equal. Also noted is whether, and to what degree, there is vertical rather than lateral movement of the hands, and whether this is symmetrical. There should be little, or no, vertical movement in diaphragmatic breathing. The results should be charted.

NOTE: Chapter 6.5 offers alternative guidelines for manual assessment of breathing patterns – see *The Manual Assessment of Respiratory Movement* (MARM) in that chapter.

E. Supine rib palpation test: ribs 2–10 (Fig. 6.2.4)

The patient is supine. The practitioner stands at waist level, facing the patient's head, with a single finger contact on each of the superior aspect of a pair of ribs (Fig. 6.2.4). The practitioner's dominant eye determines the side of the table from which he is approaching the observation of rib function (right-eye dominant calls for standing on the

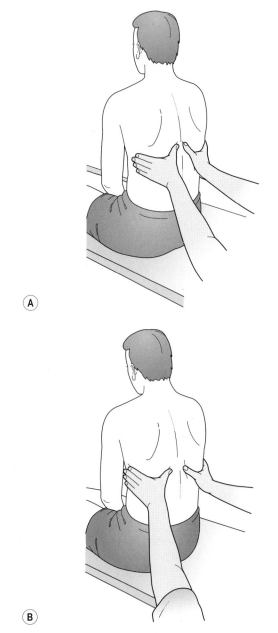

(A)

(B)

Figure 6.2.3 Assessment for lateral expansion of lower ribs.

patient's right side). The fingers are observed as the patient inhales and exhales fully (eye focus is on an area between the palpating fingers so that peripheral vision assesses symmetry of movement).

If one of a pair of ribs fails to rise as far as its pair on inhalation it is described as a depressed rib, unable to move fully to its end of range on inhalation ('locked in exhalation'). If one of a pair of ribs fails to fall as far as its

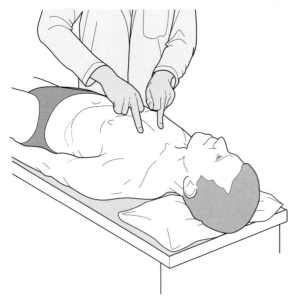

Figure 6.2.4 Assessment of rib function (ribs 2 to 10).

pair on exhalation it is described as an elevated rib, unable to move fully to its end of range on exhalation ('locked in inhalation') (see Box 6.2.1). Treatment options should include attention to overlying and attaching musculature as well as to possible articulation restriction – as described in Chapter 7.2.

In addition, with the patient prone or seated, it is useful to palpate for changes in the normal thoracic lordosis by running the fingers over the paraspinal muscles alongside the thoracic spine, assessing for areas of altered soft tissue tension and/or tenderness that suggests underlying segmental dysfunction, likely to impact on rib function (Cleland et al 2007). Identification of impaired mobility of a region of the thoracic spine may be associated with increased or decreased thoracic kyphosis, reduced range of motion, hypertonic soft tissue status accompanied by tenderness, as well as hypomobility with spring testing of the prone patient. Heiderscheit & Boissonnault (2008) note that tenderness over the rib angle, reduced excursion during respiration, and hypomobility during spring-testing over the anterior or posterior aspect of the rib, are all suggestive of rib restriction.

F.   Assessment of lower thorax/ thoracolumbar restriction

Mobility of the lower thoracic region is evaluated by means of a gentle rotational effort to assess symmetry. The diaphragm attaches internally to the structures of the lower thorax, and if these are limited in their rotational ability a degree of diaphragmatic restriction may be assumed.

Box 6.2.1 **Rib dysfunction assessment** (Hruby & Goodridge 1997, Greenman 1996)

Restrictions in the ability of a given rib, or pair of ribs, to move (rise) fully while inhaling, indicates a depressed ('locked in exhalation') status, while an inability to move fully into exhalation, indicates an elevated ('locked in inhalation') status.

As a rule, unless there has been direct trauma, rib restrictions of this sort are compensatory, and involve groups of ribs. Osteopathic clinical experience suggests that if a group of depressed ribs is located, the 'key' rib is likely to be the most superior of these: if successfully released, it will 'unlock' the remaining ribs in that group. Similarly, if a group of elevated ribs is located, the 'key' rib is likely to be the most inferior of these: if successfully released/mobilized, this rib will 'unlock' the remaining ribs in that group.

If assessment commences at the most cephalad aspect of the thorax, the 2nd rib is the most easily palpated. The ribs are sequentially assessed, and if a depressed rib is noted this is clearly the most cephalad and is the one to be treated (see Ch. 7.2). Similarly, if an elevated rib is identified the ribs continue to be evaluated until a rib with normal movement is located, and the dysfunctional rib cephalad to that is then treated.

As in all forms of somatic dysfunction, causes should be sought and addressed in addition to mobilization of restrictions using MET or other methods, as described in this text.

The patient is supine, and the practitioner stands at waist level, facing cephalad, and places his hands over the middle and lower thoracic structures, with his fingers along the rib shafts. Treating the structure being palpated as a cylinder, the hands test the preference this cylinder has to rotate around its central axis, first one way and then the other. Side-flexion mobility may also be assessed by introduction of a translational force – as illustrated in Figure 6.2.5. Ideally, a symmetrical degree of rotation and side-flexion should be noted. Mobilization methods are described in Chapter 7.3.

SUPINE ASSESSMENT OF BREATHING PATTERN

- Does the abdomen move anteriorly on inhalation? It should, slightly.
- How much of the abdomen is involved? Greatly? Marginally?
- Is there an observable lateral excursion of the lower ribs? There should be observable lateral motion.

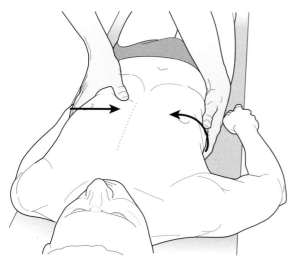

Figure 6.2.5 Assessment of rotational and side-flexion potential of lower thorax.

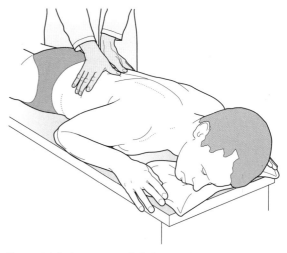

Figure 6.2.7 Assessment of rib function (ribs 11 and 12).

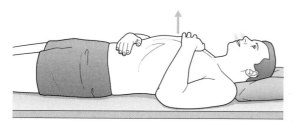

Figure 6.2.6 Paradoxical breathing – abdomen retracts, upper chest expands, on inhalation.

- Does the upper chest move forward on inhalation while the abdomen is seen to retract? If so this is evidence of paradoxical breathing (Fig. 6.2.6).

Implications: Paradoxical breathing suggests that the following soft tissues are probably shortened: scalenes, sternocleidomastoid, upper trapezius, pectoralis major, intercostal muscles. Evaluation of the possible additional overactivity/shortness in psoas and quadratus lumborum should be evaluated. Rib and general thoracic spine mobility should be evaluated.

G. Rib palpation test: ribs 11 and 12 (Fig. 6.2.7)

Assessment of ribs 11 and 12 is usually performed with the patient prone and palpation performed with a hand contact on the posterior shafts to evaluate full inhalation and exhalation motions.

The 11th and 12th ribs usually operate as a pair, so that if any sense of reduction in posterior motion is noted on one side or the other, on inhalation, both are regarded as depressed, unable to fully inhale ('locked in exhalation'). If any sense of reduction in anterior motion is noted on one side or the other, on exhalation, the pair are regarded as elevated, unable to fully exhale ('locked in inhalation').

H. Hip abduction test (Fig. 6.2.8)

Quadratus lumborum (QL) has respiratory influences via its role as a stabilizer of the 12th rib, during exhalation, as well as through direct fascial connections to the diaphragm (Palastanga et al 2002). It is assessed by palpation during the hip abduction test: side-lying (Fig. 6.2.8).

The patient should be side-lying, with the practitioner standing facing the patient's front at hip level, while simultaneously palpating gluteus medius, tensor fasciae latae (TFL), and quadratus lumborum (QL), as the patient abducts the upper leg.

In balanced abduction, gluteus medius fires first, with TFL operating later in the pure abduction of the leg. QL should not become active – other than a gentle toning – until the leg has reached between 25° and 30° abduction.

When it is overactive, QL will often fire first as abduction commences, along with TFL. This would suggest shortness in QL – something that would potentially impact on breathing function (Morris et al 2006).

Observation of the side-lying hip-abduction test may offer additional information (see Fig. 6.2.8).

- A rapid firing of QL – suggesting shortness and potential negative influence on the diaphragm – is

105

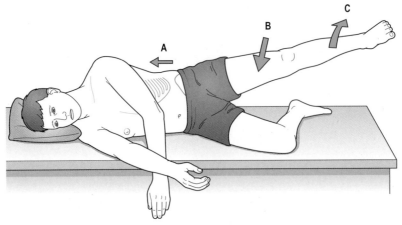

Figure 6.2.8 Hip abduction test which, if normal, occurs without 'hip hike' (**A**), hip flexion (**B**) or external rotation (**C**).

indicated by a 'hip-hike' at the start of the abduction (see 'A' in Fig. 6.2.8)

- If the abducted leg drifts forwards, the suggestion is of hip-flexor shortness (see 'B' in Fig. 6.2.8)
- If the abducted leg externally rotates this suggests shortness in piriformis (see 'C' in Fig. 6.2.8).

I.   Hip extension test

Sacrospinalis is part of the erector spinae group and is subdivided into lateral, intermediate and medial parallel columns that extend from the sacrum to the rib cage. These have multiple roles including stabilization of the vertebral column. The anchoring of many of the muscle fibres into ribs indicates the potential influence of respiratory function if these elements of the erector spinae group are hypertonic and/or shortened (Palastanga et al 2002) (Fig. 6.2.9A).

The most common activation sequence on prone hip extension is gluteus maximus and hamstrings followed by erector spinae (contralateral then ipsilateral).

If the hamstrings and/or erectors fire first, and take the prime mover role of gluteus maximus, they are considered to be overactive and probably shortened, while gluteus is inhibited (Fig. 6.2.9B).

J.   Scapulohumeral rhythm test

This test offers evidence of imbalances involving some of the accessory respiratory muscles that are likely to be over-worked and dysfunctional when a pattern of upper-chest breathing is a feature (Liebenson 1999, Courtney 2009).

- The patient is seated and the practitioner stands behind to observe.
- The patient is asked to let the arm being tested hang down and to flex the elbow to 90° with the thumb pointing upwards.

- The patient is asked to slowly abduct the arm toward the horizontal.
- A normal abduction will include elevation of the shoulder and/or rotation or superior movement of the scapula only after 60° of abduction has occurred.
- Abnormal performance of this test occurs if elevation of the shoulder, rotation, superior movement, or winging of the scapula occurs within the first 60° of shoulderabduction, indicating levator scapula and/or upper trapezius as being overactive and shortened, while lower and middle trapezius and serratus anterior are inhibited and are therefore weak.

Variation 1

- The patient performs the abduction of the arm as described above and the practitioner observes from behind.
- A 'hinging' should be seen to take place at the shoulder joint, if upper trapezius and levator are normal. If 'hinging' appears to be occurring at the base of the neck, this is an indication of excessive activity in the upper fixators of the shoulder and shortness of upper trapezius and/or levator scapula is suggested.
- The muscles that appear to be overactive should be assessed for shortness (see below) and should be searched for the presence of myofascial trigger points.

K.   Spring test for upper thoracic spine (Beal 1983) (Fig. 6.2.10)

A useful assessment for mobility of the upper thoracic spine, where restriction may relate to viscerosomatic reflex activity, involves the patient lying supine with the practitioner at the head of the table, with the palpating hand

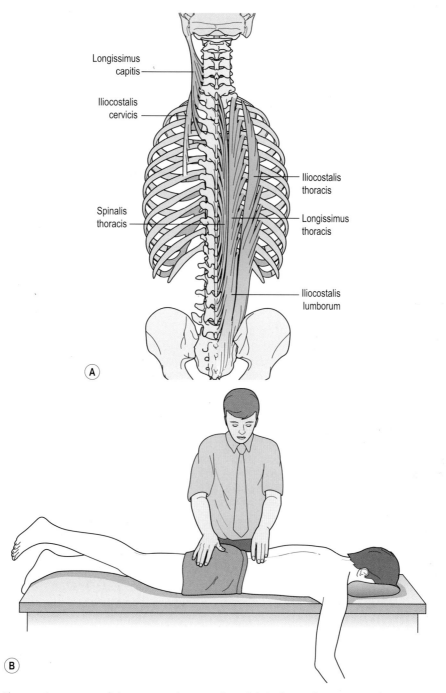

Figure 6.2.9 A The constituent parts of the erector spinae muscle and their rib attachments. **B** Janda's hip extension test for overactivity of erector spinae. *Janda 2006.*

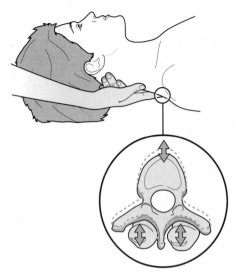

Figure 6.2.10 Upper thoracic spring test.

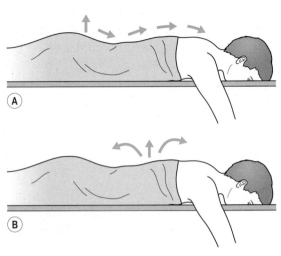

Figure 6.2.11 Breathing wave. **A** Normal movement from lower to upper spine on inhalation. **B** Restricted areas move 'en bloc' on inhalation. This pattern should revert towards normal as restricted areas are mobilized, and as breathing function improves. *Lewit 2009.*

inserted under the upper spine so that fingers lie either side of the T1 to T3 area.

A gentle springing action is introduced to evaluate freedom of motion at these articulations

Beal suggests that a diagnosis of a paraspinal viscerosomatic reflex should be based upon two or more adjacent spinal segments showing evidence of somatic restriction, involving confluent spinal muscle splinting and resistance to segmental joint motion. Less severe restrictions may relate to hypertonic local musculature (for example scalenes, upper trapezius) and/or joint dysfunction.

The findings of this assessment should be correlated with findings from rib evaluation involving the upper ribs, as described earlier.

L. The 'breathing wave' (Fig. 6.2.11)

Lewit (2009) describes the following useful protocol for evaluating the efficiency with which the spine responds to respiratory function:

- Standing to the side the practitioner observes the spinal contours as the seated or standing patient fully flexes. If there are obvious 'flat' areas of the thoracic spine (suggesting inability to flex fully), this may additionally indicate rib restrictions at those levels.
- The patient lies prone with his head in a face-hole. The practitioner is at waist level, observing from the side, eyes at the same level as the spine.
- A full inhalation is performed and the spine is observed to see whether movement commences at the sacrum and finishes at the base of the neck (an ideal, if rare, observation). More often, restricted spinal

segments 'rise' simultaneously, as a block, and movement of the spine occurs in two directions, caudally and cephalad, from the 'blocked' area. Often very little movement occurs above the T7/8 area.

- If the breathing wave starts in the upper thoracic spine this suggests an upper-chest breathing pattern. NOTE: Observation of the wave is not diagnostic, but offers evidence of the current spinal response to breathing. This 'wave' may be monitored from treatment session to treatment session, to see whether it slowly normalizes – becoming longer and starting lower, suggesting an improvement in breathing function and greater mobility of the thoracic cage and spine. The wave provides a 'snapshot' of increased, or decreased, or static, functional efficiency of the spinal and thoracic structures in response to a normal function, i.e. breathing.
- If the breathing wave is other than a movement from the sacrum to the upper thoracic area, a degree of spinal restriction probably exists, correlating with 'flat' segments observed during seated or standing flexion.

Evidence from these functional tests, as well as from the palpation assessment and observation of breathing function (see above), may suggest which postural muscles are most likely to require attention for hypertonicity shortening and/or weakness. A selection of specific assessments of the key muscles for relative shortness is described below – however it is important to note that there are numerous additional assessment protocols.

ASSESSMENT OF SHORTNESS IN ACCESSORY (AND OBLIGATORY) BREATHING MUSCLES

Frequent or continued deep and/or rapid breathing (hyperpnoea) results in progressive muscular fatigue and increasing sensations of distress. Renggli et al (2008) report that during normocapnic hyperpnoea (involving partial re-breathing of CO_2), contractile fatigue of the diaphragm and abdominal muscles develops, triggering an increased recruitment of rib cage muscles. Han et al (1993) described the action, and interaction, of these rib cage muscles, during ventilation, noting that the parasternal intercostal muscles act in concert with the scalenes to expand the upper rib cage, and/or to prevent it from being drawn inward by the action of the diaphragm, during quiet breathing. The respiratory activity of the external intercostals, however, appear to constitute a reserve system, only being recruited when increased expansion of the rib cage is required. The implications point to the need for attention to the often-neglected intercostal muscles, during breathing rehabilitation, and not only the more obvious (e.g. scalenes) muscles.

Masubuchi et al (2001) used fine-wire electrodes inserted into muscles, and high-resolution ultrasound, to compare the activity of three muscle groups, in response to various respiratory and postural manoeuvres. They demonstrated that the scalenes are the most active, and trapezius the least active, cervical accessory inspiratory muscles, while SCM is intermediate. This confirms what has long been suspected by observation and palpation – that the scalenes are the most important respiratory muscle group lying superior to the thorax. It is suggested that the relative lack of involvement of the upper trapezius (UT) muscles during respiration should not lead to them being ignored in the context of breathing rehabilitation, as they have profound effects on (and are affected by) posture – which itself impacts breathing function (Gregory 2007). See notes on upper crossed syndrome and also Figures 2.2.1, 2.2.3, 2.2.4.

Lewit (2009) simplifies the need to assess for shortness of UT by stating. 'The upper trapezius should be treated if it is tender and taut.' Since this is an almost universal state in modern life, it seems that *everyone* requires appropriate treatment of UT to encourage reduction in its probable (assumed) hypertonic state in most adults. More specifically UT has been found to be overactive (and therefore by implication shortened) in singers (Pettersen 2005) (see also Ch. 7.5) and mouth-breathing children (Ribeiro-Corre et al 2004). Of interest in relation to current mobile (cell) phone use, Lin & Peper (2009) report that:

83% of [college students] reported hand and neck pain during texting, and held their breath when receiving text messages.

Scalene dysfunction and the presence of trigger points in them ('functional pathology') were identified in more than 50% of individuals, in a series of 46 hospitalized patients who demonstrated paradoxical patterns of respiration (Pleidelová et al 2002). The implications of the presence of myofascial trigger points, in relation to breathing function, are discussed later in this chapter in regard to assessment, and again in Chapter 7.2 in regard to treatment approaches.

Barrier terminology

When describing somatic dysfunction such as muscle shortness, or joint restriction, the words 'ease' and 'bind' are often used to describe what is noted when tissues and structures are unduly tight or loose. When joint and soft tissue 'end-feel' is being evaluated, a similar concept is involved in the area being evaluated, and it is common practice to make sense of such findings by comparing sides (Kaltenborn 1985).

The characterization of features described as having a 'soft' or 'hard' end-feel, or as being tight or loose, or as demonstrating feelings of 'ease' or 'bind', may relate to chronic or acute changes, and such distinctions influence the choice of therapeutic approach or approaches, and the sequence in which these are introduced. The findings loose, tight, etc. have an intimate relationship with the concept of barriers, which need to be identified in preparation for direct methods – where action is directed towards the restriction barrier, i.e. towards bind, tightness – and indirect methods – where action involves movement away from barriers of restriction, toward ease, looseness. Such methods are described in Chapter 7.2.

Not every shortened muscle requires attention

It is seldom necessary to treat all shortened muscles that may be identified as part of a dysfunctional pattern. For example, Lewit (2009) and Simons et al (1998) report that isometric relaxation of the suboccipital muscles will also relax the sternocleidomastoid muscles; release of the thoracolumbar muscles induces relaxation of iliopsoas, and vice versa; and treatment of the scalene and sternocleidomastoid muscles, for example using muscle energy technique (MET) (as described in Chapter 7.2) also relaxes the pectorals.

The muscles described below are a selection of those most intimately involved with the biomechanical function of breathing. These muscles can become dysfunctional due to habitual overuse and misuse factors or due to trauma, as well as through the influence of emotions (see Ch. 5). Short, tight muscles predispose to the evolution of myofascial trigger points at both the motor end point (muscle belly, central points) and at the attachments (Mense &

Simons 2001) (see notes on trigger points later in this chapter and in Ch. 7.2).

The relative shortness of the following muscles should be assessed and charted: quadratus lumborum, psoas, pectoralis major, latissimus dorsi, upper trapezius, levator scapulae, scalenes, sternocleidomastoid, as well as thoracic and cervical paraspinal musculature (see Box 2.2.2, and also individual muscle assessment methods below).

Assessment for shortness of iliopsoas (Fig. 6.2.12)

Psoas is intimately associated with the diaphragm and its function which makes assessment for shortness, and rehabilitation of excessive shortness, a priority in breathing rehabilitation. See Figures 2.2.7 and 2.2.9 for a reminder of the relationship between psoas and the diaphragm.

For the test the patient lies supine with the buttocks (coccyx) as close to the end of the table as possible, the non-tested-side leg held towards the chest to produce stability in the pelvis while the tested side leg hangs freely off the end of the table, with the knee flexed.

Full flexion of the non-tested-side hip helps to maintain the pelvis in full rotation with the lumbar spine flat. This is essential if the test (Thomas test) is to be meaningful, and stress on the spine avoided.

If the thigh of the tested leg lies in a horizontal position, parallel to the floor, as well as there being a degree of 'spring' as the thigh is moved passively towards the floor, then the indication is that iliopsoas is not short.

If, however, the thigh rises above the horizontal – or is parallel with the floor but has a rigid feel – then iliopsoas

is probably short. If effort is required to achieve 10° of hip extension, this suggests iliopsoas shortening on that side.

Peelera & Anderson (2007) have noted that while there are doubts regarding the 'statistical reliability of the [Thomas test] when used to score ROM and ilio-psoas muscle flexibility about the hip joint' – it nevertheless remains a useful clinical tool.

Assessment for shortness of quadratus lumborum (Fig. 6.2.13)

The side-lying hip abduction test described earlier in this chapter offers an indication of overactivity (and therefore probable shortness) of QL. An indication of the relative shortness is obtained by means of observation:

The patient stands with her feet shoulder-width apart, and side-bends as far as comfortably possible sideways, running the hand down the side of the thigh. No forward or backward bending should be combined with side-bending in this test.

One side is compared with the other in terms of the degree of flexibility, using the knee crease as a marker. If it is not possible to reach as far to the left as it is to the right, then the quadratus lumborum (QL) muscle on the right is probably shortened. It should be possible to reach to just below the knee crease.

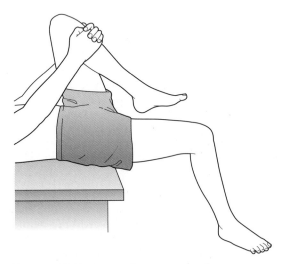

Figure 6.2.12 Thomas test for assessment of psoas shortness. The unsupported leg should lie with the thigh parallel to the floor, and should easily be moved into 10° of extension, if psoas is not short.

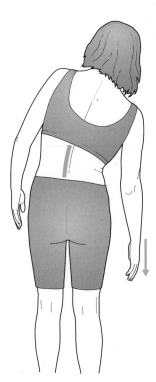

Figure 6.2.13 Assessing side-bending range as an indication of QL shortness.

Assessment for shortness in pectoralis major (Fig. 6.2.14)

The patient lies supine, with the head approximately 40 cm from the top edge of the table, and is asked to rest the arms, extended above the head, on the treatment surface, palms upwards. If these muscles are normal the arms should be able easily to rest directly above the shoulders, in contact with the surface for almost all of their length, with no arching of the back or twisting of the thorax. If an arm cannot rest with the dorsum of the upper arm fully in contact with the table surface, without effort, then pectoral fibres are probably short.

Assessment of the subclavicular portion of pectoralis involves abduction of the arm to 90° from the body. In

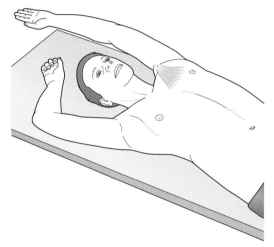

Figure 6.2.14 Observational assessment of shortness in pectoralis major. If the arm is unable to lie flat against the supporting surface, and alongside the head, in the absence of shoulder dysfunction, pectoralis major is probably shortened.

this position the tendon of pectoralis at the sternum should not be found to be unduly tense, even with maximum abduction of the arm.

Assessment for shortness of upper trapezius (Fig. 6.2.15)

The patient is supine, with the head/neck fully rotated and laterally flexed away from the tested side. The practitioner stands at the head of the table and assesses the ease with which the shoulder can be depressed (moved distally). There should be an easy springing sensation as the shoulder is pushed toward the feet, with a soft end-feel. If there is a 'solid' end-feel, the posterior fibres of upper trapezius are probably short.

With the head and neck fully rotated away from the side to be tested, and side-flexed to approximately 40°, shoulder 'springing' should be tested. If it is rigid the posterior fibres of upper trapezius are probably shortened. Half-turning the head away from the side to be assessed and using the same methodology, allows assessment of the middle fibres of upper trapezius, while rotation of the head toward the side being tested, allows assessment of the anterior fibres, using the same shoulder springing evaluation. In each instance, normal upper trapezius status is indicated if 40° to 45° of lateral flexion is possible while retaining a degree of spring when the shoulder is depressed.

NOTE: The treatment and assessment positions for the muscle are the same – as described in Chapter 7.2.

Assessment for shortness in scalenes

Hudson et al (2007) observe that human scalenes are obligatory inspiratory muscles that have a greater

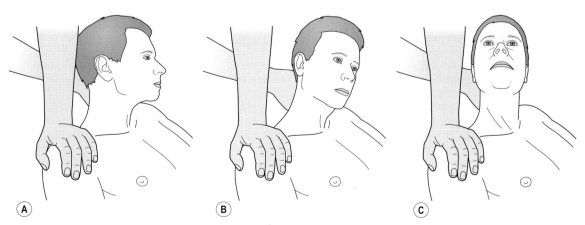

(A)   (B)   (C)

Figure 6.2.15 MET assessment of right side upper trapezius muscle. **A** Posterior fibres, **B** middle fibres, **C** anterior fibres.

mechanical advantage than the sternocleidomastoid (SCM) muscles, which are accessory respiratory muscles. They found that irrespective of respiratory tasks the scalenes and SCM are recruited in the order of their mechanical advantages – with scalenes always starting to operate earlier than SCM. The scalenes, which are prone to trigger point activity, are a controversial muscle since they seem to be both postural and phasic in nature, their status being modified by the type(s) of stress to which they are exposed. Janda (1996) reports that, 'spasm and/or trigger points are commonly present in the scalenes as also are weakness and/or inhibition.'

There is no easy test for shortness of the scalenes, apart from observation, palpation, and assessment of trigger point activity/tautness and a functional observation as follows:

The practitioner places his relaxed hands over the patient's shoulders so that the fingertips rest on the clavicles, at which time the seated patient is asked to inhale moderately deeply. If the practitioner's hands noticeably rise during inhalation, then there exists inappropriate use of scalenes, suggesting that they will have become shortened and would benefit from stretching.

Adapted from Lewit 2009

In reality, everyone with an upper-chest breathing pattern will display hypertonic scalenes.

Assessment for shortness of sternocleidomastoid

As for the scalenes, there is no absolute test for shortness of sternocleidomastoid (SCM), but observation of posture (hyperextended neck, chin poked forward) and palpation of the degree of induration, fibrosis and trigger point activity (see below), can all alert to probable shortness. This is a postural, accessory breathing muscle which, like the scalenes, will be shortened by inappropriate breathing patterns which have become habitual.

Observation is an accurate assessment tool. Since SCM is barely observable when normal, if the clavicular attachment is easily observed, or any part of the muscle is prominent, this can be taken as an indication of tightness of the muscle.

If the patient's posture involves the head being held forward of the body, it is often accompanied by cervical lordosis and dorsal kyphosis – see Chapter 2.2 for discussion of upper crossed syndrome. In such individuals weakness of the deep neck flexors and tightness of SCM can be suspected (Hudson et al 2007).

MYOFASCIAL TRIGGER POINTS: RELEVANCE AND ASSESSMENT

Myofascial trigger points (MTrPs) are palpable, punctate areas of hardening in muscle tissue ('taut bands'), that are painful on movement of the muscle, and on palpation. Light-microscopic studies have revealed contraction knots within MTrPs (Simons et al 1998) involving local thickenings of individual muscle fibres associated with contraction of sarcomeres. It is proposed by Mense (2008) that a muscular lesion damages the neuromuscular endplate (Simons 2002) and that this tissue damage results in abnormal amounts of acetylcholine (ACh) being released from the nerve terminal of the motor endplate, leading to contraction knots and other contractile effects, causing local ischemia and hypoxia – combined with a greatly increased energy consumption. A combination of increased energy demand and loss of energy (ATP) supply, creates a crisis that causes release of neuro-vasoreactive sensitizing substances. The resulting depolarization produces a contraction knot that compresses neighbouring capillaries, causing local ischemia, leading to the release of substances that sensitize nociceptors, partially explaining the tenderness of MTrPs noted on applied pressure. A variety of these sensitizing substances have been found to be present within MTrPs on dialysis analysis (Shah 2005).

In addition, Baldry (2001) has observed that hypoxia induced by hyperventilation, is a potent stimulator of bradykinin release, encouraging perpetuation of MTrP sensitization, and persistence of pain.

Lucas et al (2004) found that the presence of trigger points in myofascial structures alters activation (firing) sequences in entire kinetic chains. In addition MTrPs in the cervical, shoulder-girdle, thoracic or lumbar muscles strongly influence, and can be strongly influenced by, disturbances of ventilation mechanics, such as paradoxical respiration, or by abnormal postural patterns (Sachse 1995, Lewit 2009).

Relevance of trigger points in breathing pattern disorder

MTrPs may occur in any age group, except infants. They often appear to result from local muscle overuse and ischemia, and have been associated with localized pain problems, joint dysfunction, visceral and pelvic diseases, hypothyroidism, auto-immune diseases, infections, complex regional pain syndrome, hypoglycaemia, systemic medication effects (particularly statin drugs), metabolic or nutritional imbalances (ferritin, vitamin B12, vitamin D in particular) (Dommerholt & Huijbregts 2011).

MTrPs are a major source of pain and dysfunction generally, however the relevance of their inclusion in this chapter relates less to this than to their potential impact on respiratory function. See Figures 6.2.16 and 6.2.17.

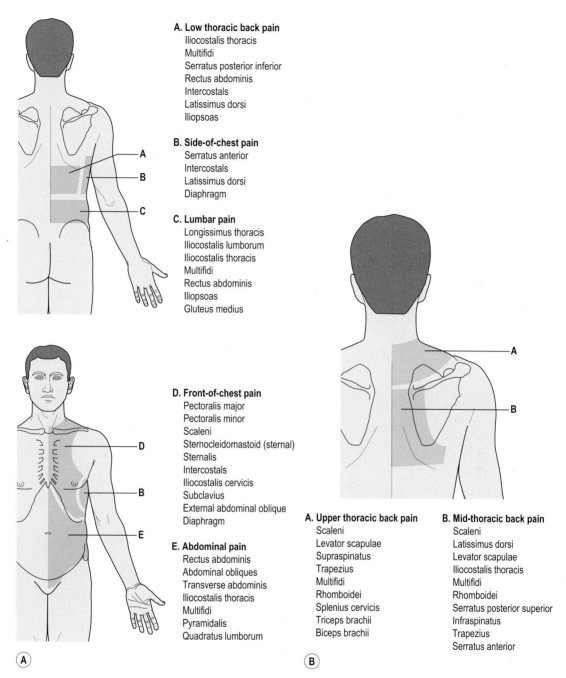

A. Low thoracic back pain
Iliocostalis thoracis
Multifidi
Serratus posterior inferior
Rectus abdominis
Intercostals
Latissimus dorsi
Iliopsoas

B. Side-of-chest pain
Serratus anterior
Intercostals
Latissimus dorsi
Diaphragm

C. Lumbar pain
Longissimus thoracis
Iliocostalis lumborum
Iliocostalis thoracis
Multifidi
Rectus abdominis
Iliopsoas
Gluteus medius

D. Front-of-chest pain
Pectoralis major
Pectoralis minor
Scaleni
Sternocleidomastoid (sternal)
Sternalis
Intercostals
Iliocostalis cervicis
Subclavius
External abdominal oblique
Diaphragm

E. Abdominal pain
Rectus abdominis
Abdominal obliques
Transverse abdominis
Iliocostalis thoracis
Multifidi
Pyramidalis
Quadratus lumborum

A. Upper thoracic back pain
Scaleni
Levator scapulae
Supraspinatus
Trapezius
Multifidi
Rhomboidei
Splenius cervicis
Triceps brachii
Biceps brachii

B. Mid-thoracic back pain
Scaleni
Latissimus dorsi
Levator scapulae
Iliocostalis thoracis
Multifidi
Rhomboidei
Serratus posterior superior
Infraspinatus
Trapezius
Serratus anterior

Figure 6.2.16 AB Possible tissues and structures affected by trigger points in listed muscles.

Identifying MTrPs

The ability to reliably palpate a taut band or to elicit a twitch response in a muscle varies and depends on the palpation skills and training of the examiner and the depth and size of the muscle. Gerwin et al (1997) found that inter-rater reliability improves when examiners are well trained before testing. Sciotti et al (2001) demonstrated that four blinded experienced examiners who 'trained extensively together prior to the study' were able

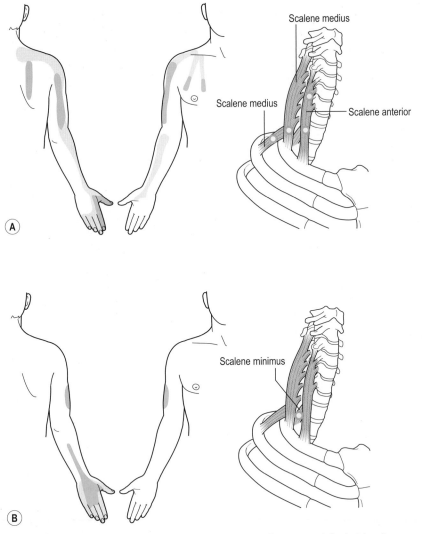

Figure 6.2.17 AB Scalene trigger points produce patterns of common complaint potentially deriving from any of the scalene muscles.

to reliably (80% agreement) identify the location of latent MTrPs in the upper trapezius muscle.

Diagnostic features of MTrPs (Simons et al 1998, Simons 2002, Simons 2004)

In osteopathic medicine, the acronym 'STAR' is a reminder of the characteristics of somatic dysfunction:

- **Sensitivity** – is almost always present on movement and/or applied pressure
- **Texture change** – dysfunctional tissues, including the skin (Box 6.2.2) may 'feel' tense, fibrous, swollen, hot, cold or display other 'differences' from normal

- **Asymmetry** – common, but not always present
- **Range of motion reduced** – involving muscles and/or joints.

The locality, but not the nature or etiology, of a problem is confirmed when two or three of these features are identified. In a blind study Fryer et al (2004) confirmed that when thoracic paraspinal muscles palpated as 'abnormal' (tense, dense, indurated) the same tissues also had lowered pain threshold (using an algometer).

Sikdar et al (2008) demonstrated that myofascial trigger points can be visualized using diagnostic ultrasound and sonoelastography. Myofascial trigger points are hypoechoic on two-dimensional ultrasound and appear stiffer than the surrounding muscle on vibration sonoelastography.

Box 6.2.2 Skin palpation methods (drag, etc.) for myofascial trigger points

The skin overlying areas of reflexively active tissue has a heightened sympathetic tone and increased sweat activity (Lewit 2009). This increased hydrosis results in a sense of hesitation as a finger or thumb is very lightly passed across the skin. The degree of pressure required is minimal, with skin touching skin being all that is necessary (a 'feather-light' touch).

Movement of a single palpating digit should be purposeful, not too slow, and certainly not very rapid. Around 5–7 cm per second is a satisfactory speed.

A sense of 'drag' which suggests a resistance to the easy passage of the finger across the skin surface is felt for. This can be sensed as 'dryness', a 'sandpapery' feel, or a slightly harsh or rough texture. These may all indicate increased presence of sweat.

Once located, deeper pressure should elicit an area of discomfort, or, if over an active trigger point, an exquisitely sensitive area, which may refer pain elsewhere. Additional characteristics of skin overlying trigger points include the following (and see Fig. 6.2.18):

- Skin more adherent to underlying fascia, elicited by 'skin-rolling' or comparing bilateral skin 'pushes' which evaluate 'slideability' of local skin areas

- Skin loses local elasticity which is evaluated by introducing a sequential stretching of the skin, taking it to its elastic barrier and comparing with immediately adjacent area, and so on until an area is noted where elasticity is markedly reduced (this would also be an area of 'drag')

- There would be a variation in temperature compared with surrounding tissue, commonly warmer (indicating relative hypertonicity), but sometimes colder if tissues are ischemic (Barral 1988)

- A goose flesh appearance is observable in facilitated areas when the skin is exposed to cool air, the result of a facilitated pilomotor response

- A palpable sense of 'drag' is noticeable as a light touch contact is made across such areas, due to increased sweat production resulting from facilitation of the sudomotor reflexes

- There is likely to be cutaneous hyperesthesia in the related dermatome, as the sensitivity is increased (for example to a pin prick) due to facilitation

- An 'orange peel' appearance is noticeable in the subcutaneous tissues when the skin is rolled over the affected segment, due to subcutaneous trophoedema.

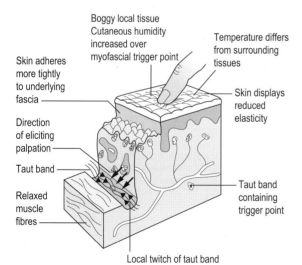

Boggy local tissue
Cutaneous humidity increased over myofascial trigger point

Temperature differs from surrounding tissues

Skin adheres more tightly to underlying fascia

Skin displays reduced elasticity

Direction of eliciting palpation

Taut band

Taut band containing trigger point

Relaxed muscle fibres

Local twitch of taut band

Figure 6.2.18 Altered physiology of tissues in region of myofascial trigger point. *Reproduced with kind permission from Chaitow & DeLany 2000.*

When MTrPs are present there may be a history of a regional aching pain complaint, with onset related to acute, chronic or repetitive muscle overload. Associated pain intensity is usually related to movement or positioning but may become continuous when severe. Diagnostic findings commonly involve:

- A painful limit to stretch range of motion
- Presence of a palpable taut band housing an exquisitely tender nodule.

Pressure on this is likely to elicit pain that is familiar to the patient and often a pain response (jump sign).

Figures 6.2.16a and 6.2.16b illustrate areas of the body that might be affected by trigger points in the listed muscles, with a potential to influence respiratory function. Trigger points might be located anywhere in the listed muscles, but most commonly near the belly/motor end-point, and close to attachments.

Figure 6.2.17 shows symptomatic areas affected by trigger points in the scalene muscles. Treatment options are discussed in Chapter 7.2.

CONCLUSION

This chapter has highlighted assessment approaches in identification of biomechanical as well as functional changes associate with BPD. The particular relevance to a person's breathing pattern of such dysfunction, revealed via assessment, will be individual to them. It is suggested that breathing rehabilitation protocols should include strategies aimed at improving the biomechanical, as well as functional status of the structures – osseous and soft-tissue – that are most involved in the processes of respiration.

REFERENCES

Baldry, P., 2001. Myofascial pain and fibromyalgia syndromes. Churchill Livingstone, Edinburgh.

Barral, J.P., 1988. Visceral manipulation. Eastland Press, Seattle.

Beal, M.C., 1983. Palpatory testing for somatic dysfunction in patients with cardiovascular disease. J Am Osteopath Assoc 82, 822–831.

Bradley, D., 1998. Hyperventilation syndrome: breathing pattern disorders and how to overcome them. Kyle Cathie, London.

Chaitow, L., DeLany, J., 2000. Clinical applications of neuromuscular techniques. Volume 1: Upper body. Churchill Livingstone, Edinburgh.

Chaitow, L., DeLany, J., 2010. Clinical applications of neuromuscular techniques. Volume 2: Lower body, second ed. Churchill Livingstone, Edinburgh.

Chila, A., 1997. Fascial-ligamentous release. In: Ward, R. (Ed.), Foundations for osteopathic medicine. Williams and Wilkins, Baltimore.

Cleland, J.A., Childs, J.D., Fritz, J.M., 2006. Inter-rater reliability of the history and physical examination in patients with mechanical neck pain. Arch. Phys. Med. Rehabil. 87 (10), 1388–1395.

Cleland, J.A., Childs, J.D., Fritz, J.M., et al., 2007. Development of a clinical prediction rule for guiding treatment of a subgroup of patients with neck pain: use of thoracic spine manipulation, exercise, and patient education. Phys. Ther. 87 (1), 9–23.

Courtney, R., 2009. The functions of breathing and its dysfunctions and their relationship to breathing therapy. International Journal of Osteopathic Medicine 12, 78–78.

Dommerholt, J., Huijbregts, P.A., 2011. Myofascial trigger points: pathophysiology and evidence-informed diagnosis and management. Jones & Bartlett, Boston.

Dommerholt, J.C., Bron, C., Franssen, J., 2006. Myofascial trigger points: an evidence-informed review. J Manual Manipulative Ther 14, 203–221.

Flynn, T., Whitman, J., Magel, J., 2001. Orthopaedic manual physical therapy management of the cervical-thoracic spine & ribcage. Evidence in Motion, Louisville, KY.

Fryer, G., Morris, T., Gibbons, P., 2004. Relation between thoracic paraspinal tissues and pressure sensitivity measured by digital algometer. Journal Osteopathic Medicine 7 (2), 64–69.

Gerwin, R., Shannon, S., Hong, C.Z., et al., 1997. Interrater reliability in myofascial trigger point examination. Pain 69, 65–73.

Greenman, P., 1996. Principles of manual medicine. Williams and Wilkins, Baltimore.

Gregory, S., 2007. Evaluation and management of respiratory muscle dysfunction in ALS. Neuro-Rehabilitation 22, 435–443.

Han, J., Gayan-Ramirez, G., Dekhuijzen, R., 1993. Respiratory function of the rib cage muscles. European Respiratory Journal 6 (5), 722–728.

Heiderscheit, B., Boissonnault, W., 2008. Reliability of joint mobility and pain assessment of the thoracic spine and rib cage in asymptomatic individuals. J. Man. Manip. Ther. 16 (4), 210–216.

Hruby, R., Goodridge, J., 1997. Thoracic region and rib cage. In: Ward, R. (Ed.), Foundations of osteopathic medicine. Williams & Wilkins, Baltimore.

Hruby, R., Hoffman, K., 2007. Avian influenza: an osteopathic component to treatment. Osteopath Med Prim Care 1, 10.

Hruska, R., 1997. Influences of dysfunctional respiratory mechanics on orofacial pain. Dent Clin North Am. 41, 211–227.

Hudson, A., Gandevia, S., Butler, J., 2007. The effect of lung volume on the co-ordinated recruitment of scalene and sternomastoid muscles in humans. J Physiol 584 (1), 261–270.

Janda, V., 1996. Evaluation of muscular balance. In: Liebenson, C. (Ed.), Rehabilitation of the spine. Williams and Wilkins, Baltimore.

Janda, V., Frank, C., Liebenson, C., 2006. Evaluation of muscular imbalance. In: Liebenson, C. (Ed.), Rehabilitation of the spine, second ed. Lippincott Williams and Wilkins, Baltimore.

Kaltenborn, F., 1985. Mobilization of the extremity joints. Olaf Norlis Bokhandel, Universitetgaten 24, N-0162 Oslo 1, Norway.

Knott, M., Tune, J.D., Stoll, S.T., et al., 2005. Lymphatic pump treatments increase thoracic duct flow. JAOA 105, 447–456.

Kuchera, M., Goodridge, J., 1997. Lower extremity. In: Ward, R. (Ed.), American Osteopathic Association: Foundations for Osteopathic Medicine. Williams and Wilkins, Baltimore.

Lewit, K., 2009. Manipulative Therapy: Musculoskeletal Medicine. Churchill Livingstone, Edinburgh.

Liebenson, C., 1999. Re-education of faulty respiration. Journal of Bodywork and Movement Therapies 3 (4), 225–228.

Lin, I.M., Peper, E., 2009. Psychophysiological patterns during cell phone text messaging: a preliminary study. Appl Psychophysiol Biofeedback 34 (1), 53–57.

Lindgren, K., Leino, E., Manninen, H., 1989. Cineradiography of the hypomobile first rib. Arch. Phys. Med. Rehabil. 70 (5), 408–409.

Lindgren, K.-A., 1997. Conservative treatment of thoracic outlet syndrome: a 2-year follow-up, Arch Phys Med Rehabil 78, 373–378.

Lucas, K., 2004. Latent myofascial trigger points: their effects on muscle activation and movement efficiency. Journal of Bodywork & Movement Therapies. 8 (3), 160–166.

Masubuchi, Y., Abe, T., Yokoba, M., 2001. Relation between neck accessory inspiratory muscle electromyographic activity and lung volume. Journal Japanese Respiratory Society 39 (4), 244–249.

Mense, S., 2008. Muscle pain: mechanisms and clinical significance. Dtsch Arztebl Int 105 (12), 214–219.

Mense, S., Simons, D., 2001. Muscle pain; understanding its nature, diagnosis and treatment. Philadelphia, Lippincott Williams & Wilkins, Baltimore.

Morris, C., Chaitow, L., Janda, V., 2006. Functional examination of low back syndromes. In: Morris, C. (Ed.), Low back syndromes. McGraw-Hill, New York.

Palastanga, N., Field, D., Soames, R., 2002. Anatomy and human movement, fourth ed. Butterworth-Heinemann, Oxford, pp. 478–479.

Peelera, J., Anderson, J., 2007. Reliability of the Thomas test for assessing range of motion about the hip. Physical Therapy in Sport 8, 14–21.

Pettersen, V., 2005. Muscular patterns and activation levels of auxiliary breathing muscles and thorax movement in classical singing. Folia Phoniatr Logop. 57 (5–6), 255–277.

Pleidelová, J., Balážiová, M., Porubská, V., 2002. Frequency of scalenal muscle disorders. Rehabilitacia 35 (4), 203–207.

Pryor, J.A., Prasad, S.A., 2002. Physiotherapy for respiratory and cardiac problems, third ed. Churchill Livingstone, Edinburgh.

Renggli, A., Verges, S., Notter, D., 2008. Development of respiratory muscle contractile fatigue in the course of hyperpnoea. Respiratory Physiology & Neurobiology 164, 366–372.

Ribeiro-Corre, E., Marchiori, S.C., Silva, A.M.T., 2004. Electro-myographic muscle activity in mouth and nasal breathing children. J Craniomandibular Prac 22, 45–50.

Riley, G.W., 2000. Osteopathic success in the treatment of influenza and pneumonia 1919. JAOA 100, 315–319.

Ross, J., Bereznick, D., McGill, S., 2004. Determining cavitation location during lumbar and thoracic spinal manipulation: is spinal manipulation accurate and specific? Spine 29 (13), 1452–1457.

Sachse, J., 1995. The thoracic region's pathogenetic relations and increased muscle tension. Manuelle Medizin 33, 163–172.

Sciotti, V., Mittak, V.L., DiMarco, L., 2001. Clinical precision of myofascial trigger point location in the trapezius muscle. Pain 93, 259–266.

Shah, J., 2005. An in vivo microanalytical technique for measuring the local biochemical milieu of human skeletal muscle. J Appl Physiol 99, 1977–1984.

Sikdar, S., Shah, J.P., Gilliams, E., et al., 2008. Assessment of myofascial trigger points (MTrPs): a new application of ultrasound imaging and vibration sonoelastography. Conf Proc IEEE Eng Med Biol Soc 2008, 5585–5588.

Simons, D., Travell, J., Simons, L., 1998. Myofascial pain and dysfunction: the trigger point manual, Vol. 1 second ed. Williams and Wilkins, Baltimore.

Simons, D., 2002. Understanding effective treatments of myofascial trigger points. Journal of Bodywork and Movement Therapies 6 (2), 81–88.

Simons, D., 2004. New Aspects of Myofascial Trigger points - etiological and clinical. Journal of Musculoskeletal Pain 12 (3/4), 15–21.

Smith, R.K., 1920. One hundred thousand cases of influenza with a death rate of one-fortieth of that officially reported under conventional medical treatment. Journal American Osteopathic Association 20:172–175. Reprinted in 2000: Journal American Osteopathic Association 100, 320–323.

Vance, C., 2003. Enhance patient compliance by targeting different learning styles. Podiatry Today 16 (8), 28–29.

Ward, R.C., Hruby, R.J., Jerome, J.Z., 2002. Foundations for osteopathic medicine, third ed. Lippincott Williams & Wilkins, Baltimore.

Chapter | **6.3** |

Physiotherapy assessment approaches

Dinah Bradley

Physiotherapy has been involved in the assessment and treatment of chest problems, whether from organic disease or from functional or idiopathic causes, for many decades. Early published physiotherapy literature including Thompson & Thompson (1968), Cluff (1984), Innocenti (1987) and Holloway (1992) formed the backbone of future directions in physiotherapy management.

Breathing Works©, an independent physiotherapy service, has developed professional assessment and treatment guidelines for managing symptomatic breathing pattern disorders, known as the BradCliff® Method. The approach has been to further advance assessment strategies, patient educational material, stress reduction techniques, physical coping skills, and exercise plans to help patients restore confidence and health (Clifton-Smith & Rowley 2011).

PHYSIOTHERAPY ASSESSMENT

The physiotherapy approach described below in treating people with breathing pattern disorders may be summarized as 'maximum involvement with minimum intervention' (Hough 2001). Many patients have already been tested exhaustively – sometimes by painful or invasive investigations – and often arrive with nervous expectations of yet more. Self-confidence may have evaporated and secondary problems emerged. Avoidance behaviours and phobias may have flourished, along with feelings of extreme anxiety. The cascade of symptoms is shown in Box 6.3.1.

Symptomatic breathing dysfunction affects emotions. While there are prescribed rituals to deal with well-understood major upheavals such as death, divorce or trauma, those who experience the frightening or worrying

Box 6.3.1 **Cascade of symptoms**

Original cause (emotional or physical)
↓
Tension and anxiety
↓
Hyperventilation
↓
Acute hyperventilation attack
↓
Anticipation anxiety
↓
Avoidance behaviours/phobias

Box 6.3.2 **Smokers**

Inhalations from cigarettes, cigars and pipes reinforce upper-chest breathing patterns. While not wanting to encourage smokers to breathe abdominally (drawing smoke into the depths of the lung):
- Smokers can be offered smoking cessation programmes
- Marijuana smokers, who tend to prolong hyperinflation, must be discouraged from doing this
- Those who choose to continue can be encouraged to breathe in lightly and very shallowly.

symptoms of chronically disordered breathing are often poorly understood. They suffer without the automatic social support of more tangible life events and are often labelled as hypochondriacs or 'highly strung'. Thus the 'low-tech' approach makes a refreshing change for most patients. Management includes assessment and treatment involving detailed explanations of breathing pattern disorders, the physiological consequences of 'overbreathing' and building an individual integrated recovery programme based on:

- Breathing awareness and retraining
- Tension release through talk and relaxation
- Stress perception and management
- Enjoyable graduated exercise prescriptions
- Rest/sleep guides (Bradley 2012).

The environment

An airy, quiet room with a relaxed atmosphere is recommended for assessment and treatment. A welcoming sense of safety, confidentiality and privacy is essential, with comfortable chairs and treatment bed. Space for extra family members or friends should be provided if requested, and a box of tissues and drinking water should be on hand. An hour should be allotted for the first appointment.

Physiotherapy assessment

Patient referrals can arrive from many sources: specialist medical consultants, general practitioners, psychologists, practice nurses, community health workers, speech therapists or dentists, or patients may refer themselves. Some provide a detailed picture, while others offer only scant information with little or no background information. Clear communications with referral agents are essential.

When patients self-refer, and present with no records of previous tests or health problems, it is recommended that permission should be sought from these patients to liaise with their general practitioners/physicians.

CAUTION: If any patients have unexplained chest pain, breathlessness, or dizziness, the therapist must report to and check with the patient's doctor before assessment, in order to rule out more sinister causes.

Detailed history

Prescribed medications should be recorded to establish current treatments and conditions, and possible side-effects. For example, beta-blockers may have been prescribed to patients experiencing stress/adrenalin-induced cardiac arrhythmias. These medications can cause bronchospasm, exacerbating hyperventilation.

Past medical history

Past health problems may provide clues and should be listed; for example 'chesty' as a child, sinus problems, facial trauma, history of allergy, anaemia, diabetes, migraine, gastro-esophageal reflux disease (GERD), emotional or physical trauma, 'panic' attacks, anxiety and depression, past surgeries and number of hospital admissions.

Current health problems such as irritable bowel, headaches, constipation, sleep disturbances, premenstrual or menopausal hormone difficulties, chronic fatigue or fibromyalgia, tinnitus and orofacial or temporomandibular joint (TMJ) pain should be noted.

Socially acceptable drug use (e.g. tobacco, caffeine and alcohol) should be recorded (Box 6.3.2). Recreational drug use or past or present history of addiction as possible contributing factors to present health status should be discussed. Referral on to relevant agencies and websites may be offered if the patient requests help. Check your local agencies.

As sleep is the barometer of overall health, sleep disturbances or disorders the patient may be experiencing should be recorded. The commonest sleep-related disorder is insomnia; others include obstructive sleep apnoea (OSA), snoring, or shift work sleep adjustments.

A chance to talk about symptoms and give a subjective view to an empathetic ear will help establish rapport and trust: for some patients it may the first time they have really been listened to – a case of literally 'getting it off one's chest'.

History taking is also an excellent time to note autonomic disturbances (e.g. clammy hands, sweating, dilated pupils, postural tension/restlessness, rapid speech) indicating sympathetic dominance (Nixon & Freeman 1988).

Social history

Sensitive enquiries will help reveal stress-related events/triggers. Occupation, job satisfaction, redundancy issues, marital status, whether the patient's domestic life is calm, complicated or isolated should be noted.

Record how many days off work or school the patient has had in the last 6 months. This is a useful statistic to keep, for long-term outcome measures.

Sensitive topics may surface such as abuse, emotional or sexual problems. Be prepared to listen, and if the patient wishes, further expert help can be offered from specialist counsellors. See also Chapter 6.4.

History of tests/investigations

An inventory of tests and investigations gives a clear picture to the therapist of the number of interventions the patient has endured and what coexisting problems may have been revealed (e.g. anaemia), or ruled out (e.g. brain tumour). Possible interventions include blood tests, X-rays, lung function tests, sleep studies, scans, neurology or cardiology tests.

Alternative therapies

Natural remedies or dietary changes which may currently be impacting on the patient's health profile need to be recorded and openness encouraged in discussing these. Orthodox medicine's reluctance to recognize or offer treatment options to people with chronic breathing pattern disorders often drives sufferers to seek alternatives – sometimes drastic, and often very expensive, which may have no accountability or research data to back up claims. CAUTION: There is also the risk of harm caused by dangerous combinations of prescribed medication with herbal remedies. As with all drugs, whether prescription or naturopathic, make sure that your patients understand exactly what they are swallowing, and why.

Questionnaires

Nijmegen Questionnaire

As yet there is no 'gold standard' laboratory test to clinch the diagnosis of chronic HVS. However, the Nijmegen Questionnaire (see questionnaire on p. 145 in Ch. 6.5) is the next best thing, and provides a non-invasive test of high sensitivity (up to 91%) and specificity up to 95% (Van Dixhoorn & Duivenvoorden 1985). This easily administered, internationally validated (Vansteenkiste et al 1991) diagnostic questionnaire is the simplest, kindest, and, to date, most accurate indicator of acute/chronic hyperventilation. It also has great educative value as patients often for the first time appreciate the widespread nature of their symptoms.

Retesting at a later date is helpful in showing patients their progress as their symptoms decrease or vanish. It is common for chronic hyperventilators to concentrate on the most worrying symptom (i.e. chest pain) and ignore others. Retesting can help patients to accept that faulty breathing affects all systems and in fact they have 'a welter of bodily symptoms' (Lum 1985).

The results also help establish:

- Whether the initiating triggers causing hyperventilation syndrome/breathing pattern disorders (HVS/BPDs) have been resolved; the patient will then only have to deal with the 'bad breathing' habit and the musculoskeletal and motor pattern changes they have been left with.
- If the initiating triggers are ongoing or unresolved; the patient may need further psychological help. Shared care with a psychiatrist, psychologist, or psychotherapist may be offered to this group of patients.
- An appreciation by the therapist as to what symptoms the patient is struggling against.

The Rowley Breathing (RoBE) Self-Efficacy Scale

This self-administered scale is a functional indicator of how a patient's breathing pattern disorder is affecting or altering their normal daily life (Rowley & Nichols 2006). While the Nijmegen scale tells the patient and therapist about symptoms, the RoBE Scale records improvements or regressions in function (e.g. are they able to take part in sport again?). See Chapter 9 to view the scale, and information sheet for practitioners on how to use and interpret this questionnaire.

The Hospital Anxiety and Depression (HAD) Questionnaire (Zigmond & Snaith 1983)

This is also a simply administered score which helps identify anxiety or depression levels. Co-treatment with a counsellor or psychologist may be indicated if patients agree to added help (see Ch. 9). CAUTION: Suicidal thoughts or intentions must be reported at once to the patient's doctor, or relevant crisis management team if the patient is under psychiatric care.

Clinical observation of rate and patterns of breathing

After observing unobtrusively the patient's posture/body language while history taking, note should be taken of the following:

1. Resting respiratory rate (normal adult range is 10–14 per minute) (West 2000).
2. Nose or mouth breather?
3. Resting breathing pattern:
   a. Effortless upper chest/hyperinflation?
   b. Accessory muscle use?
   c. Frequent sighs/yawns?
   d. Breath holding ('statue breathing')?
   e. Abdominal/pelvic splinting?
   f. Chaotic/combinations of the above?
   g. Repeated throat clearing/air gulping?

These observations can be made discreetly while taking the patient's radial pulse.

Nasal problems (see also Ch. 2.3)

One of the most frequent findings in patients with HVS/BPD is chronic mouth breathing. To check nasal airflow:

Hold a small pocket mirror under the patient's nostrils and note the exhaled moisture pattern on the surface. Two areas of condensation should appear, indicating airflow from both nostrils. If one nostril is blocked, note which one.

To further check for partial or complete obstruction, use a sinus rinse bottle or nose pipe to check flows from right to left and vice versa.

Check this website for more information. http://www.fammed.wisc.edu/research/past-projects/nasal-irrigation (Accessed June 2013).

Obstruction

If partial or complete obstruction is revealed (reduced or absent saline solution flow), discuss with the patient and their doctor the option of scheduling a mini series CT scan to establish the source of the problem. Referral on to an otorhinolaryngeal (ORL) specialist may be required to sort out these problems before starting effective breathing retraining.

Children with sleep disordered breathing (SDB) may have obstructive sleep apnoea (OSA) or snore due to enlarged tonsils and adenoids. This group would not benefit from breathing retraining until these problems are addressed by an appointment with a paediatric ORL or sleep specialist.

Snoring

In adults, OSA and snoring are the most common SDB problem and can flourish if a patient is overweight. Excess weight on the outside of the throat increases pressure on the inside of the throat, which in turn narrows or intermittently collapses the upper airways. If alcohol, tranquilizers or sleeping pills are used prior to going to sleep, these can excessively relax throat muscles as well, making people more susceptible to OSA.

Enlarged tonsils or nasal obstruction may also be a factor and require ORL specialist assessment. An appointment at a sleep clinic for help with lifestyle changes or assessment for use of a CPAP (continuous positive airway pressure) device would be advised (Gay 2006).

Seasonal rhinitis

Children with seasonal rhinitis may benefit from saline nasal rinsing to help clear their upper airways and assist nose breathing (Garavello et al 2011).

Some chronic mouth breathers simply have 'soggy' noses through disuse which respond well to saline/bicarbonate nasal washes (Rabago & Zgierska 2009). This aids the mucociliary linings to slough off excess mucus build-up and restore normal function. The addition of bicarbonate of soda adds to the effectiveness by acting rather like Teflon® (non-stick), coating the nasal linings to aid drainage (see example recipe in Ch. 9).

Mouth breathing

Patients with mild to moderate OSA who hyperventilate and are mouth breathers, have been shown to improve their symptoms with restoration of nose/diaphragm breathing by day, to influence nose/abdominal breathing while sleeping. Specific oropharyngeal exercises have also been shown to reduce snoring, and OSA (Gulmaraes et al 2009) in mild to moderate cases, and is an alternative – and novel–way to treat OSA. See http://www.youtube.com/watch?v=RB3nCDA1uic (Accessed June 2013)

Breath-hold tests

While no standardized test yet exists, breath-hold times are recorded by many clinicians as a part of HVS/BPD assessment. Failure to hold beyond 30 seconds is considered by some a positive diagnostic sign of chronic hyperventilation (Gardner 1996). In practice, chronic hyperventilators seldom hold beyond 10–12 seconds before gasping. It makes a useful marker to test at regular intervals, and note improved breath-holding times (see Chs 7.6 and 8.2 for more on this topic).

Musculoskeletal inspection/observation

Observe and draw on a body chart (Fig. 6.3.1) any areas of pain, tension and other symptoms such as numbness, paresthesia or skin colour changes.

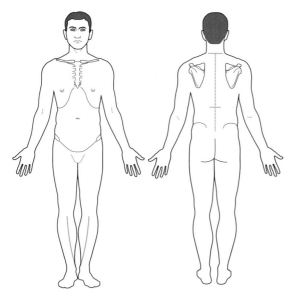

Figure 6.3.1 Body map.

Note jaw, facial and body tension, tremor, tics or twitches. Note chest wall abnormalities, such as:

- pectus carinatum (anterior sternal protrusion)
- pectus excavatum (depression or hollowing of the sternum)
- kyphosis (abnormal forward anteroposterior spinal curvature)
- scoliosis (lateral spinal curvature)
- kyphoscoliosis (a combination of the former two).

Adaptive upper thoracic and shoulder-girdle muscle changes

Check and record active and passive ranges of motion of the cervical and thoracic spine, scapular movement and the glenohumeral joints to reveal excessive overuse of upper chest and the respiratory accessory muscles.

Check and note abdominal wall and pelvic tension/splinting.

Box 6.3.3 describes some of the factors thought to contribute to occupational overuse syndrome and repetitive strain injury.

Three key upper thoracic trigger points are shown in Figures 6.3.3–6.3.5. See also Chapter 6.2 for more examples.

Selection of appropriate ventral and dorsal upper chest and neck trigger points and recording the subjective response by the patient on the Numeric Pain Scale (Box 6.3.4, Jensen et al 1986) to palpation of these points provides a repeatable objective measure of:

Box 6.3.3 Work-related breathing problems
(Fig. 6.3.2)

Thoracic outlet nerve and blood vessel compression due to musculoskeletal changes from persistent upper-chest breathing has been implicated in the development of occupational overuse syndrome (OOS)/repetitive strain injury (RSI) – the blight of the electronic age. Schlieffer & Ley (1994) have presented a hyperventilatory model of psychological stress as a contributing factor to the current epidemic of musculoskeletal problems in repetitive VDU/computer work.

They found that under stressful conditions (high workload demands, long hours, boredom, and fatigue), sedentary breathing exceeds metabolic requirements for oxygen, and hypocapnia results. At the cellular level, relatively mild reductions in arterial CO_2 result in a rise in pH (alkalosis). Under such conditions, heightened neuronal activity, increased muscle tension and spasming, paresthesiae, and a suppression of parasympathetic activity, and consequent sympathetic dominance of the autonomic nervous system, result in amplified responses to catecholamines. These hyperventilatory-induced stress reactions have been implicated as an important factor in work-related overuse and stress injuries.

While there are excellent OOS prevention schemes, with on-site ergonomic checks and strategies, few include breathing awareness/retraining as part of overall stress reduction. Schleifer & Ley's findings indicated a positive correlation between work-related hyperventilation and onset of symptoms. More recent research has shown links in overbreathing, neck and arm pain triggered by digital phone use and texting.

In addition to breathing retraining, mobilizing exercises to reduce thoracic outlet restrictions, and neural stretches can be taught in liaison with occupational safety and health officers and GPs.

- The intensity of chest wall pain at assessment
- Reduction in chest wall pain in response to breathing retraining and employment of muscle stretch/release and relaxation techniques.

While no move to deactivate trigger point pain by compression is part of the BradCliff® treatment plan, rechecking at regular intervals monitors progress and motivates patients to persevere with breathing retraining, body awareness of tension, and return of elasticity to their muscles. It also serves as a useful marker for the patients themselves to check as part of symptom recognition (Chaitow & DeLany 2008).

For details of the BradCliff® Angle Test (xyphycostal border) see Chapter 7.6.

Patients who have tight 'switched on' abdominal muscles, either from psychosocial tensions, or overdoing 'abs' training may have a reduced xyphocostal angle,

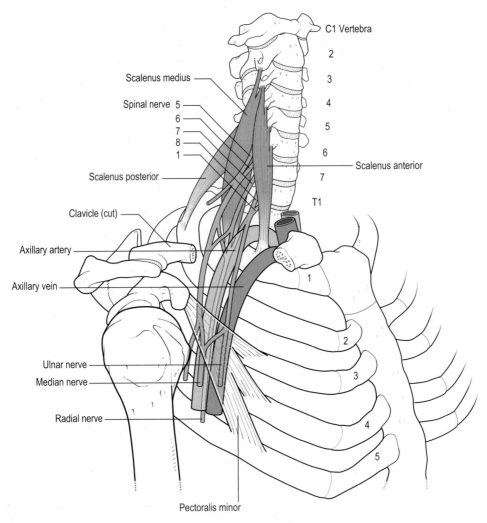

Figure 6.3.2 Thoracic outlet.

Box 6.3.4 **The Numeric Pain Rating Scale** (Jensen et al 1986)

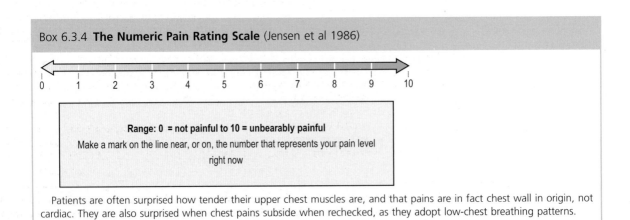

Range: 0 = not painful to 10 = unbearably painful
Make a mark on the line near, or on, the number that represents your pain level
right now

Patients are often surprised how tender their upper chest muscles are, and that pains are in fact chest wall in origin, not cardiac. They are also surprised when chest pains subside when rechecked, as they adopt low-chest breathing patterns.

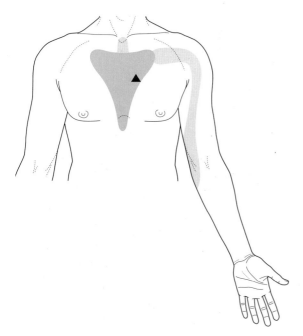

Figure 6.3.3 The pattern of pain referral from a trigger point (or points) in the sternalis muscle. *From Baldry 1993.*

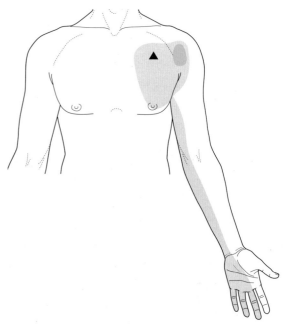

Figure 6.3.5 The pattern of pain referral from a trigger point (or points) in the pectoralis minor muscle. *From Baldry 1993.*

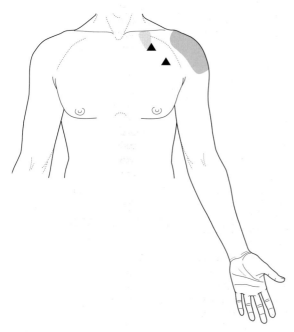

Figure 6.3.4 The pattern of pain referral from a trigger point (or points) in the clavicular section of the pectoralis major muscle.

restricting normal diaphragm excursion (normal ranges are between 75–90 degrees).

Oximetry

An oximeter is a small battery-operated hand-held device allowing for non-invasive instant feedback of arterial oxygen (O_2) saturations. It is recorded as SpO_2 to differentiate from arterial blood gas (ABG) saturations of haemoglobin with oxygen (SaO_2) analyses obtained from arterial puncture (Hanning & Alexander-Williams 1995). Measured as a percentage, pulse oximetry is reasonably accurate at values above 75%. Desaturation is indicated at values below 95% in black skinned people, 92% in white people, or a drop of 4% (Durbin 1994). Oximeters may be fooled by the presence of anaemia, hypotension, hypovolaemia, peripheral vascular disease or vasopressor drugs. Nicotine stains and nail varnish both compromise finger sensor readings.

Normal resting SpO_2 levels are between 95% and 98% (West 2000).

With patients who demonstrate breathing pattern disorders, there are two purposes in using an oximeter:

1. As a safety measure to check patients with concurrent cardiac or respiratory disease. For example, unexplained chest pain, breathlessness with hypoxaemia may indicate pulmonary embolus.

Box 6.3.5 **Oxygen carrying capacity**
(Carroll 1997)

Overall oxygen carrying capacity is calculated by multiplying 1.34 ml (the amount of oxygen 1 g of haemoglobin carries) by the haemoglobin level and the SpO_2 reading.

For instance, if patient X's haemoglobin is 15 g/dL, SpO_2 saturations 97%, the calculation would be: $1.34 \times 15 \times 0.97 = 19.5$ ml/dL, within the normal range of 19–20 ml/dL. Shortness of breath would not be caused by low oxygen carrying capacity.

Patient Y, also with SpO_2 sats of 97%, who has a low haemoglobin level of 11 g/dL, by the same calculation ($1.34 \times 11 \times 0.97 = 14.3$ ml/dL) would experience shortness of breath from reduced availability of oxygen to the tissues.

SpO_2 values should be interpreted in context with the patient's total haemoglobin levels where possible.

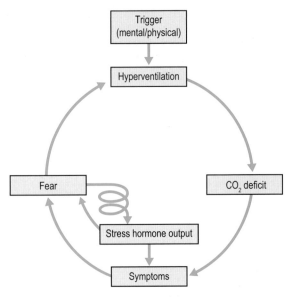

Figure 6.3.6 Atypical breathing problems.

2. As a teaching aid, it is a positive way of showing patients in otherwise good health they have plenty of available O_2 and can easily afford to reduce their respiratory rate and volume. Chronic overbreathers tend to be well above 95%, the minimum normal level. A high proportion are 100% saturated, much to their surprise. (See Box 6.3.5.)

Capnography (see also Ch. 7.7)

Hospital physiotherapists may have access to a capnograph. This device measures end tidal CO_2 levels from exhaled air (collected via nasal prongs), which resembles those of arterial values. Fluctuating CO_2 levels, or those below 32 mmHg (4.3 kPa) would suggest chronic hyperventilation (Timmons & Ley 1994). Outcome measures may also be provided (Hough 2001).

Peak expiratory flow rate (PEFR)

A peak flow meter is a simple, inexpensive device which measures the highest flow of air out of the lungs, from peak inspiration, in a fast single forced breath out. This reflects airflow resistance, the elasticity of the supporting lung tissues and ease of breathing. Its uses are those listed below:

- As a kinder and less risky alternative to the hyperventilation provocation test (HVPT) (see Ch. 6.4 p. 134).
- The best of three blows in quick succession may elicit light-headedness or familiar tingling, linking the relationship between overbreathing and symptoms to the patient.

- Revealing 'normal lung power' often encourages those who frequently feel 'air hunger' or chest tightness.
- Reductions in normal expected flows would indicate the need for spirometry/further investigations for more accurate measures.
- Establishing a baseline for people with asthma, or chronic airflow limitation at the start of treatment.

Another use is for patients who have been on repeated or prolonged courses of oral steroids, for whatever reason, and who may therefore have reduced skeletal muscle strength. The diaphragm is not exempt.

Breathing retraining with diaphragm strengthening and inspiratory muscle training (IMT) (McConnell 2011, Cochrane Review 2009) may show an improvement within 2–6 weeks. A simply measured outcome is a repeat PEFR after a month of retraining.

Education

The time spent on history taking and data gathering is an excellent opportunity for explanations of the mechanical and physiological consequences of breathing dysfunction. At the summing up of findings, the therapist can complete a fuller teaching session with the help of visual aids (e.g. diagrams of the chest walls, lungs, diaphragm, nasopharynx, typical and atypical breathing patterns (Fig. 6.3.6)).

Discretion as to how much detail to go into at first should be considered, since too much information may 'go in one ear and out the other'. Highly stressed patients often have poor concentration. Getting straight to quietness and simple physical coping skills, with biomechanical explanations being left until later may be the better option.

After collating all the relevant findings, a personalized treatment plan can be created, with patient involvement. Find out what your patient's expectations are, as well as their commitment to their new plan and possible lifestyle changes (reduce caffeine intake, prioritize obligations for example.) Treatment with clear measurable and attainable goals can then get underway.

See Chapter 7.3 for physiotherapy rehabilitation strategies.

REFERENCES

Baldry, P., 1993. Acupuncture, trigger points and muscular pain. Churchill Livingstone, Edinburgh.

Bradley, D., 2012. Hyperventilation syndrome/breathing pattern disorders. Random House NZ.

Carroll, P., 1997. Pulse oximetry: at your fingertips. RN (Feb), 22–27.

Chaitow, L., DeLany, J., 2008. Clinical applications of neuromuscular techniques. Vol 1: Upper body, second ed. Churchill Livingstone, Edinburgh, p. 110.

Clifton-Smith, T., Rowley, J., 2011. Breathing pattern disorders and physiotherapy: inspiration for our profession. Physical Therapy Reviews 16 (1), 75–86.

Cluff, R.A., 1984. Chronic hyperventilation and its treatment by physiotherapy: discussion paper. Journal of the Royal Society of Medicine 77, 855–862.

Cochrane Review, 2009. IMT Asthma Review. Ram, F.S.F., Wellington, S.R., Barnes, N.C. Inspiratory muscle training for asthma. Cochrane Database of Systematic Reviews 2003, Issue 3. Art. No.: CD003792. DOI: 10.1002/14651858. CD003792.<IMT asth09.pdf>

Durbin, C.G., 1994. Monitoring gas exchange. Respiratory Care 39, 123–137.

Garavello, W., Romagnoli, M., Sordo, L., et al., 2011. Hypersaline nasal irrigation in children with symptomatic seasonal allergic rhinitis: A randomized study. Pediatric Allergy and Immunology 14 (2), 140–143, April 2003.

Gardner, W.N., 1996. The patho-physiology of hyperventilation disorders. Chest 109, 516–534.

Gay, P., Weaver, T., Loube, D., et al., 2006. Evaluation of positive airway pressure treatment for sleep related breathing disorders in adults. SLEEP 29 (3), 381–401.

Gulmaraes, K., Drager, L., Genta, P., et al., 2009. Effects of oropharyngeal exercises on patients with moderate obstructive sleep apnoea syndrome. American Journal of Respiratory Critical Care Medicine 179, 962–966.

Hanning, C.D., Alexander-Williams, J.M., 1995. Pulse oximetry: a practical view. British Medical Journal.

Holloway, E., 1992. The role of the physiotherapist in hyperventilation. In: Timmons, B.H., Ley, R. (Eds.), Behavioral and psychological approaches to breathing disorders (Ch. 11). Plenum Press, New York, London.

Hough, A., 2001. Physiotherapy in respiratory care, third ed. Nelson Thornes Publishers, pp. 278.

Innocenti, D.M., 1987. Chronic hyperventilation syndrome. Cash's textbook of chest, heart and vascular disorders for physiotherapists, fourth ed. Faber and Faber, London, pp. 537–549.

Jensen, M.P., Karoly, P., Braver, S., 1986. The measurement of clinical pain intensity: a comparison of six methods. Pain 27, 117–126.

Lum, L.C., 1985. Psychogenic breathlessness and hyperventilation. Update 12 July, pp. 99–111.

McConnell, A., 2011. Breathe strong perform better. Human Kinetics Publishing.

Nixon, P.G., Freeman, L.J., 1988. The 'think test': a further technique to elicit hyperventilation. Journal of the Royal Society of Medicine 81, 277–279.

Rabago, D., Zgierska, A., 2009. Saline nasal irrigation for upper respiratory conditions. Am Fam Physician 2009. Nov 15;80 (10), 1117–1119.

Rowley, J., Nichols, D., 2006. Development of the RoBE self-efficacy scale for people with breathing pattern disorders. NZ Journal Physiotherapy 34 (3), 131–141.

Schlieffer, L., Ley, R., 1994. End tidal CO_2 as an index of psychophysiological activity during VDU data entry work, and relaxation. Ergonomics 37 (245), 261–266.

Thompson, B., Thompson, H., 1968. Forced expiratory exercises in asthma and their effects on FEV1. New Zealand Journal of Physiotherapy 3 (15), 19–21.

Timmons, B.H., Ley, R., 1994. Behavioural and psychological approaches to breathing disorders. Plenum, London.

Van Dixhoorn, J., van Duivenvoorden, H., 1985. Efficacy of Nijmegen questionnaire in recognition of hyperventilation syndrome. Journal of Psychosomatic Research 29, 199–206.

Vansteenkiste, J., Rochette, F., Demendts, M., 1991. Diagnostic tests of hyperventilation syndrome. European Respiratory Journal 4, 393–399.

West, J.B., 2000. Respiratory physiology: the essentials. Lippincott, Williams and Wilkins, Philadelphia.

Zigmond, A.S., Snaith, R.P., 1983. The Hospital Anxiety and Depression Scale. Acta Psychiatrica Scandinavica 67, 361–370.

Chapter | **6.4**

Psychological assessment of breathing problems

Chris Gilbert

As discussed in Chapter 5, a breathing pattern can be disrupted by emotional stimuli which are strictly internal and sometimes unknown to the person, so this type of assessment is hard to quantify. Yet the breathing pattern can be chronically altered by an emotional bias which has become an 'attitude' in both senses of the word: a state of mind with a predisposition to respond in a certain way, or a 'way of holding oneself' (American Heritage Dictionary 2000). Besides applying to posture, this could be applied to breathing style. The psychologically minded clinician can make headway sometimes by inquiring about chronic emotional states which might be congruent with a particular breathing pattern (see Bloch et al 1991, covered in Chapter 5).

PHYSIOLOGICAL MONITORING OF THE BREATHING PATTERN

Biofeedback involves both detecting and displaying some physiological variable, completing an information loop for the person being monitored. However, biofeedback instruments are, first, monitors of physiological activity, and can be used without the information loop for measurement only. Some body variables are relatively stable and not so easily changed by transient emotions. Breathing, however, is easily altered by conscious intent as well as shifting attitudes, and directing a person's attention to his/her breathing will certainly alter it. So assessing breathing pattern should be unobtrusive or else the pattern will show the effects of being observed. Distraction or covert measurement will yield a better sample of natural breathing.

Below are five ways that breathing pattern can be measured fairly easily so that indicators of breathing rate, inhale/exhale ratios, presence of pauses, steadiness of breathing, and involvement of upper chest vs. abdomen can be obtained while the person is distracted or in some way not attending to the information being gathered (Fig. 6.4.1).

1. **Strain gauge:** This is a stretchable band, tube or line placed around the circumference of the chest or abdomen, or both. Change in electrical resistance from changing the length of the sensor translates into rise and fall of a value as the subject inhales and exhales. With two separate sensors and channels, the ratio of thoracic to abdominal breathing can be ascertained.

2. **Surface electromyography (EMG):** Adhesive electrodes are placed over the muscles of interest, usually upper trapezius or scalene muscles, to follow the muscle as it participates in exhalation and inhalation. Like the strain gauge method, monitoring specific muscles also indicates relative dominance of thoracic or abdominal breathing. The signal is displayed on a video monitor, as a sound, as a moving light or LEDs, or as digits on a display.

3. **Air temperature at the nostril:** By placing the sensor of a fast-response digital thermometer in the air stream from a nostril, temperature will be seen to vary as much as 5.5 °C between exhalation and inhalation. Display can be a moving line on a video screen, a fluctuating sound, moving light or numerical display. This method shows clearly the duration of the exhalation.

4. **Heart rate variability:** This requires an ECG setup or a photoplethysmograph sensor linked to software for analyzing this variable. Normally the heart rate rises and falls in synchronization with the breathing cycle, so that the displayed output resembles the breathing trace from the previous three methods.

5. **End-tidal CO_2,** measured with a capnometer, rises as an exhalation proceeds and reaches a peak just before inhalation begins. The trace, displayed as changes in numbers or a line on a screen, contains dynamic breathing information similar to the other methods in addition to CO_2 level for each exhalation, which can indicate adequacy of respiration and presence of hypo- or hyperventilation.

For most of these measures there is a range defining 'normal', so that some evidence for a breathing disorder can be obtained with a brief sample, provided it is not influenced by the patient's attempt to do 'good breathing'. With EMG, a clear involvement of the trapezius, sternocleidomastoid or scalene muscles will confirm observation of excessive thoracic breathing (see Figs 6.4.2 and 6.4.3).

Air temperature at the nose will reveal regularity and rate of breathing. A strain gauge shows the relative participation of thoracic and abdominal areas if two strain gauges are used; if not, then only regularity and rate. Heart rate variability shows the response of the heart rate to breathing, an index of autonomic balance, but can usually be used as a quick measure of breathing rate also, even when only heart rate is being measured. Finally, end-tidal CO_2 readings for each breath show normality of CO_2 relative to hypo- or hyperventilation; this display will also contain information about rate and regularity of breathing. These measures are obviously redundant with each other, but if one wishes to use simple equipment to obtain objective measures of breathing, one or two of these five would suffice.

In monitoring natural breathing with any of these methods, baseline information about breathing style can be obtained under the conditions at the time of measurement. Yet many instances of dysfunctional breathing patterns will be intermittent, specific to particular conditions such as being in the workplace, at a computer, in tense social situations, or being in an anxious or angry mood.

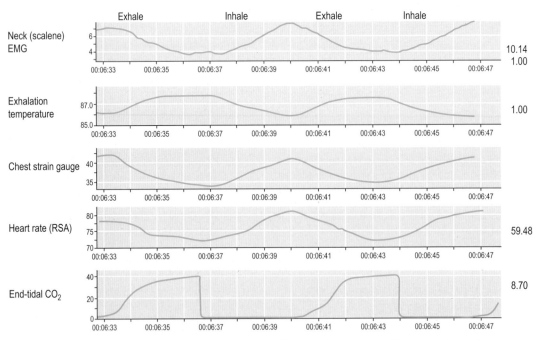

Figure 6.4.1 Five ways to monitor breathing. 14-second record of five simultaneous breathing traces. Top to bottom: muscle tension in scalene muscles; temperature at the nostril; thoracic circumference; heart rate synchronized with breathing; exhalation of CO_2.

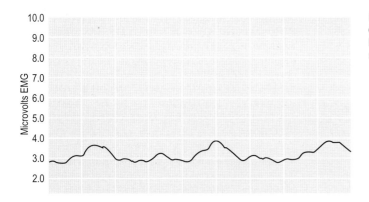

Figure 6.4.2 EMG tracing of scalene muscle (side of neck) during normal breathing (three breaths) with abdominal expansion and shoulders relaxed.

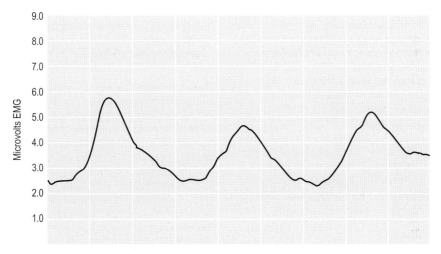

Figure 6.4.3 EMG tracing of scalene muscle (three breaths) with abdominal movement restricted; accessory muscles recruited.

Determining the chronicity of the disordered breathing pattern calls for more questioning. Without ambulatory monitoring, assessment during real-life conditions may not be possible, but sometimes asking the patient to recall the details of those conditions is enough to bring out the aberration in breathing.

Two breathing assessment questionnaires are useful in this regard: the Nijmegen Questionnaire (NQ) and the Self-Evaluation of Breathing Questionnaire (SEBQ). The first has a 28-year history (van Dixhoorn & Duivenvoorden 1985) and seeks to evaluate the likelihood that certain symptoms indicate a chronic hyperventilation pattern. The SEBQ is newer (Courtney & Greenwood 2009, Courtney et al 2011) and includes more items inquiring about perception of dysfunctional breathing and lack of air. They are both one page long, easy to score and understand, and

yield a good sampling of reported symptoms related to disordered breathing, though they are not specific to hyperventilation. Both the SEBQ and the NQ are covered thoroughly in Chapter 6.5, and the complete questionnaires are available in that chapter's appendices.

Psychological factors include subjective expectations, memories and persistent attitudes, along with consequent observable behaviours. A breathing pattern represents some combination of reflexive and intentional input plus a constant stream of emotional shading reflecting many things, including one's feelings about the breathing itself. Just as candid photos of people represent how they usually look more accurately than does a posed photo, observing natural breathing requires diverting the patient's attention from voluntary control of breathing. How a person breathes in response to 'Now just breathe naturally for me' is likely to be very different from covert observation of someone breathing in the waiting room.

The following are some possibilities to consider when faced with an aberrant breathing pattern plus perhaps any results from a breathing questionnaire.

1. How does the patient interpret the breathing problem? Is it considered dangerous, annoying, distracting, embarrassing or does it represent an attempt to feel better? 'Take a deep breath' can become an all-purpose coping method for any emotional stress.
2. Does the breathing problem occur continuously in many diverse settings and conditions or is it episodic? If the latter, are the triggering conditions known? Normalizing breathing in a clinical setting may not generalize to a high-pressure workplace or a stressful social situation.
3. What capacity does the patient have to change any aspect of the breathing voluntarily, on demand? To some people, slowing one's exhalation or switching from abdominal to thoracic breathing seems as unattainable as ear-wiggling.
4. How psychologically minded is the person? Is he/she likely to consider emotional influences on their breathing pattern, or simply scoff at the question and just wish the problem to be fixed?
5. Is there a general pattern of being bothered by signs of anxiety – for instance, uneasiness about heart palpitations, sweating or restlessness?

Regarding this last issue, the Anxiety Sensitivity Index has proved useful for examining this aspect of the mind-body interface.

THE ANXIETY SENSITIVITY INDEX

The Anxiety Sensitivity Index (ASI) is a 16-item scale that focuses on apprehension about the symptoms of anxiety itself (see Box 6.4.1 for sample test items). A key trait in most panic patients is anxiety about the symptoms of

being anxious. This self-referential problem is often called a 'vicious circle' and is akin to 'fear of fear'. Whether the attention is focused on accelerated heart rate, sweating, dyspnoea, light-headedness or some other bodily sign of anxiety, some people react very strongly to these symptoms, and they tend to be high scorers on the ASI.

Reiss et al (1986), originators of the ASI, suggested that anxiety sensitivity functions as an amplifier of anxiety. In their words:

…anxiety sensitivity may be a predisposing factor in the development of fears and other anxiety disorders. According to this view, people who believe that anxiety has few negative effects are more able to tolerate anxiety-provoking stimuli. In contrast, people who believe that anxiety has terrible effects, such as heart attacks and mental illnesses, may tend to have anxiety reactions that grow in anticipation of severe consequences. Anxiety sensitivity implies a tendency to show exaggerated and prolonged reactions to anxiety-provoking stimuli.

Reported symptoms are not necessarily 'objective' data just because they are physical. Sturges et al (1998) gave female college students the ASI and then a hyperventilation challenge task consisting of eight 15-second intervals of hyperventilation, separated by 10-second periods in which they tried to estimate their heart rates. Skin conductance was also monitored. Subjects rated both the magnitude of their physiological sensations and their subjective degree of distress. Those who had high scores on the ASI judged their heart rate changes as larger, and their anxiety as more intense, than those with low scores on the ASI. However, the actual changes in heart rate and skin conductance did not differ between the two groups; the difference was due to biased perception alone. 'Anxiety sensitivity' somehow amplified the bodily changes in the minds of the subjects. Factor analysis has shown that simply having higher general anxiety is not responsible for high ASI scores; the questionnaire taps a specific kind of anxiety which might be termed a 'body phobia.'

The ASI has been found to distinguish panic and hyperventilation syndrome from other anxiety disorders. It is more specific to panic and to hyperventilation than standard anxiety tests such as the State-Trait Anxiety Inventory or Hamilton Anxiety Inventory, which do not discriminate between panic and generalized anxiety disorder, obsessive-compulsive disorder, and simple phobias. According to some studies (e.g. Cox et al 1996), the ASI contains four factors:

1. Fear of cardiorespiratory distress and gastrointestinal symptoms
2. Fear of cognitive/psychological symptoms
3. Fear of symptoms visible to others (social fear)
4. Fear of fainting and trembling.

Box 6.4.1 **Sample items from the anxiety sensitivity index**

'It scares me when my heart beats rapidly.'

'When I am nervous, I worry that I might be mentally ill.'

'It is important for me to stay in control of my emotions.'

If, for example, a person is interpreting the mental fogginess accompanying hyperventilation to mean that he is losing his mind, this could be addressed with explanations and reassurance about the limits to the deficit. Another person may be unconcerned about the mental fogginess but quite anxious about the palpitations as possible warning signs of a heart attack. This could also be dealt with by education and reassurance. So the test responses, ideally, can direct the psychological treatment as surely as a blood test would direct treatment in the medical realm.

Adding the ASI to an evaluation takes only a few minutes and provides additional data about the person who has the problem, as opposed to data about the problem itself (objective data such as respiration rate, CO_2 readings, reported symptoms, etc.). A high score compared with the ASI norms suggests that a subjective factor is amplifying the symptom picture. Seeing one's abnormally high score on a brief test like the ASI can spark new insight in a person and encourage rethinking the significance of anxiety symptoms. The 'vicious circle' concept is usually familiar to patients in some form, so suggesting that their anxiety is in part a response to their fear of being anxious can deflate the whole symptom complex, including anxious breathing.

Anxiety sensitivity is also associated with deficient coping resources for emotional distress (Kashdan et al 2008), and this is associated with magnification and persistence of anxiety symptoms, including disordered breathing and its effects. Processing and expressing negative feelings is a skill that some people lack, leaving them less able to regulate their emotional life, and this pattern correlates with the ASI. Helping such a person to regulate breathing is part of the solution, but regulating the effect behind the symptom may be as important.

Patients with breathing complaints may be missing the deeper reason for the symptoms as they seek a more simple solution. Similarly, indigestion due to poor eating choices, or arm pain due to muscle overuse, can be reduced by behaviour changes rather than medicine. Sometimes referral to a mental health specialist will be a better treatment choice than attempting to improve the breathing pattern. Anxiety sensitivity is a complex cognitive-emotional trait that may show limits to the patient's coping strategies for self-regulation of emotion, so that focus is placed on the somatic aspect of anxiety rather than catastrophic thinking in general.

RESPIRATORY SINUS ARRHYTHMIA (RSA)

This term refers to the cyclic rise and fall of the heart rate in rhythm with breathing. Most people tend to consider a steady, unvarying heartbeat a good sign, perhaps because skipped beats, palpitations, extra beats and a racing heart are all deviations from clock-like steadiness. The truth is actually the opposite: a heartbeat that is steady like a metronome is not a sign of good health, and if chronic, usually indicates autonomic dysfunction and increased risk of cardiovascular disease (Thayer et al 2010). Yoo et al (2011) found that low variability correlates with the Framingham risk score, and thus increased risk of coronary heart disease. (The term 'heart rate variability' – or HRV– is used when describing the RSA activity quantitatively.)

In a relaxed, healthy person, the heart rate normally rises during inhalation and drops with exhalation. The range of variation in beats per minute can range from fewer than 5 to more than 30, but averages between 8 and 14. This variability is often used as an index of general vagal tone, since when the autonomic nervous system is properly balanced there is a waxing and waning of parasympathetic influence with each breath. Stress and hyper-vigilance reduce the parasympathetic component, leaving the autonomic nervous system unbalanced and biased toward action and danger. Deep, slow breathing amplifies the variability; atropine, a parasympathetic inhibitor, will abolish it.

Much basic physiological research is being done in this area and some applied research as well (Lehrer et al (2004) for asthma, Hassett et al (2007) for fibromyalgia, and Zucker et al (2009) for PTSD symptoms). Inflammation and depression have also shown response to improved HRV. The general assumption is that learning to increase HRV promotes a healthier balance between sympathetic and parasympathetic dominance. Many chronic disorders which involve autonomic imbalance seem to respond to the slow steady breathing involved in HRV training.

Although low HRV cannot be said to reflect a breathing pattern disorder in the narrow sense, its long-term nature has important health implications, and can be improved by improving the breathing pattern. Monitoring HRV can involve elaborate electrocardiographic equipment, but any device which can display heart rate and updates rapidly can give rough biofeedback, and simply palpating the pulse will give an indication of whether the heartbeat is rising and falling in line with the breathing rhythm. A popular hardware/software package is made by Heartmath for both clinical and lay use; it is widely used for biofeedback of HRV, with a photoplethysmograph sensor instead of ECG leads. While its precision and diagnostic utility are limited, it can provide a starting point and does show changes in HRV according to breathing and relaxation. If ECG equipment is available, software to derive HRV measures extend its use to either brief or overnight assessment.

PSYCHOPHYSIOLOGICAL MONITORING

Many breathing pattern problems represent a too-tight coupling between the emotional life and breathing. This

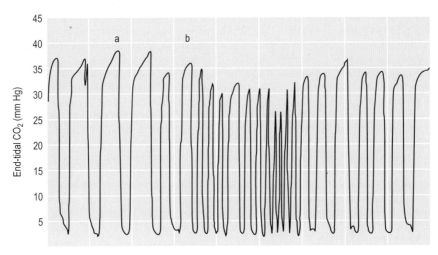

Figure 6.4.4 Capnogram showing drop in 36-year-old male patient's end tidal CO_2 while relaxing **(a)** and **(b)** starting to think (with frustration) about a missed job promotion. Trace duration was 90 seconds. Each wave represents a breath: peaks are end-points of exhalations.

interaction conflicts with innate breathing regulation in the same way that eating can be disrupted by psychological factors. Voluntary regulation of the breath (trying to 'breathe well') may be opposed by emotional factors which can, for instance, serve as a brake on free abdominal expansion. The works of Wilhelm Reich and Alexander Lowen address this issue thoroughly (Gilbert 1999).

Assessing the psychological influences on breathing behaviour can be simple or complicated (see Fig. 6.4.4). Simply observing the change in breathing from a stressful state to a relaxed state can be informative to both parties; if there is a large adjustment in a good direction (slower, more abdominal, more regular), this shows good response of the system to calming down. Lack of response to suggested relaxation does not mean that relaxation 'doesn't help'; it may mean that the person is not feeling relaxed, but rather immobile and tense.

The descriptions in Chapter 5 of using hypnosis to discover hidden triggers for hyperventilation shows what can be done, but this is usually impractical. Inquiry about possible sources of a persistent breathing problem, especially when more direct breathing training has failed, is a reasonable step for any clinician to consider. Rather than limit the inquiry to talking and listening, if possible it is very useful to monitor breathing during the discussion using one of the instruments described earlier, so that the clinician is attending to the bodily as well as the verbal responses. For instance: while monitoring breathing pattern in some way:

1. Inquire about history of near-suffocation such as near-drowning, a pillow over the face, a frightening asthma episode or any near-strangulation. Such experiences can establish a deep and life-long, sometimes phobic anxiety about breathing, and hypersensitivity to relevant cues and conditions.

2. Inquire about whether either breath-holding or overbreathing actually feel better. Either of these can be a default mode of breathing during stress, linked with paying close attention, feeling threatened, angry, frustrated, paralysed, etc.

3. Ask about what associations occur when talking about the breathing problem. With no understanding of the larger context, the breathing disruption may become the target of concern when it is only a symptom of overall arousal. Something associated with past trauma, such as a smell, sound, body position, image or situation can trigger a recurrence of panicky irregular breathing.

4. If a blood relative has a history of heart or severe asthma attack, being aware of the genetic link may make the patient feel extra vulnerable to chest pain or difficulty breathing.

5. History of panic attacks will put the person's sense of control in doubt, and if the episode included feelings of breathlessness, overbreathing could easily be a response to onset of anything resembling pain. Fear of losing control in public, with subsequent embarrassment and vulnerability, may not be mentioned until asked specifically (see Box 6.4.2).

Hyperventilation provocation test

When a patient presents with symptoms typical of hyperventilation but is sceptical about the explanation for them,

---

Box 6.4.2   Understanding panic attack 'triggers'

A 32-year-old woman with panic attacks and hyperventilation was being monitored by capnometry while discussing a recent panic attack. She was asked to recount, with eyes closed, the context in which the attack occurred. On the way to visit a friend she had begun to feel chest tightness, difficulty breathing and light-headedness. She began to worry about being able to control her car, and as she continued driving toward the friend's house, this worry escalated into panic over the possibility of crashing. She stopped the car, tried to calm her breathing and racing heart, and finally felt able to drive back home.

Recalling and describing this whole episode dropped her CO_2 by about 20%, especially as she described pulling the car over and becoming convinced that she could not drive safely. She could not state what set off the incident, but assumed it came 'out of the blue' or else was connected somehow with driving. She denied any uneasiness about the woman she was visiting, or the neighbourhood, or the car itself. She speculated that her panicky breathing might be connected with the chest tightness from the last time she had panicked.

To pursue the question of what triggered her attack, I asked her to visualize each stage of the trip and briefly mention the associations she had to these images. The capnometer was recording, and intervals of silence permitted adequate samples of her breathing.

As she spoke more about driving toward the woman's house, her breathing became faster and the CO_2 level dropped from 39 to 28–30 in about a minute. As I mentioned this to her, she reported feeling some chest tightness and rapid heartbeat again. Suddenly she remembered that her friend sometimes took care of a relative's dog, chaining it in the back yard. This had major psychological meaning for her because she had once walked into someone else's back yard and was attacked by a dog. This connection became clear to her for the first time; it was as if her 'warning system' was operating beneath her awareness. The mere possibility of the friend keeping a dog that day had set off anticipatory hyperventilation, and her attention went to the resulting symptoms instead of to the real cause.

Understanding this was a revelation to her and led to greater understanding of the concept of 'triggers' activating her panicky state. Without this understanding, teaching her to control her breathing while approaching her friend's house might not have been successful, because it would be opposed by the 'hidden alarm' being activated.

---

one popular diagnostic procedure is the 'provocation test'. The principle is to ask the person to breathe both fast and deeply for a minute or two, and then to resume normal breathing. This is usually done with no monitoring, but a capnometer if available adds validity and provides objective information to the patient. If the provoked hyperventilation reproduces some of the symptoms that the person has been concerned about (dizziness, mental fog, weakness, anxiety, palpitations, tingling lips and fingers) and they subside once the breathing becomes normal again, this offers a rational explanation for the symptoms. At CO_2 levels below 30 mmHg the average person is likely to feel some of the changes above, and almost certainly under, 20.

Doing this requires caution, however; hyperventilation increases cardiac risk because of its vasoconstrictive effects on smooth muscle, including the bronchi, esophagus, gastrointestinal tract, cerebral blood vessels and coronary arteries. If there is any reason to suspect a compromised cardiovascular system, a risk of stroke, or possibility of seizure, provoking hyperventilation may not be wise. Vigorous hyperventilation does stress the cardiovascular system and can trigger anginal pain or worse in those who are susceptible. (This effect has led to its use by cardiologists for diagnosing latent angina and vasospasm of coronary vessels (Sueda et al 2002)). If uncertain about this, one can substitute what might be called the hyperventilation provocation *suggestion* test. To do this, simply propose to the patient the act of breathing fast and deep for a short time to see what happens. If the response is apprehension, refusal or obvious discomfort (perhaps accompanied by hyperventilation!) the patient probably knows already that symptoms might be provoked, in which case demonstration would be superfluous.

The advantage of deliberate hyperventilation lies in demonstrating that the symptoms can be terminated by restoring normal breathing, and this can be quite convincing if the symptoms were considered unpredictable and uncontrollable. Some patients will be surprised, intrigued and grateful.

The extreme form of this provocation test was developed by Peter Nixon, a London cardiologist. With patients complaining of cardiac symptoms suggestive of hyperventilation as a source, he would first identify through interview a strong emotional issue that he suspected was stimulating overbreathing. Next he would ask the patient to hyperventilate, and then during recovery of normal breathing, exhort the patient to think and focus on the emotional issue. This led sometimes to dramatic catharsis, flashbacks and abreactions, but did increase the potential for insight about symptom etiology (see Nixon & Freeman 1988).

REFERENCES

American Heritage Dictionary, 2000, fourth ed. Houghton Mifflin, Boston, MA.

Bloch, S., Lemeignan, M., Aguilera, N., 1991. Specific respiratory patterns distinguish among human basic emotions. International Journal of Psychophysiology 11 (2), 141–154.

Courtney, R., Greenwood, K.M., 2009. Preliminary investigation of a measure of dysfunctional breathing symptoms: the Self Evaluation of Breathing Questionnaire (SEBQ). International Journal of Osteopathic Medicine 12, 121–127.

Courtney, R., Greenwood, K., Cohen, M., 2011. Relationships between measures of dysfunctional breathing in a population with concerns about their breathing. Journal of Bodywork and Movement Therapies 15, 24–34.

Cox, B.J., Parker, J.D.A., Swinson, R.P., 1996. An examination of levels of agoraphobic anxiety sensitivity: confirmatory evidence for multidimensional construct. Behaviour Research and Therapy 34, 591–598.

van Dixhoorn, J., Duivenvoorden, H.J., 1985. Efficacy of Nijmegen Questionnaire in recognition of the hyperventilation syndrome. Journal of Psychosomatic Research 29, 199–206.

Gilbert, C., 1999. Breathing: the legacy of Wilhelm Reich. Journal of Bodywork and Movement Therapies 3 (2), 97–106.

Hassett, A.L., Radvanski, D.C., Vaschillo, E.G., et al., 2007. A pilot study of the efficacy of heart rate variability (HRV) biofeedback in patients with fibromyalgia. Applied Psychophysiology and Biofeedback 32 (1), 1–10.

Kashdan, T.B., Zvolensky, M.J., McLeish, A.C., 2008. Anxiety sensitivity and affect regulatory strategies: individual and interactive risk factors for anxiety-related symptoms. Journal of Anxiety Disorders 22 (3), 429–440.

Lehrer, P.M., Vaschillo, E., Vaschillo, B., et al., 2004. Biofeedback treatment for asthma. Chest 126 (2), 352–361.

Nixon, P.G., Freeman, L.J., 1988. The 'think test': a further technique to elicit hyperventilation. Journal of the Royal Society of Medicine 81 (5), 277–279.

Reiss, S., Peterson, R.A., Gursky, D.M., et al., 1986. Anxiety sensitivity, anxiety frequency and the prediction of fearfulness. Behaviour Research and Therapy 24, 1–8.

Sturges, L.V., Goetsch, V.L., Ridley, J., et al., 1998. Anxiety sensitivity and response to hyperventilation challenge: physiologic arousal, interoceptive acuity, and subjective distress. Journal of Anxiety Disorders 12 (2), 103–115.

Sueda, S., Hashimoto, H., Ochi, N., et al., 2002. New protocol to detect coronary spastic angina without fixed stenosis. Japanese Heart Journal 43 (4), 307–317.

Thayer, J.F., Yamamoto, S.S., Brosschot, J.F., 2010. The relationship of autonomic imbalance, heart rate variability and cardiovascular disease risk factors. International Journal of Cardiology 28;141 (2), 122–131.

Yoo, C.S., Lee, K., Yi, S.H., et al., 2011. Association of heart rate variability with the Framingham risk score in healthy adults. Korean Journal of Family Medicine 32 (6), 334–340.

Zucker, T.L., Samuelson, K.W., Muench, F., et al., 2009. The effects of respiratory sinus arrhythmia biofeedback on heart rate variability and posttraumatic stress disorder symptoms: a pilot study. Applied Psychophysiology & Biofeedback 34 (2), 135–143.

Questionnaires and manual methods for assessing breathing dysfunction

Rosalba Courtney, Jan van Dixhoorn

INTRODUCTION

The assessment of breathing dysfunction includes the evaluation of the patient's symptoms using questionnaires, and of their breathing pattern through the use of instrumentation, or by direct observation and palpation.

Questionnaires or breathing pattern evaluation are often used as the sole basis for assigning to the patient the diagnostic label of dysfunctional breathing. This may not be an appropriate use of these tools. Dysfunctional breathing is not precisely defined and cannot be established on the basis of a single measurement. Subjective symptoms of breathing discomfort may have relatively little correlation with objective signs of breathing dysfunction. Breathing is a dynamic system which is under the influence of many factors. These are of a physical and pathological nature, as well as from psychic and emotional origin and also may be part of social and behavioural patterns. Respiratory disturbances or breathing pattern disorders can arise from a host of causes. Information gleaned from questionnaires and breathing pattern assessments need to be interpreted with attention to the particular context in which they appear, in light of other clinical findings and with an attempt to understand other possible causes of the patient's symptoms and breathing pattern abnormalities.

Questionnaires and assessment of breathing patterns, however, do provide a useful place from which to start to understand the patient, and when used together with other assessment tools, can inform the practitioner about the functionality of a patient's breathing. This chapter will discuss two questionnaires, the Nijmegen Questionnaire (NQ) and the Self-Evaluation of Breathing Questionnaire

(SEBQ), located in the appendices to this chapter, as well as a manual procedure to assess the global quality of respiratory movement called the Manual Assessment of Respiratory Motion (MARM). Alternative/additional evaluation approaches are to be found in the other chapters in Section 6.

The Nijmegen Questionnaire was originally devised to evaluate the symptoms of hyperventilation syndrome and is the questionnaire most commonly used to identify and evaluate dysfunctional breathing. In recent years this questionnaire has also been used to evaluate medically unexplained (respiratory) symptoms whose origins are likely to be rooted in psychic and emotional stress and are variably connected to hypocapnia (Katsamanis et al 2011, Gevirtz 2007, Han et al, 2004). However, it has always been clear that there is a large overlap with symptoms of stress/anxiety. NQ may therefore be helpful to identify the presence of symptoms mediated by general distress as well as symptoms of respiratory distress.

The SEBQ can be a useful complement to the NQ in evaluating breathing dysfunction. It was designed to evaluate a broader range of breathing symptoms than the NQ. It can be useful for monitoring both the extent of respiratory discomfort and the distinct qualities of these uncomfortable breathing sensations.

The efficiency with which the mechanical act of breathing is performed is an important aspect of breathing functionality. Inefficient patterns of breathing can contribute to dyspnoea, musculoskeletal dysfunction and impact on the efficiency of circulatory and homeostatic processes. The MARM is a manual procedure that can be used to quantify the distribution of breathing movement. It has two aspects: the area or extent of breathing movement and the location of breathing on a vertical axis (upper-thoracic, costo-abdominal, abdominal).

Efficient breathing is dependent on the coordination and balanced use of many breathing muscles. The efficiency of particular muscular coordination patterns is dependent on a person's posture, activity level and disease. Breathing patterns considered dysfunctional in some situations may be appropriate in others. During increased activity or at times of increased respiratory drive it is considered normal for the breathing to become more thoracic-dominant, and for there to be increased recruitment of the accessory muscles of respiration (De Troyer & Estenne 1988). In patients with restrictive lung disease or in the advanced stages of chronic obstructive pulmonary disease a thoracic upper chest breathing pattern may be the best adaptation to severe lung pathology (Cahalin et al 2002). Efficient breathing also involves appropriate timing and volume adjustments that are sensitive and responsive to changes in the person's internal and external environment but not excessively chaotic or irregular. Context can be an important factor in differentiating normal from abnormal breathing patterns, i.e. disease, ventilatory drive, states of activity compared with states of rest.

QUESTIONNAIRES

Generally speaking people with breathing dysfunction have more respiratory discomfort than those whose breathing is efficient and functional (Courtney et al 2011a). They may also have complaints in other systems whose function is closely inter-related with breathing such as the cardiovascular or autonomic nervous systems (Wilhelm et al 2001).

The SEBQ focuses on evaluating respiratory symptoms while the NQ evaluates the broader range of symptoms whose presence often accompanies breathing dysfunction.

The Nijmegen Questionnaire (NQ)

(see Appendix 1, at end of this chapter)

Normal and abnormal values

NQ consists of 16 items, to be answered on a five point scale, ranging from 'never', counted as zero, to 'very often', counted as 4. The total score ranges from 0 to 64 (Doorn et al 1983). Completion of the questionnaire is quick, and only takes a few minutes. The items were chosen to represent a range of symptoms:

- Stress and arousal (e.g. feeling anxious, tense, having palpitations)
- Presumed consequences of hypocapnia (e.g. dizziness, blurred vision, tingling and stiffness around mouth and in hands)
- Difficulty breathing (e.g. inability to take a deep breath, tightness in the chest).

However, items presumed to result from hypocapnia could be the result of stress and high sympathetic tone as well.

For its practical use, it is of importance to establish a criterion for the presence or absence of dysfunction and abnormal level of complaints. On average, a normal, healthy individual has a sum score of 11 ± 7, men score somewhat lower than women (Han et al 1997). These data imply that most normal individuals have scores that range from 4 to 18. Note however, that these values have been obtained in Belgium and the UK. In China, by contrast, the normal average value is 5. To define a criterion for dysfunction we used data from over 2000 patients who were referred for treatment with breathing and relaxation therapy, about one quarter of whom were labelled as having 'hyperventilation complaints' (Dixhoorn 2012). Average NQ value of the latter group was 29.5. When taking these patients as the reference for those who most probably would have breathing dysfunction it appears that a value of 20 or higher differentiates them from normal. So, a value of NQ > 19 denotes the presence of (respiratory) distress and dysfunction. The higher the score, the more distress is present. Values below 20 are considered within the normal and functional domain.

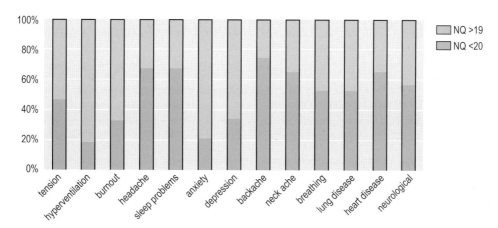

Figure 6.5.1 Distribution of normal (NQ 1–19) versus abnormal NQ scores (NQ 20–64) for different patient groups.

Distress and respiratory distress

However, high NQ scores do not appear to be exclusively present among patients with 'hyperventilation complaints'. The other 1500 patients had stress-related, but not necessarily respiration-related complaints: headaches, sleep problems, fatigue, burnout, anxiety, neck or back ache, voice problems or chronic pain. Some had medical diseases but were referred for the stress complaints. Given this large diversity in conditions and complaints, average NQ value for the group as a whole was elevated (Thomas et al 2005). Thus, contrary to what may be commonly thought, high NQ scores are not specific for 'hyperventilation complaints'.

Figure 6.5.1 shows the distribution of normal versus elevated scores (NQ>19) for the different categories. It is clear that the percentage of patients with high NQ varies considerably, between 80% (hyperventilation complaints and anxiety) and 30–40% (headache, neck ache, sleep problems, heart disease). There is no category where patients with high NQ are absent, even though the problem does not seem to have a respiratory component. This corroborates the fact that NQ does measure both general and respiratory stress. However, when a particular problem has minimal respiratory components, fewer patients have elevated scores. Interestingly, not all patients within the category 'breathing', having problems with nasal breathing, coughing, breathing during speech or effort etc., show an elevated NQ.

Responsive to treatment

The advantages of the NQ is that it is responsive to treatment effect and that it is short. Thus, it can be administered repeatedly over the course of treatment to assess progress. Among the 2000 patients, referred for breathing therapy, those who responded well and had a clear reduction in their main complaint, showed on average near

normal values at the end of treatment. This applied to patients with 'hyperventilation complaints', but equally to all other patients. By contrast, when treatment was less or not successful, the NQ score decreased slightly but on average it remained elevated and above 19. Therefore, the NQ seems a useful evaluation tool in the treatment of patients with stress-related and unexplained problems. When the NQ does not normalize, treatment strategy should be re-evaluated. As to a cut-off score, it appears that a decrease of at least 10 points, calculated for hyperventilation patients with Jacobson's formula for 'reliable change index', indicates a clinically significant change (Jacobson & Traux 1991). This applies when the initial NQ score is clearly elevated.

Not all patients with medically unexplained symptoms have elevated NQ scores. In those cases NQ reflects treatment outcome less well, and it is difficult to obtain a decrease of 10 points or more. For instance, patients with asthma have on average slightly elevated NQ scores, around 19 in one study (Holloway & West 2007). Their response to breathing therapy (Papworth method) was positive and the final NQ score normalized (around 11–12). Nevertheless, the criterion of at least 10 points decrease was not reached by most of them. Thus, the clinician should evaluate the meaning of changes in NQ scores individually (Holloway & West 2007).

Sub scores

It is sometimes useful to inspect the individual items in the NQ. For instance, among asthma patients it was found that the relatively modest elevation on NQ is caused by high scores on the respiratory items, but relatively low scores on the other items. Thus, when the sum score appears to be unexpectedly low, given the nature of the complaints, the advice is to inspect the individual items. Another reason to select the respiratory items is in comparing the NQ to the MARM (see later in this chapter). In one data set, the sum score of NQ correlated only slightly with MARM and this was due to a correlation with the respiratory items (Courtney et al 2011b).

The Self-Evaluation of Breathing Questionnaire (SEBQ) (see Appendix 2 at end of this chapter)

The SEBQ is a recently developed questionnaire whose items were drawn from the various descriptions in the scientific and popular literature of respiratory symptoms and breathing behaviours proposed to be associated with breathing dysfunction (Courtney & Greenwood 2009). The most current versions of the SEBQ (Version 3), appearing in Appendix 2, contains 25 items to be answered on a three-point scale, ranging from 'never', counted as zero, to 'very frequently/very true', counted as 3. One study of 180 individuals found that scores on this version of the SEBQ range from 0–64. This study also found that the SEBQ has a high level of test re-test reliability (ICC=0.88, 95%CI=84–91). Mean values in this study were 16, with smokers scoring 51% higher than non-smokers and sufferers of respiratory disease scoring 69% higher than those without respiratory disease (Mitchell 2011).

The SEBQ is useful as a means of evaluating the quality and quantity of uncomfortable respiratory sensations, and the person's perception of their own breathing, and may help to give insight into the origins of the discomfort.

Research into the language of dyspnoea (or breathing discomfort) has established that the different types of dyspnoea or uncomfortable respiratory sensation have their origins in different receptors and different pathophysiological processes and that people given similar breathing challenges or suffering with similar diseases will use the same sort of words to describe their sensations or respiratory difficulty or discomfort (Simon et al 1989, Simon & Schwartzstein 1990, Elliot et al 1991).

Analysis of the SEBQ using a statistical technique called factor analysis showed that this questionnaire can differentiate two distinct categories or dimensions of breathing discomfort. The first of these dimensions, called 'lack of air', is related to 'air hunger' (as described below) and the second of these, related to the work, or effort of breathing, is called a perception of 'inappropriate or restricted breathing'. The two dimensions of the SEBQ may represent strongly related, but distinct, aspects of breathing perception and dysfunction representing biochemical and biomechanical mechanisms, and also sensory and cognitive aspects of interoception. The clinical assessment of these two dimensions may prove useful for understanding more about the nature of a person's breathing dysfunction, so that treatment can be individualized.

The SEBQ category called 'lack of air' contains items such as 'I feel short of breath', 'I can't catch' my breath', 'I

feel breathless on physical exertion' and 'I feel that the air is stuffy'. These qualities or verbal descriptors of dyspnoea are very similar to those identified by other researchers as 'air hunger' or 'urge to breathe'. Research has shown that sensations of 'air hunger' are primarily related to the activation of chemoreceptors and also influenced by neuro-mechanical interactions primarily involving feedback from the medulla. The feeling of 'air hunger' is produced when CO_2 is increased, or when tidal volumes are decreased and relieved when CO_2 levels are lowered and tidal volumes increased (Lansing 2000). Studies of patients with suspected hyperventilation syndrome have shown that the dyspnoea symptoms have no relationship to low CO_2 levels (Hornsveld & Garssen 1996).

The SEBQ category called 'perception of inappropriate or restricted breathing' contains descriptors such as 'I cannot take a deep and satisfying breath' and 'My breathing feels stuck or restricted' that convey a sense of restricted or otherwise unsatisfied respiration. These types of sensations arise, as least in part, from receptors in the chest wall and muscles of breathing and also represent the qualities of dyspnoea that arise when the motor output of the respiratory system is not able to match the expectations generated in the sensory cortex by corresponding discharges from the motor cortex (Beach & Schwatrzstein 2006). These types of sensations are reported in situations where the work of breathing is made more difficult such as when the chest wall is strapped (O'Donnell et al 2000) or when there is impaired function of the respiratory muscles and rib cage and when neuromuscular coupling and respiratory muscle functioning is impaired because the lungs are hyperinflated (Lougheed et al 2006).

The two dimensions identified in the SEBQ also describe different aspects of interoception with the first being related to the sensory and often using the words, 'I feel', and the second indicating the more cognitive or evaluative aspects of interoception. It is interesting that the sensations related to the urge to breathe or SEBQ 'lack of air' category come from the medulla, and the sensations related to the work of breathing and using the words 'I notice' arise from the cortex.

Comparing the SEBQ and the NQ

The symptoms measured by the NQ represent a cluster of complaints long recognized to exist together in people whose breathing disorders accompany stress, anxiety and hyperarousal and in many instances also to acute or chronic hypocapnia (hyperventilation complaints). The NQ does not enquire as extensively as the SEBQ into the different qualities of respiratory discomfort.

In patients given both questionnaires, the NQ scores were found to correlate with the SEBQ total score and with Factor 1 of the SEBQ – 'Lack of air' but not with Factor 2 of the SEBQ – 'Perception of inappropriate or restricted breathing'. This suggests that the SEBQ is useful as an additional questionnaire to the NQ for differentiating symptoms arising from the biomechanical aspects of breathing dysfunction and from the cognitive/evaluative aspects of interoception.

It has been suggested that the weak association between dysfunctional breathing symptoms and hypocapnia may be partly explained by the fact that these arise from other causes such as tense breathing patterns (Hornsveld & Garssen 1997). This assertion is supported by the presence of a separate biomechanical and evaluative dimension to dysfunctional breathing symptoms in the SEBQ, as well as by the mediating role of MARM in the presence of breathing discomfort.

Practical uses of the SEBQ

The two dimensions of the SEBQ may represent strongly related, but distinct, aspects of breathing perception and dysfunction, and might prove to be useful as a means for differentiating breathing symptoms that are more connected to medullary and biochemical mechanisms from those that have a greater contribution from dysfunction of the neuromuscular aspects of breathing. This can guide the practitioner in performing further evaluation with manual techniques, capnometry or of the person's psychological state and stress level.

Research to establish normative values for the SEBQ has not been formally undertaken. However, in one study examining the relationships between measures of dysfunctional breathing, it was found that individuals with NQ scores below 20 had a mean score of 11 for the SEBQ (Courtney et al 2011a).

MANUAL TECHNIQUES FOR EVALUATING BREATHING PATTERN

In the research setting, instrumentation is used to determine breathing pattern whilst in the clinical environment, the cheaper and less time-consuming methods of observation and palpation are the mainstay of breathing pattern assessment.

The main types of instrumentation used to evaluate the breathing pattern are respiratory induction plethysmography (RIP), magnetometry and a new technique called optoelectronic plethysmography. These types of instrumentation which can collect a large number of volume, movement and timing measures enable a sophisticated and precise assessment of breathing pattern, but their cost is prohibitively expensive for the average clinician.

In the clinical environment, the practitioner who is evaluating breathing pattern dysfunction relies primarily on their senses and powers of observation. By observing the patient's posture, demeanour and speech pattern it is frequently possible to begin to recognize breathing pattern disorders. In looking more closely at breathing itself, clinicians who are so inclined can easily identify the heaving chest and increased shoulder movement of excessive thoracic breathing, and the chest wall rigidity and tense respiratory muscles of the person with stressed and effortful breathing. The accurate recording and reporting of these observational and palpatory findings requires standardized techniques. The following section focuses on the Manual Assessment of Respiratory Motion (MARM), one of the few validated manual techniques that quantifies some aspects of breathing pattern.

The Manual Assessment of Respiratory Movement (MARM)

The MARM is similar to manual assessments of lateral rib cage motion, long used by manual therapists to assess diaphragm function. However, the MARM also interprets and quantifies this motion in relationship to other aspects of global respiratory motion. The MARM procedure was first developed and applied in a follow-up study of breathing and relaxation therapy with cardiac patients in the 1980s. Patients who were treated solely with exercise rehabilitation showed clear differences in MARM values, as compared to those who had additional breathing retraining therapy, and these were evident up to 2 years after rehabilitation (Dixhoorn 1994). Later tests have shown that the MARM has good (ICC=0.85, p=0.0001, CI 0.78, 0.89) inter-examiner reliability and is better able to determine changes in extent of thoracic breathing in response to changes in posture and verbal instruction than respiratory induction plethysmograph (Courtney et al 2008).

Performing the MARM

In performing the MARM the examiner sits behind the subject and places their hands at the posterior and lateral aspect of their rib cage. The whole hand rests firmly and comfortably so as not to restrict breathing motion. The examiner's thumbs are approximately parallel to the spine, pointing vertically, and the hands are comfortably open with fingers spread so that the little fingers of both hands approach a horizontal orientation. The 4th and 5th fingers reach below the lower ribs so that they can feel abdominal expansion. With this particular hand position the examiner brings their attention to the breathing motion of the whole rib cage and abdomen in the lateral, vertical and anterior/posterior directions (see Fig. 6.5.2). An assessment is then made of the extent of overall vertical motion, relative to the overall lateral motion, in order to determine whether the motion is predominantly upper rib cage, lower rib cage/abdomen or relatively balanced.

Recording the MARM

The examiner then records the findings using two lines drawn in one half of a circle to form a pie chart (see

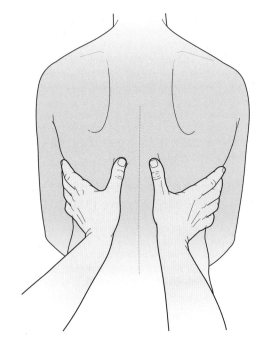

Figure 6.5.2 Performing the MARM.

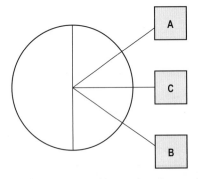

Figure 6.5.3 The MARM graphic notation. See text for explanation of lettering.

Fig. 6.5.3). The upper line (A in Fig. 6.5.3) represents motion occurring in the upper rib cage combined with extent of motion in the vertical direction. The lower line (B in Fig. 6.5.3) represents motion in the lower rib cage combined with extent of movement in the lateral direction for the rib cage and downward push of the diaphragm to the abdomen. In deciding where to put these two lines the examiner needs to keep in mind the global or spherical nature of breathing motion. A horizontal line (C in Fig. 6.5.3) represents the middle of this globe. The upper line will be further from the horizontal and closer to the top if there is more vertical and upper rib cage motion. The lower line will be further from the horizontal and closer to the bottom if there is more lateral and lower rib cage/ abdomen motion. Finally the examiner can also report on

their sense of the overall magnitude and freedom of rib cage motion by placing lines further apart to represent greater overall motion and closer for less motion.

Calculating MARM variables

MARM variables are calculated by measuring angles determined from the two lines drawn by examiners, with the top taken to be 180 degrees and the bottom at 0 degrees. An upper line (A) represents the 'highest point of inhalation' and is made by the examiner's perception and estimation of the relative contribution of upper rib cage, particularly the extent of vertical motion of the sternum and upper rib cage. The lower line (B) represents the 'lowest part of inhalation' and this corresponds to the examiner's perception and estimation of the relative contribution of lower rib motion and abdominal motion, particularly the extent of sideways and downward expansion. With more thoracic breathing the upper line A is placed higher and when breathing is more abdominal with greater involvement of the lower rib cage and abdominal cavity, line B is placed lower. Thus, two kinds of variables are derived: firstly, the distance between the two lines representing the extent or area of breathing movement. This can also be called 'volume' because it will increase when breathing is deeper and decreases when inhalation is shallower. However, absolute values of the MARM 'area' variable have little correlation with measures of tidal volume. More accurately it represents the extent or area of the trunk that is involved in breathing movement. The second set of MARM variables concerns the location of breathing on the vertical axis: upper body, middle or lower part. The two lines can be averaged, where an average value of 90 represents the middle position. Higher values represent more upper thoracic breathing and lower values represent more abdominal breathing. Two derivatives are firstly MARM 'balance' where the two parts above and below the midline are subtracted. A value of zero represents the middle position or perfect balance. A positive value indicates thoracic dominant breathing, a negative value representing less thoracic mobility and more diaphragmatic activity. The second derivative is percentage of rib cage motion, a measure that corresponds to one of the respiratory induction plethysmography (RIP) parameters. Both are linear transformations and express the location of breathing on a vertical axis.

The MARM measurement variables are:

1. Area = angle formed between upper line and lower line (area AB)
2. MARM average = $(A + B)/2$
2a) Balance = difference between angle made by horizontal axis (C) and upper line (A) and horizontal and lower line (AC-CB)
2b) Percent rib cage motion = area above horizontal/ total area between upper line and lower line × 100. (AC/AB×100)

The MARM and balanced breathing

It appears that functional breathing consists of a balance between upper and lower compartments of breathing. This would result in average values of 'percent rib cage' of around 50, of 'balance' of around zero and of 'average' of 90. The diaphragmatic, abdominal and rib cage muscles all have optimal length tension relationships and coordination patterns that make breathing most efficient when all muscle groups are equally involved (De Troyer and Estenne 1988). This suggests that 'optimal' breathing occurs when there is an even distribution of breathing effort between the two main functional compartments of the body involved in breathing, i.e. upper rib cage and lower rib cage/abdomen. Such a balance also provides the greatest flexibility of the respiratory system to respond to any internal or external alterations to respiratory drive. An uneven breathing distribution, without good reason, may be considered to be unnecessary, effortful and dysfunctional.

Using the MARM to assess functionality of breathing

An important assumption is that healthy functioning includes variability of biological systems, including respiration. So, functional breathing is responsive, variable and flexible (Dixhoorn van 2007). This can be tested by asking the patient to voluntarily change their breathing or by observing the changes in breathing that come about as posture changes (Courtney et al 2011b). For instance, the person can be asked to breathe normally and more deeply, to breathe with emphasis on upper thoracic or more abdominal inhalation, or to breathe in an upright or easy sitting posture. The position of the upper and lower lines of the MARM are then used to assess the range of responses. A larger range, calculated as the difference between the highest and the lowest value across the protocol, may then indicate greater functionality.

MARM testing protocol and normal values

Data on normal values are available from therapists, which can be compared to COPD patients and patients with stress and tension complaints (Table 6.5.1).

Table 6.5.1 MARM values for different groups

Category	MARM average	MARM area
Breathing therapists (n = 67)	90.5 ± 6.9	58 ± 15.8
Physiotherapists (n = 16)	90.8 ± 7.9	44 ± 10.7
COPD patients (n = 35)	103.2 ± 20.8	42.3 ± 17.9
Stress and tension patients (n = 62)	112 ± 10.2	20.4 ± 5.4

It appears that therapists indeed have average values of 90. The difference between experienced and non-experienced breathers does not lie in the average value, but in the area of breathing involvement. Experienced breathers show on average a larger area of involvement. As a rule of thumb, an average value of 90 and an area value of 60 appears to be more or less optimal.

By contrast, COPD patients have similar MARM area values as physiotherapists but their average MARM is higher, indicating more thoracic breathing. In particular, the standard deviation is much higher. This results from the fact that many have normal or even below normal values, whereas only a subgroup have high values. Thus, not all COPD patients show upper thoracic breathing and many handle their breathing problem adequately, when in an unchallenged situation. Moreover, the presence of high values and upper thoracic breathing appears unrelated to the severity of the COPD.

Patients with stress and tension however, do show an upper thoracic breathing pattern, with a small area of movement. The breathing movement is relatively restricted, indicated by the average value of the area of involvement (20.4) and the standard deviation, which are 2–3 times smaller than in all others. It implies that stress and anxiety result in a more or less homogeneous breathing pattern. Average MARM is markedly elevated, even in contrast to COPD patients. This confirms the idea that dysfunctional and thoracic-dominant breathing results more from stress and tension than from somatic causes. The cut-off value to differentiate normal from abnormal values can be calculated, using Jacobson's formula (Jacobson & Traux 1991), by comparing the breathing therapists to the stress patients. When average MARM value is 100 or higher, it can be classified as abnormal. For MARM area the cut-off value that indicates an abnormally small area of involvement is 30 or lower.

Using the MARM to assess other aspects of breathing

The MARM can be used to assess asymmetry between the two sides of the body. In case of scoliosis or sideways distortion of the spinal column there is a marked difference in breathing movement between the left and right sides of the body and this can be registered clearly by the examiner's two hands. Such asymmetry is unlikely to be adequately assessed by instrumentation such as RIP.

CONCLUSION

Breathing dysfunction is difficult to define precisely and cannot be assessed by one single measure. It involves breathing discomfort as well as inappropriate breathing movement. There can be a host of causes and it is sensitive to excess stress and tension. It can occur with and without somatic pathology and produces additional stress and tension, which aggravates symptoms. Three assessment procedures are presented. They are complementary to each other. Each of them indicates the presence of breathing dysfunction and is a reason to take further steps.

REFERENCES

Beach, D., Schwatrzstein, R.M., 2006. The genesis of breathlessness. In: Booth, S., Dudgeon, D. (Eds.), Dyspnoea in advanced disease: a guide to clinical management. Oxford University Press, Oxford.

Cahalin, L., Braga, M., Matsuo, Y., et al., 2002. Efficacy of diaphragmatic breathing in persons with chronic obstructive pulmonary disease. A review of the literature. Journal of Cardiopulmoary Rehabilitation 22, 7–21.

Courtney, R., Greenwood, K., Cohen, M., 2011a. Relationships between measures of dysfunctional breathing in a population with concerns about their breathing. Journal of Bodywork and Movement Therapies 15, 24–34.

Courtney, R., Greenwood, K.M., 2009. Preliminary investigation of a measure of dysfunctional breathing symptoms: the Self Evaluation of Breathing Questionnaire (SEBQ). International Journal of Osteopathic Medicine 12, 121–127.

Courtney, R., Van Dixhoorn, J., Cohen, M., 2008. Evaluation of breathing pattern. Comparison of a manual assessment of respiratory motion (MARM) and respiratory induction plethysmography. Applied Psychophysiology and Biofeedback 33, 91–100.

Courtney, R.C., Greenwood, K.M., Dixhoorn, J., et al., 2011b. Medically unexplained dyspnea partly moderated by dyfunctional (thoracic dominant) breathing pattern. Journal of Asthma 48, 259–265.

De Troyer, A., Estenne, M., 1988. Functional anatomy of the respiratory muscles. Clinics in Chest Medicine 9, 175–193.

Dixhoorn, J., 2012. Nijmegen Questionnaire in the evaluation of medically unexplained symptoms, including hyperventilation complaints. Biological Psychology (in press).

Dixhoorn, J.V. 1994. Two year follow up of breathing pattern in cardiac

patients. In: Proceedings 25th Annual meeting, Wheat Ridge, CO, USA. Association for Applied Psychophysiology and Biofeedback.

Dixhoorn Van, J., 2007. Whole-Body breathing: a systems perspective on respiratory retraining. In: Lehrer, P.M., Woolfolk, R.L., Sime, W.E. (Eds.), Principles and practice of stress management. Third ed. Guilford Press, New York.

Doorn, P., Folgering, H., Colla, P., 1983. Een vragenlijst voor hyperventilatieklachten. De Psycholoog 18, 573–577.

Elliot, M.W., Adams, L., Cockcroft, A., et al., 1991. The language of breathlessness: use of verbal descriptors by patients with cardiorespiratory disease. Am Rev Respiratory Diseases 144, 826–832.

Gevirtz, R. (Ed.), 2007. Psychophysiological perspectives on stress related and anxiety disorders. Guilford Press, New York.

Han, J., Stegen, K., Simkens, K., et al., 1997. Unsteadiness of breathing in patients with hyperventilation syndrome & anxiety disorders. Euro Respiratory Journal 10, 167–176.

Han, J., Zhu, Y., Li, S., et al., 2004. Medically unexplained dyspnea, psychological characteristics and role of breathing therapy. Chinese Medical Journal 117, 6–13.

Holloway, E., West, R.J., 2007. Integrated breathing and relaxation training (Papworth Method) for adults with asthma in primary care: a randomised controlled trial. Thorax 62, 1039–1042.

Hornsveld, H., Garssen, B., 1996. The low specificity of the hyperventilation test. Journal of Psychosomatic Research 41, 435–449.

Hornsveld, H.K., Garssen, B., 1997. Hyperventilation syndrome: an elegant but scientifically untenable concept. Neth J Med 50, 13–20.

Jacobson, N.S., Traux, P., 1991. Clinical significance: a statistical approach to

defining meaningful change in psychotherapy research. J Consult Clin Psychol 59, 12–19.

Katsamanis, M., Lehrer, P.M., Escobar, J.I., et al., 2011. Psychophysiological treatment for patients with medically unexplained symptoms: a randomized controlled trial. Psychosomatics 52, 218–229.

Lansing, R.W., 2000. The perception of respiratory work and effort can be independent of the perception of air hunger. Am J Respir Crit Care Med 162, 1690–1696.

Lougheed, D., Fisher, T., O'Donnell, D., 2006. Dynamic hyperinflation during bronchoconstriction in asthma: implications for symptom perception. Chest 130, 1072–1081.

Mitchell, A., 2011. Test/retest reliability and determinants of the Self Evaluation of Breathing Questionnaire. Masters of Osteopathy Research, Unitec Institiute of Technology.

O'Donnell, D.E., Hong, H., Webb, K., 2000. Respiratory sensation during chest wall restriction and dead space loading in exercising men. Journal of Applied Physiology 88, 1859–1869.

Simon, P., Schwartzstein, M., 1990. Distinguishable types of dyspnea in patients with shortness of breath. Am Rev Respiratory Diseases 142, 1009–1014.

Simon, P., Schwartzstein, R., Weiss, J., et al., 1989. Distinguishable sensations of breathlessness induced in normal volunteers. Am Rev Respiratory Diseases 140, 1021–1027.

Thomas, M., Mckinley, R.K., Freeman, E., et al., 2005. The presence of dysfunctional breathing in adults with and without asthma. Prim Care Respir J. 14, 78–82.

Wilhelm, F.H., Gertivz, R., Roth, W., 2001. Respiratory dysregulation in anxiety, functional, cardiac, and pain disorders: assessment, phenomenology, and treatment. Behavioral Modification 25, 513–545.

APPENDIX 1   The Nijmegen Questionnaire

Nijmegen Questionnaire	Never 0	Rare 1	Sometimes 2	Often 3	Very often 4
Chest pain					
Feeling tense					
Blurred vision					
Dizzy spells					
Feeling confused					
Faster or deeper breathing					
Short of breath					
Tight feelings in chest					
Bloated feeling in stomach					
Tingling fingers					
Unable to breathe deeply					
Stiff fingers or arms					
Tight feelings round mouth					
Cold hands or feet					
Palpitations					
Feelings of anxiety					
Total: /64*					

*Patients mark with a tick how often they suffer from the symptoms listed. A value of NQ > 19 denotes the presence of (respiratory) distress and dysfunction. The higher the score, the more distress is present. Values below 20 are considered within the normal and functional domain.

APPENDIX 2   The Self-Evaluation of Breathing Questionnaire

Scoring this questionnaire: (0) never/not true at all; (1) occasionally/a bit true; (2) frequently/mostly true; and, (3) very frequently/very true

1) I get easily breathless out of proportion to my fitness	0	1	2	3
2) I notice myself breathing shallowly	0	1	2	3
3) I get short of breath reading and talking	0	1	2	3
4) I notice myself sighing	0	1	2	3
5) I notice myself yawning	0	1	2	3
6) I feel I cannot take a deep or satisfying breath	0	1	2	3
7) I notice that I am breathing irregularly	0	1	2	3
8) My breathing feels stuck or restricted	0	1	2	3
9) My ribcage feels tight and can't expand	0	1	2	3
10) I notice myself breathing quickly	0	1	2	3
11) I get breathless when I'm anxious	0	1	2	3
12) I find myself holding my breath	0	1	2	3
13) I feel breathless in association with other physical symptoms	0	1	2	3
14) I have trouble coordinating my breathing when speaking	0	1	2	3
15) I can't catch my breath	0	1	2	3
16) I feel that the air is stuffy, as if not enough air in the room	0	1	2	3
17) I get breathless even when resting	0	1	2	3
18) My breath feels like it does not go in all the way	0	1	2	3
19) My breath feels like it does not go out all the way	0	1	2	3
20) My breathing is heavy	0	1	2	3
21) I feel that I am breathing more	0	1	2	3
22) My breathing requires work	0	1	2	3
23) My breathing requires effort	0	1	2	3
24) I breathe through my mouth during the day	0	1	2	3
25) I breathe through my mouth at night while I sleep	0	1	2	3

Courtney, R., Greenwood, K.M., 2009. Preliminary investigation of a measure of dysfunctional breathing symptoms: the Self Evaluation of Breathing Questionnaire (SEBQ). International Journal of Osteopathic Medicine 12, 121–127.

Chapter | **6.6**

Capnography assessment

Laurie McLaughlin

This chapter outlines capnography as an assessment tool assisting in identifying specific breathing abnormalities. Measuring the CO_2 levels at the end of an exhaled breath gives insight as to whether the person's respiratory system is meeting metabolic demands. Information is also gathered about respiratory rate and rhythmicity, helping to focus and individualize management strategies while evaluating their effectiveness. Following standardized protocols can also be helpful in comparing among and within individuals.

CAPNOGRAPHY BASICS

The balance of carbon dioxide (CO_2) production and elimination is measured by the partial pressure of CO_2 in the blood. It gives important information about metabolism, cardiopulmonary function and breathing behaviour. The gold standard measurement is through arterial blood gases (Gardner 1996). That test is invasive, requiring a blood sample through an arterial puncture and a laboratory to perform the tests. It gives information about the CO_2 level only at that moment in time. Since CO_2 levels can change on a breath by breath basis (Levitsky 2007), knowing about one moment in time can limit detection of transient or situational hypocapnia (Gardner 1996) which is a feature of poor breathing behaviour. However, continuous values can be obtained using capnometry or capnography that test CO_2 levels in exhaled air. The reading at the end of exhale, termed End Tidal CO_2 (ETCO$_2$) is most representative of the alveolar air. The ability to measure ETCO$_2$ in the patient's breath in such a convenient non-invasive way is considered by some to be an important, even fundamental, advance in modern health care (Jaffe 2008). It has been suggested that ambulatory monitoring of ETCO$_2$ should become a new gold standard (Hornsveld & Garssen 1997).

The molecular structure of CO_2 is such that it absorbs infrared light. CO_2 concentration is determined in the capnometer/capnograph by an infrared photo detector where the intensity of light transmission with and without the exhaled air is compared. Infrared light absorption increases as CO_2 concentration increases and can therefore be measured and converted to a CO_2 measure. The sensor can be at the patient's airway (mainstream) which can only be used in intubated patients or at the monitor (sidestream), which can not only be used when someone is intubated but also allows for CO_2 monitoring in non-intubated patients. Measurement error is possible as readings can be affected by moisture, ambient temperature, barometric pressure and altitude. Calibration against a reference gas may be necessary to ensure measurement accuracy.

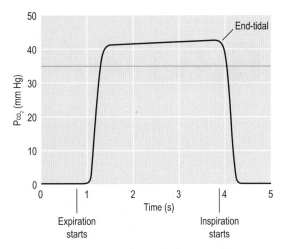

Figure 6.6.1 Capnogram. The y-axis shows partial pressure of carbon dioxide ($PaCO_2$) in millimeters of mercury (mmHg). This may also be shown as $ETCO_2$ (end tidal carbon dioxide). The x-axis shows time in seconds. *Levitsky 2007.*

Capnometry measures the rise and fall of CO_2 concentration in a numeric format continuously throughout the breath. When these values are plotted over time by a capnograph, a waveform or capnogram is created.

During inspiration, the reading will show 'zero' as CO_2 contributes only 0.3 mmHg to the total pressure of 760 mmHg in ambient air. At the onset of expiration, there is a delay before the graph rises as the air being exhaled occupies the anatomical dead space where there has been no gas exchange and is essentially room air, therefore registering 'zero'. This is followed by a sharp upswing as the CO_2 values increase. The next phase is almost horizontal, representing the alveolar or expiratory plateau which reaches a peak at the end of the plateau. This peak value is the $ETCO_2$ and is highly correlated with the alveolar CO_2 in people with healthy lungs. The $ETCO_2$ can be lower if the person does not complete the breath as there can be a mix of air from the passageways where there has been no gas exchange. Inspiration causes a sharp downward swing back to baseline. See Figure 6.6.1.

By representing the values in both numeric and graphic formats, capnography assists in confirming that the measurement is End Tidal. Without seeing the waveform one cannot be certain that a given value is actually End Tidal.

$ETCO_2$ is a good clinical estimate of arterial CO_2 provided cardiovascular function is normal, ensuring the lungs are well perfused and well ventilated such that ventilation and perfusion are matched. With lung disease, there will be greater perfusion than ventilation, resulting in some of the blood passing through the capillary bed not ventilating its CO_2. In cardiac pathology there will be less perfusion than ventilation so there will be alveoli with no CO_2 diffusing into them. In both instances there will

be a lower $ETCO_2$ reading than there is in the arterial blood. In these cases capnography readings will be less reliable. However, the lack of reliability can be remedied by comparing $ETCO_2$ readings to arterial blood gases to establish a baseline. Provided that the difference has been allowed for through comparison, capnography can still be a useful tool in these situations (http://www.capnography.com (Accessed June 2013)).

Capnography is used most typically in critical care settings to monitor ventilation status, confirm and verify endotracheal tube placement, monitor effectiveness of CPR and to assist in procedural sedation (Scarth & Cook 2012, Grmec & Mally 2004, Hinkelbein et al 2008). Validation studies comparing capnography with other measures of CO_2 have found it to be an accurate, time-sensitive measure of CO_2 levels (Cinar et al 2012). Barten & Wang (1994) compared End Tidal CO_2 and arterial CO_2 in patients with hypocapnia and found they were not significantly different (d = 0.7 mmHg, p = 0.174). When the patient's problem resulted in respiratory or metabolic acidosis there was a significant difference between arterial CO_2 and $ETCO_2$ (d = 6.0 mmHg, p = 0.005). However, both groups were still highly correlated (greater than 0.9). These findings suggest that there is relative accuracy when $ETCO_2$ levels are low (as in hypocapnia) but in metabolic pathologies causing acidosis (such as uncontrolled diabetes or excessive aerobic exercise where the numerator of the Henderson–Hasselbalch equation is altered) or in situations of *under*breathing (such as lung or neural pathology) where there is *hyper*capnia, the high $ETCO_2$ levels can be seen to be less accurate, giving lower readings than the true arterial CO_2 levels. Given the high correlation, even in people with serious pathology, the absolute value may not be attainable without comparing with blood gases, but the trend will depict whether breathing is improving or not (Martin 1992).

There are many different portable capnographs on the market, some of which can be worn while ambulatory while others require a computer interface. Reliability has been established in a number (Hildebrandt et al 2010, Craig et al 2010).

Most capnographs are geared to medical applications, not functional breathing habits, and are often used as a 'spot-check' with average readings and a representative waveform. Educational capnography is facilitated when continuous waveforms over 20–30 seconds can be visualized and historical information is available. This helps to identify dysfunctional breathing triggers and track the response to breathing interventions.

CLINICAL SETTING

When evaluating breathing, the underlying goal is to determine whether learned breathing habits are compromising the individual's physiology. One needs to sort out whether breathing habits precipitate negative functional effects, or result in physical, emotional, psychological or cognitive symptoms.

It is important to gather information about the individual's general health in addition to specific symptom details. Some physical conditions can alter ETCO$_2$ readings such as heart or lung pathology and must be taken into consideration when interpreting findings. Various factors can facilitate poor breathing habits such as pregnancy, menses, asthma, trauma or pain states. To truly customize evaluation it is essential to have a clear idea of the triggers and resultant symptoms that could contribute to or result from poor breathing (remembering that symptoms can arise from *any* body system)(see Chs 1, 3 and 4).

Capnography testing

Screen interpretation: normal/examples of abnormal (Figs 6.6.2 to 6.6.6)

Capnography is used to monitor ETCO$_2$ in order to establish whether it is within normal limits (35–45 mmHg), respiratory rate and whether that falls within the normal range of 8–14 breaths per minute, as well as whether the waveforms are smooth or choppy. The breath is meant to be smooth and rhythmical so that it can function in its role as a pump. Even people with normal ETCO$_2$ and respiratory rates can have symptoms if their pattern is choppy.

Examples of poor pattern

When using capnography for testing, there are a number of different approaches that can be used. Standardized tests can be a way of establishing the connection between

how the person being tested breathes and associated feelings and emotions. It is also helpful to use as a standardized outcome measure for data collection purposes comparing within and among subjects. Since breathing is very individual and context dependent it is also useful to customize testing along with standardized tests to include specific situations or environments, be they internal or external, in order to isolate specific problematic breathing behaviours.

Standardized tests

Set the capnograph along with the computer at table height and have the patient place a nasal cannula in their nostrils before attaching the cannula to the sampling

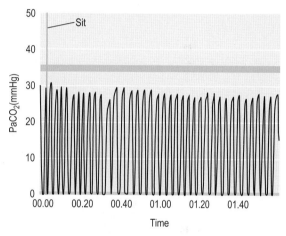

Figure 6.6.3 This capnogram shows low ETCO$_2$ and a fast respiratory rate (20 breaths per minute).

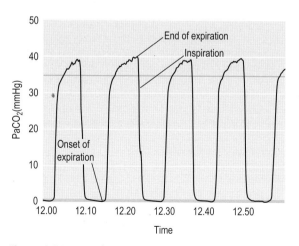

Figure 6.6.2 Normal capnogram. Blue horizontal line at 35mmHg here and in Figs 6.6.3 to 6.6.6 indicates low end of normal range.

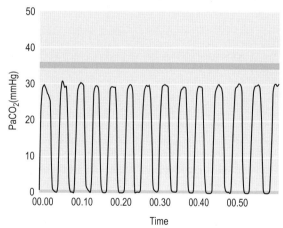

Figure 6.6.4 This capnogram shows a normal respiratory rate of 14 breaths per minute and a smooth pattern but an ETCO$_2$ of 30 mmHg indicating that too large a volume of air is being inhaled.

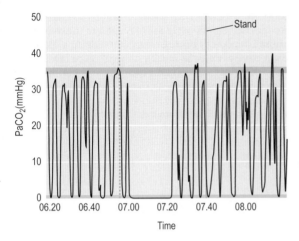

Figure 6.6.5 This capnogram shows apnoea or a period of breath holding.

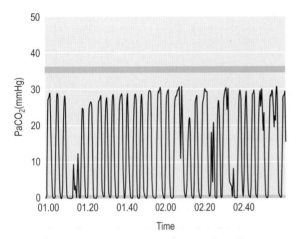

Figure 6.6.6 This capnogram shows a combination of low CO_2, a fast respiratory rate as well as poor pattern as evidenced by wave forms that do not fully complete the cycle. These are described as aborted breaths.

hose. The sampling hose is attached to a filter and then to the capnograph which is in turn connected to the computer. Arrange the patient's position so the screen is not visible. People generally change their breath as soon as they see the graph – to get a more accurate idea of the breathing baseline it is best initially if this information is hidden. With the CapnoTrainer® from Better Physiology Ltd, there is a recording function so that the session can be recorded and archived for future reference. It is also possible to identify the onset of any new challenge with an event marker that shows on the graph to

assist with interpretation during post-testing reviews. When recording the findings from standardized challenges, the average $ETCO_2$ reading should be captured once the pattern has stabilized after several breaths in a row. Respiratory rate should be noted as well as any indications of poor pattern (gasping, apnoea, aborted breaths, etc.). The person being tested should be informed that testing can be stopped at any time if discomfort is experienced. It is important to ask the subject to pay attention to their symptoms and to report any changes experienced during the testing.

1. Initially get a baseline in sitting. Once the breathing has stabilized for several breaths in a row – roughly 20 seconds – record.
2. Ask the individual to stand, and once the reading has stabilized, record the reading.
3. After resuming a seated position, and when the screen shows a stable series of breaths, ask the individual to take 10 deep breaths in and out through their nose. This will purposefully reduce CO_2 levels. Symptoms should be monitored in order to see if a lower CO_2 status reproduces any symptoms. Following this, attention should be paid to the screen images of the waveforms to note how rapidly – or slowly – recovery occurs to CO_2 levels evident prior to the deep breathing exercise. Someone who breathes well will increase the CO_2 levels towards normal with each breath, taking very few to re-establish their norm. Many poor breathers will get 'stuck' and struggle to return to their normal level. Recording the length of time it takes for recovery can be a useful objective measure. Typically, return to pre-test levels occurs within the first 40 seconds (Tawadrous & Eldridge 1974).
4. Once the breathing pattern and CO_2 levels have recovered, a rate challenge can be introduced. Have the individual breathe at 20 breaths per minute for a period of 2 minutes. Again monitor and record any symptom reproduction along with the $ETCO_2$ values. Stop the test if the patient becomes uncomfortable. If their CO_2 levels markedly drop, time the recovery period as this can be an indicator of whether they have difficulty recovering when under challenge. It is also important to watch for gasping or other indicators of struggle.
5. Next – have the individual talk for a period of 2 minutes. CO_2 levels tend to drop with prolonged speech (Hoit & Lohmeier 2000) and people who do a great deal of talking in their work such as teachers or call centre employees can be vulnerable to lowered CO_2 values. The test can be accomplished by encouraging them to tell you something about themselves or have them read from a standardized passage. The screen readings during speech will be

unreliable, so the actual reading occurs in the first few breaths once they have stopped talking. This will indicate whether the subject is able to maintain $ETCO_2$ during speech.

6. Finally, have the individual lie supine, comfortably supported. Since there are no postural demands one would expect the CO_2 readings to be the highest in this position. Once this test is completed breathing retraining can often be initiated in the supine position.

Test interpretation

Once data have been captured from the standard tests, interpretation is required to determine whether the person is a chronic overbreather, situational overbreather or less commonly a dissociative overbreather. When the findings at baseline are below 35 mmHg and stay low throughout the standardized tests, the individual can be considered to be a chronic overbreather. In the author's experience, this appears quite commonly in people diagnosed with fibromyalgia, chronic pain, chronic fatigue, etc. These findings can also indicate poor chest mechanics. When there is tightness within the chest wall or poor diaphragm and abdominal muscle coordination/activation, breathing mechanics can be altered to such a degree that normal breathing is not possible, and all the readings in the standardized tests are low. This type of presentation can be seen in patients with, for example, spinal pain. There are many studies outlining the altered muscle function that occurs in response to spinal pain (Kolar et al 2012, Radebold et al 2001, Hodges et al 2007, O'Sullivan & Beales 2007). Since the postural muscles affected are also breathing muscles, it is not surprising that breathing can be compromised. Once normal chest wall and diaphragm excursion is re-established with manual techniques and motor control retraining, the readings on the standardized tests commonly improve. Alternatively, breathing retraining itself has been shown to improve pain and function in patients with spinal pain (McLaughlin et al 2011).

When some of the tests are normal and others fall below 35 mmHg the individual is considered a situational overbreather. As the title implies, there are certain situations where breathing becomes problematic and may not be evident with standardized tests. A combination of interviewing, checklist information such as the Nijmegen Questionnaire (van Dixhoorn & Duivenvoorden 1985), and customized testing (see below) to see if symptoms are reproduced with lowered $ETCO_2$ levels, may be required in order to reach this conclusion. Situational overbreathing can be considered more of a breathing behaviour issue rather than one of poor chest mechanics. Management involves identifying problematic breathing behaviours, triggers and contexts through testing and interviewing. Once the problem areas are identified, treatment is aimed at education around these areas to facilitate awareness and set the stage for learning better breathing behaviours.

Occasionally, people can use overbreathing to detach from reality and will test low in end tidal CO_2. This is something that can be seen in people with a history of trauma or anxiety associated with certain situations. Using breath in this way can be situational or chronic. This concept is discussed more fully in Chapter 5, and may require collaboration with a mental health professional.

Customized testing

Breathing is context dependent. Thoughts, beliefs or emotions such as fear or stress create an internal environment or context that can precipitate a change in breathing. It is important to customize testing and subsequently for training to be specific to these triggers. Simply asking the individual to replicate the pattern of breathing experienced in particular situations can be a good way to start.

When identifying a person's breathing issues, it is best to replicate the problematic situation as closely as possible. This can be accomplished by physical activity such as use of a treadmill or bike if the person reports difficulty when exercising, or sitting behind the wheel of a car if a driving anxiety is reported, or by using the imagination where a past situation is imagined in which symptoms have been experienced. This is sometimes called a 'think test' (Nixon & Freeman 1988). Alternatively, intentional overbreathing can be used to replicate the poor physiology to determine whether symptoms are reproduced and if the individual gets 'stuck' when attempting to normalize following hypocapnia.

Think test (Case study 6.6.1)

Once the patient is connected to the capnograph, ask the individual to close their eyes and imagine a situation where symptoms are being experienced. Monitor the CO_2 readings to see if they fall. Watch how the breathing mechanics change so that you can help the patient recognize how changing breathing mechanics in response to triggers can contribute to their symptoms.

Intentional overbreathing

This should be avoided with patients with cardiac pathology, asthma or anaemia. It is also best to avoid in people with a history of panic attacks unless you are an appropriately trained and licensed health care professional. Ensure the patient is advised to stop the test if they become uncomfortable. You may wish to have a paper bag available. The use of paper bag rebreathing is widespread and while it is often used without difficulty, it can pose risks to people with hypoxia – such as those with cardiac pathology (Callaham 1989). This technique must be used with caution. See note on this in Chapter 7.7.

Case study 6.6.1 **Think test**

A male patient described having symptoms during exertion and with confrontational situations. He tested well on all of the standardized tests yet when placed on a treadmill or when doing a 'think test' remembering a stressful situation, his pattern became choppy and his ETCO$_2$ dropped to 30mmHg. He reported that he was experiencing his symptoms (palpitations, shortness of breath and leg cramps) at the same time as his CO$_2$ levels dropped. Interestingly, he had been diagnosed with high blood pressure. Once he changed his breathing, his blood pressure returned to the normal range and he no longer required medication.

Ask the patient to increase breath volume initially, and gradually the breathing rate, to bring the ETCO$_2$ down to the low to mid-twenties for a period of 2 minutes. Have the patient pay attention to the sensations in the body as well as to thoughts and emotions, to see if any of their symptoms surface. Once the test is complete, time the recovery period to see if they are able to come out of it easily or whether they become stuck. Post-overbreathing, people tend to show improvements in the first 10–20 seconds post-test and reach pre-test levels in approximately 40 seconds (Tawadrous & Eldridge 1974).

IN SPORT AND FITNESS

During exercise the production of CO$_2$ increases; however, arterial carbon dioxide levels should stay in the 35–45 mmHg range. Balance is maintained in the Henderson–Hasselback (HH) or pH equation by increasing the volume of air passing through the lungs per unit time through increasing volume, rate or typically both. The increased cellular activity and therefore lactic acid production is buffered by the bicarbonates (numerator of the HH equation) resulting in either glucose being re-synthesized or being broken down into CO$_2$ and H$_2$O (oxidized). Normally a balance between lactic acid production and utilization is maintained and buffers stay constant (Thomson et al 1997). However, when exercise is sufficiently vigorous, cardiac output is unable to keep up with the oxygen demand forcing the cells into anaerobic metabolism. This results in a sudden increase in lactic acid. When the acid production exceeds the utilization, the bicarbonate buffers become depleted and are not restored into the system quickly enough to maintain the ratio between bicarbonates and CO$_2$.

This results in lactic acidosis or a lowering of the pH. In order to raise the pH, a reflex kicks in to increase breathing volume and blow off CO$_2$ thus maintaining the ratio. The lungs then ventilate air faster than the heart perfuses them thereby efficiently and effectively restoring acid–base balance (Thomson et al 1997).

Capnography can be used to give specific physiological input to help with training and optimizing performance. Testing ETCO$_2$ during exercise can give indications about physical endurance and fatigue and therefore levels of fitness. The drop in ETCO$_2$ signals the point at which anaerobic exercise has begun. The athlete can use this information to learn to 'stay in the zone' and improve performance.

Anaerobic testing protocol

(Litchfield 2012)

1. Take a baseline of ETCO$_2$, while sitting on an exercise bike, without pedalling.
2. Introduce light pedalling, almost work-free, for 3 minutes.
3. Increase workload to a higher level for 3 minutes.
4. Increase the workload, 3 minutes at a time, until ETCO$_2$ drops.
5. Stop the exercise, and record ETCO$_2$ for a final 3 minutes.

Interpretation

- If ETCO$_2$ drops early on, buffers have been depleted quickly which can mean that the person is not in good shape (for example a fibromyalgia patient would reach this just walking around the grocery store!) or if noted in an athlete this might indicate overtraining.
- If the drop in ETCO$_2$ occurs only after major exercise output, it confirms that not only is the person in good cardiovascular shape, but also that they have not diminished their buffer pool through overbreathing during exercise or other activities.
- If recovery is delayed, there may be a dysfunctional breathing habit where exercise is a trigger for poor breathing.

CONCLUSION

Capnography can help to confirm that a breathing problem exists as well as isolating the specific aspect of breathing that is problematic. Once both the patient and the practitioner have clarity around the problem areas it becomes easier to focus on a management strategy. Capnography has the added benefit of being an outcome measure where it can be used before and after any intervention providing information about treatment efficacy.

REFERENCES

Barten, C.W., Wang, E.S.J., 1994. Correlation of end-tidal CO_2 measurements to arterial $PaCO_2$ in nonintubated patients. Annals of Emergency Medicine 23 (3), 560–563.

Callaham, M., 1989. Hypoxic hazards of traditional paper bag rebreathing in hyperventilating patients. Annals of Emergency Medicine 18 (6), 622–628.

Cinar, O., Acar, Y., Arziman, I. et al, 2012. Can mainstream end-tidal carbon dioxide measurement accurately predict the arterial carbon dioxide level of patients with acute dyspnea in ED. American Journal of Emergency Medicine 30, 358–361.

Craig, J., Kapteyn, M., Thomas, K. et al., 2010. Investigating the inter-rater and intra-rater reliability of capnography based on varied levels of training. Student Project, McMaster University.

Gardner, W.N., 1996. The pathophysiology of hyperventilation disorders. Chest 109, 516–534.

Grmec, S., Mally, S., 2004. Prehospital determination of tracheal tube placement in severe head injury. Emergency Medicine Journal 21, 518–520.

Hildebrandt, T., Espelund, M., Olsen, K., 2010. Evaluation of a transportable capnometer for monitoring end-tidal carbon dioxide. Anaesthesia 65, 1017–1021.

Hinkelbein, J., Floss, F., Denz, C., et al., 2008. Accuracy and precision of three different methods to determine PCO2 (PaCO2 vs. PetCO2 vs. PtcCO2) during interhospital ground transport of critically ill and ventilated adults. Journal of Trauma 65, 10–18.

Hodges, P., Sapsford, R., Pengel, L., 2007. Postural and respiratory functions of the pelvic floor muscles. Neurology and Urodynamics 26, 362–371.

Hoit, J., Lohmeier, H., 2000. Influence of continuous speaking on ventilation. Journal of Speech, Language and Hearing Research 43, 1240–1251.

Hornsveld, H., Garssen, B., 1997. Hyperventilation syndrome: an elegant but scientifically untenable concept. Netherlands Journal of Medicine 50, 13–20.

Jaffe, M., 2008. Infared measurement of carbon dioxide in the human breath: 'breathe through' devices from tyndall to the present day. Anesthesia and Analgesia 107, 890–904.

Kolar, P., Sulc, J., Kyncl, M., et al, 2012. Postural function of the diaphragm in persons with and without chronic low back pain. Journal of Orthopedic and Sports Physical Therapy 42 (4), 352–362.

Levitsky, MG., 2007. Pulmonary physiology, seventh ed. McGraw–Hill, Toronto ON Canada.

Litchfield, P., 2012. Respiratory fitness and dysfunctional breathing workshop. Santa Fe NM USA.

Martin, L., 1992. All you really need to know to interpret arterial blood gases. Lea & Febiger, Philadelphia.

McLaughlin, L., Goldsmith, C., Coleman, K., 2011. Breathing evaluation and retraining as an adjunct to manual therapy. Manual Therapy 16, 51–52.

Nixon, P., Freeman, L., 1988. The 'think test': a further technique to elicit hyperventilation. The Royal Society of Medicine 81 (5), 277–279.

O'Sullivan, P.B., Beales, D.J., 2007. Changes in pelvic floor and diaphragm kinematics and respiratory patterns in subjects with sacroiliac joint pain following a motor learning intervention: A case series. Manual Therapy 12, 209–218.

Radebold, A., Cholewicki, J., Polzhofer, B., et al., 2001. Impaired postural control of the lumbar spine is associated with delayed muscle response times in patients with chronic idiopathic low back pain. Spine 26 (7), 724–730.

Scarth, E., Cook, T., 2012. Capnography during cardiopulmonary resuscitation. Resuscitation doi:10.1016/j.resuscitation.2012.04.002.

Tawadrous, F., Eldridge, F., 1974. Posthyperventilation breathing patterns after active hyperventilation in man. Journal of Applied Physiology 37 (3), 353–356.

Thomson, W.S.T., Adams, J.F., Cowan, R.A., 1997. Clinical acid–base balance. Oxford University Press, New York NY.

van Dixhoorn, J., Duivenvoorden, H., 1985. Efficacy of Nijmegen questionnaire in recognition of the hyperventilation syndrome. Journal of Psychosomatic Research 29 (2), 199–206.

Indirect approaches to breathing regulation

Jan van Dixhoorn

INTRODUCTION

Breathing is largely dependent upon many factors, both physical and mental, which determine its rate, depth and shape. Given this dependency, the use for breathing regulation seems quite limited. In fact, a sceptical point of view is not uncommon and exists, for example, in the medical profession. Moreover, in some awareness schools, such as the Feldenkrais Method® (see Ch. 8.3) and the Alexander Technique, there is little or no use for breathing modification. When certain determinants are a structural cause of a particular way of breathing, then the efforts to change breathing will be barely successful and will only lead to increased strain. When such factors are of a modifiable nature (see Chs 7.1b, 7.2 and 7.3), for instance, due to increased mental or physical stress, then the attempt to change respiration may be more successful, but may still lead to increased strain: the original stress plus the effort to change breathing. This sceptical view can be countered by referring to available outcome data of breathing (see chapters in Section 7, particularly Chs 7.1b, 7.4, 7.6 and 7.7), but the argument remains valid. In this chapter we propose to consider the immediate context of breathing patterns and use it explicitly by influencing breathing indirectly, rather than attempting to impose a 'better form' of breathing.

Indirect regulation assumes that an important function of breathing is to reflect the individual's condition. It is like a mirror and is an indicator of one's physical or emotional state. From this perspective, the first thing in working with breathing is to respect this function. For instance, during physical exercise, breathing deepens to meet the increasing gas exchange requirements. When this leads to dyspnoea, indirect regulation would aim to lower the exercise intensity, or to have the subject focus on the quality of movement, whereas direct regulation would aim to confront the dyspnoea and consciously change the pattern of breathing.

There are many ways to modify breathing voluntarily, which are widely recognized and practised. Thus, there are two opposing perspectives. To deal with both points of view, both reflecting reality, instructions were developed which have been crafted to change the immediate determinants of breathing and also to change breathing indirectly, alongside direct breathing instructions (van Dixhoorn 2007). Both these direct and indirect breathing instructions include instructions for posture and focus of attention. Furthermore, it is important to leave the outcome of an instruction open, and to respect the outcome of any breathing intervention, accepting the resulting change as the best possible at the moment, rather than sticking to a preconceived idea of what optimal breathing should be. Given the multitude of determinants it is not possible to know what respiratory pattern is optimal at any given time. Finally, a basic procedure is required where the therapist tries a few approaches and carefully observes the responses. Interventions should be interrupted regularly to allow the system to process the induced changes and to observe the responses at each stage.

SYSTEMS VIEW

Within psychophysiology, respiratory measures function mainly as dependent variables, reflecting the state of the individual. Within *applied* psychophysiology however, respiration also functions as an independent variable, a potential influence on one's state. Breathing is the only major vital function that is open to conscious awareness and modification. The individual is able to voluntarily modify breathing patterns in order to change mental or physical tension states. Thus, there is a dual relationship between breathing and the state of the system, represented in Figure 7.1a.1. The arrows from respiration towards physical or mental tension states represent the regulatory role of breathing; the arrows towards respiration represent its role as indicator. The idea is that direct, regulatory instructions for breathing are quite possible and effective, but mainly temporary, and that a lasting effectiveness resides in an influence upon the mental/physical tension state. When there is a change in that state, breathing will change in due course, by way of its indicator role, and it will be more responsive to regulatory practice. Thus, one stops the regulatory practice, observes how the system responds, and how breathing continues afterwards. The resulting change may be small, but this tends to continue because its determinants have changed. Continuous practice is not required.

This way of alternating regulatory practice and stopping it is in our view the 'basic procedure' of breathing therapy. It has several advantages. It conveys to the client the idea that breathing is variable and flexible. Contrary to what many think and expect to be taught, there is not one particular way of 'proper breathing'. Also, it conveys the idea that to notice responses and changes in breathing may already be sufficient and helpful to understand and deal with respiratory discomfort. When breathing discomfort arises, one should be attentive to the context, before one practises some counter-effective breathing tactic. Acknowledging the fact that respiration responds to emotion, posture, mental focus, imagery, etc. neutralizes the cognitive interpretation that respiratory discomfort always means that something is wrong with breathing, or the system that breathing is a part of (see Fig. 7.1a.1).

This model represents a systems view of respiration. It underlines the complexity of breathing instruction which should include both mental and physical components, in addition to specific instructions for breathing. One consequence of the model is that proper breathing instruction consists of two parts: one in which breathing is consciously modified or regulated and one in which this regulation is consciously stopped. This is comparable to Jacobson's procedure of Progressive Muscular Relaxation, to consciously tense a muscle in order to learn to consciously stop muscle tension (Jacobson 1938). One cannot ask the subject to stop breathing, but it is possible to stop a conscious regulatory practice. The purpose is to observe how the system responds to the regulation, and whether there is a small, but durable and stable effect on breathing after regulation has stopped. The instruction that regulates breathing is more like an invitation to the system to respond favourably, than a dominant influence. It is important to teach a specific skill to practise, but it is equally important to have the subject stop practising it.

The message to the patient is that the purpose is not to practise a particular form of breathing as much as possible, but to observe what happens after one has practised. An instruction is not a model of good breathing but it is a stimulus to the system that hopefully yields a meaningful response.

The systems view provides a context which serves as a background for the many techniques of direct breathing regulation. There is no doubt that regular practice is beneficial and often necessary. However, it is important that the practice is not too single-minded and goal-directed, but remains open to the diversity of outcomes. Such open evaluation is an important check as to whether the particular technique is still beneficial. For instance, slow, deep breathing is not natural, but is useful to practise periodically. Breathing 6–8 times a minute has a profound restorative effect on the autonomic nervous system (Bernardi et al 2001), as well as a mobilizing effect on the musculoskeletal system involved in breathing. It may also affect the mental state. Thus, to determine which effect is beneficial and relevant at the moment, it is necessary to check the outcome with an open mind. Global evaluation (subjective experiences, checklists, observable changes in posture, movement or facial expression) is preferred, but instrumental multi-channel recordings are also possible. The latter is more objective but has limited parameters.

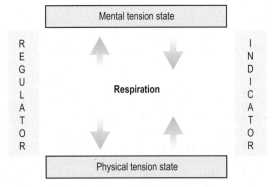

Figure 7.1a.1 Model of double relationship between respiration and its determinant. Arrows on the left: voluntarily induced changes in breathing influence physical/mental tension state. Arrows on the right: changes in physical/mental tension state influence breathing.

Rationale of indirect regulation

There are a number of arguments to use direct modification only temporarily, and to add indirect regulation. One of them is that breathing consciously and voluntarily tends to slow and deepen respiration and reduce variability. This may be a consequence of the effort to control air flow, such as occurs when breathing through a mouthpiece (Tobin et al 1983), or because the patient has the idea that slow, deep, regular breathing is the best. Simply counting one's own respiration reduces variability (Conrad et al 2007). However, natural breathing is variable and reducing variability may not be beneficial (Donaldson 1992). It may also reduce the expressive function of breathing, for instance blocking an emotional sigh and heaving of the chest, because one tries to maintain regular abdominal breathing. In addition, slow and deep breathing tends to increase minute volume. With deeper breathing, the relative contribution of dead air space becomes less, effective ventilation therefore increases and frequency has to reduce much more to retain minute ventilation. Thus, effective minute ventilation tends to increase. This is the case in particular when mental tension that accompanies a higher breathing rate is relatively high. In case of hypoventilation and lung disease, increased ventilation is beneficial and the advice to inhale slowly is proper, but in cases involving anxiety problems, breathing regulation may result in hyperventilation and consequent increase of complaints due to hypocapnia (Terai & Umezawa, 2004). In cases of asthma, the balance between over- and under-breathing is particularly tricky (Jeter et al 2012).

Another argument to limit the time for direct regulation is that sensorimotor control of proximal muscles is far less differentiated than control of distal muscle groups. The area of cortical representation is larger for the periphery. It is easy to clench only one hand, more difficult to raise only one shoulder and very difficult to breathe with one half of the rib cage. Given the relatively undifferentiated control of the trunk muscles, where breathing movement takes place, the tendency is to perform breathing instructions with undue effort. This applies in particular to novices and anxious or stressed subjects (Terai & Umezawa 2004). Instead, the instructions and manual techniques that were developed for indirect regulation use peripheral movements, with arms, legs and head, to facilitate changes in respiratory pattern. Facilitation results from the skeletal connection between rib cage, spinal column and periphery (van Dixhoorn 1997, van Dixhoorn 2007). With inhalation the rib cage lifts and rolls cranially and this is facilitated by slight increase of lordosis in the lumbar area and slight decrease of cervical lordosis. Thus, in the sitting position, opening the knees slightly enhances inhalation, as does external rotation of the arms and hands (also see Brugger's position, described and illustrated in Ch. 9). This is discussed in the practical example in the text below.

A third argument resides in the views from neuroimaging research. In the past decade it has become clear that brain regions implicated in the regulation of emotion are both responsive to breathing-related bodily changes, and important in influencing the appearance and persistence of breathing-related symptoms (Rosenkranz & Davidson 2009). Thus, to reduce the sensations of dyspnoea, laborious breathing and/or enhance the sensations of breathing freely, openly, effortlessly and unrestricted, it is not only important to change breathing patterns, but also to facilitate its generalization in the central regulation of emotion in the brain. The idea is that this is helped by indirect regulation and by allowing time for processing the effects of regulation in the period when regulation is stopped. In this time period, the patient's experiences can be expressed, their interpretation and meaning discussed, their emotional implications elaborated. Consequently, we recommend that the breathing pattern intervention be evaluated using a different posture than was used during the original intervention, in order to emphasize the effects in an open, global way: is there a change in posture, mood, general tension, mental quiet and, lastly, breathing?

PRACTICAL EXAMPLE OF INDIRECT INSTRUCTIONS IN THE SITTING POSITION

In this section a detailed example is presented, quoted from a manual that is published internally for the benefit of students of breathing therapy (van Dixhoorn 2010). It is a primary text of instructions, which has the purpose of being followed and practised. The best way to understand the concept is by experiencing the reality it describes. Indirect approaches are suitable in all positions (supine and prone, side-lying, standing and sitting). We choose to elaborate the sitting position for its ease to practice in daily life as well as in the treatment room.

Sitting position

A stool or chair without arm rests is required with a flat, uncushioned and horizontal surface. The height is such that the feet can fully rest on the floor. The instruction is to have the feet apart and in front of the knees, while looking straight ahead with the hands resting on the upper thighs.

Comment: the upper legs do not necessarily have to be horizontal, but the feet have to be able to rest fully. When the heels do not touch the ground fully, a lower stool is required, or some support, like a large book or a folded bath towel, can be put under the feet. The feet are in front of the knees. This position is essential because it induces a more passive way of sitting.

Option: position of feet

It is an option to make a point of this position by having the client place their feet alternately in front and behind the knees, each time with feet fully in contact with the floor. Have the client repeat these two positions and observe the consequences that this has on the way one sits. After allowing sufficient time for the client to make a number of comparisons involving foot position, ask the client, with the feet in front, to stand up. This is likely to be difficult. Then repeat it with the feet behind the knees. This will be easier. The point to make is that regardless of all possible differences in the way one sits, with the feet in front one sits as if one is remaining, while with the feet behind, it is possible to get up rapidly. Thus, one sits physically, and also mentally. Moreover, the procedure brings attention to the ischial tuberosities ('sitting bones'), the feet and the supporting surface.

Step 1. Move forward and backward

Observe posture but do not make any comment. Is the back erect or slumped? Is the weight in front or behind the sitting bones? Is the client restless or still, is the head directed to the front, as if looking towards the horizon, with the eyes directed more up or more down? Then have the client move slowly a little to the front and back, while the head remains directed straight ahead. Ask for this to be done a number of times, slowly, and have the client observe the shift of weight in the sitting bones. 'Observe the moment that you are sitting in front, to the back or right on top of your sitting bones. Find the position in which you are sitting fully on the sitting bones, stay there and sit easily, with a bit of slump, but don't lean back.' Observe the changes while moving to the front and back. Notice and remember, whether the upper body really moves, and with how much effort, and whether the head remains horizontal. Notice how much effort the movement entails and how the spinal column changes in shape.

Comment. The idea is twofold. Mentally, the instruction brings attention to the supporting surface. As a result, the body and the mind 'sit', that is, the body rests on the surface. The client sits more at ease and quietens mentally. Muscle tension that is required to sit more or less upright can diminish slightly. Physically, slowly moving forward and back may facilitate a more functional upright sitting posture. The spinal column changes in form, feels the support of the pelvis and may arrange its balance in a more functional, easy way. As a result the body sits better upright and the head is balanced better.

Step 2. Stay front/back and breathe

Then ask the individual to move forward, remain in that position and observe how this position feels. How does breathing feel in this position? After a couple of breaths, move backwards, remain there and compare. Repeat this a few times and have the client return to the middle. Observe how the movement is performed and how the posture may have changed; ask how it feels. Then, repeat this step and ask the individual to observe the changes in

breathing when in the two positions. Ask literally, 'Do you notice that breathing responds to your posture?' but do not go into discussions as to what feels pleasant or unpleasant, natural or unnatural, normal or abnormal, proper or improper, etc.

Comment. The point of self-observation is to have the client acknowledge that breathing responds to posture. It is not a question of preference, but of neutral observation, that posture determines breathing to a certain extent. Conversely, functional breathing adapts to this determinant and reflects the postural attitude. One can encourage the client to observe, accept and follow the changes in breathing, to go along with it and not try to continue breathing in one way, regardless of the posture. For instance, most clients think that relaxed breathing is abdominal and that the chest is not involved. However, in the forward position, the chest tends to be lifted and to participate in breathing. This is acceptable and functional.

Another issue is the change one notices after the procedure. Sitting and breathing may become noticeably easier, more comfortable, requiring less effort. The procedure entails sitting and breathing in two contrasting positions. It poses a small challenge to respiration, requiring it to adapt. The rib cage is involved in this adaptation and may become a little more flexible afterwards.

Step 3. Move forward/backward and lumbar spine (Fig. 7.1a.2)

Ask the client to again move forward and back, and to observe the weight shift in the sitting bones, while keeping the head directed forward, at a horizontal level. Now, observe the lumbar spine and lower back. Is there any movement in the sense of a form change? One may place a hand at the thoracolumbar junction. This helps both client and therapist to increase information regarding what actually takes place. The intended movement is not pelvic rolling and extending/flexing the spine from the pelvis and lower back. When the body moves backward, if the lumbar spine were to remain stiffly erect, the backward tilt would result in toppling over. Functional accommodation of the lumbar spine therefore demands slight curving of the lumbar spine (flexion). The more the body goes backward, the more the lower spine needs to curve and become round (i.e. moving into flexion) in order to keep the body in balance. Conversely, when moving forward, the lower spine tends to extend and flatten in order to carry the ribcage and head forward. Thus, one asks the client to notice whether any change occurs in the shape of the lumbar spine. 'Go forward, stay there and feel the lumbar spine. Is it more round or more straight? Go backward, stay there and observe the lumbar spine. Is it more round or more straight?' Repeat this a number of times, until the client clearly perceives that the spine tends to extend when going forward and to become rounder when going backwards. Then stop, let the client go to the middle and observe how one sits and feels while breathing.

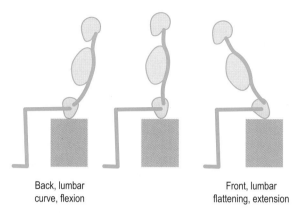

Back, lumbar curve, flexion

Front, lumbar flattening, extension

Figure 7.1a.2 Spinal form changes in three sitting positions.

Comment. We focus in this step on the spinal column. Step 1 shows the form change in the body during movement front and back. The issue now is the organization of the movement and the flexibility of the spinal column. When the client becomes aware that the lumbar spine actually changes form and participates in the movement, the result is two-fold. This kind of precise and concrete self-observation requires a lot of attention. Thus, there is less room for cognitive interpretation and mental perseveration[1] (Brosschot et al 2010). One becomes more quiet mentally and also physiologically. This is facilitated when there is avoidance of any hint as to what is good or bad and the individual simply, neutrally, compares the spine in the two positions. Secondly, when the spine becomes more flexible, the organization of the movement improves and the movement becomes easier. Thus, afterwards, sitting is more relaxed, breathing is easier, and possibly better distributed. (See Chapter 6.5 for 'MARM' relating to 'distribution'.)

Step 4. Coupling forward/backward to breathing

We return to Step 2 and ask the client to move forward and backward a couple of times, notice the weight shift, keep the head directed forward and then go forward and stay there. How does this position feel now compared to the first time, and how is breathing? When breathing involves more of the chest we encourage it, ask the individual to accept and mentally follow that breathing movement. Then we ask for movement that is a little further forward and back again. We observe the involvement of the lumbar spine as well as the lower ribs. We repeat this a few times until we can see the lower ribs and lumbar spine contracting together. Then we ask the client to go to

the middle and backwards and stay there. How does this position feel and where can breathing movement be felt? We request movement to go a little further back and forth, and observe whether the backwards movement is initiated by lumbar flexing as well as widening of the lower ribs.

Now we include direct breathing instruction. When the client goes forward and stays there, we ask about the effect on breathing. Then we encourage inhalation, together with lifting of the chest and the sternum while at the same time moving the trunk a little further forward. When exhaling, a small degree of backward movement is requested. This is repeated until it becomes clear to the individual that upper thoracic inhalation facilitates extension of the spine, while moving forward. Going backwards is facilitated by exhaling and letting the chest and sternum sink.

Comment. The issue now is the coordination of the rib cage and lumbar spine. When this is successful, breathing movement as well as spinal movement will have increased in flexibility. Spinal extension and elevation of the ribs facilitate each other. Their combination results in a pattern of 'functional upper thoracic breathing', in which 'gasping' and excessive use of the auxiliary respiratory muscles of the neck and shoulders are avoided, while still increasing the use of the upper chest. This use is supported by all the changes in posture that occur in daily life. Usually, distribution of breathing movement involves improved posture that is more easily upright so that any sense of dyspnoea becomes less anxious and more manageable.

Often, the use of the chest feels uncomfortable and may be interpreted as 'wrong'. It is important to remain neutral and focus on the actual sensation. Feeling uncomfortable may result from a combination of an unusual sense, the strange sensation of really using the ribs, with the idea that abdominal breathing should be there at all times and is favourable. However, when one practises, gets used to the sensation and observes its benefit on posture and respiratory ease afterwards, most people enjoy and appreciate it. Nevertheless, a large part of breathing regulation in this way consists of mental coaching and cognitive restructuring.

Option: opening and closing the knees

When the lumbar area is resistant to movement, and there is hardly any flattening and extension during forward motion, one factor may be the use of the legs. Opening the knees facilitates moving forward as well as lumbar extension. Some subjects do not move the knees at all, others close them while moving forward and open the knees moving backwards. In these cases it is an option to add the following: let the subject sit still, in the middle, and have them open and close the knees slightly, a couple of times. Then have them sit forward and do the same, and have them sit backward and repeat it. Next, ask them to slowly move forward and at the same time open the knees a little, while closing the knees during backward

---

[1]Perseveration: The persistence of a repetitive response after the cause of the response has been removed, or the response continues to different stimuli.

movement. Observe whether the movements are synchronous, and possibly guide and pace the movements verbally.

Option: holding the head

Some subjects have trouble keeping the head directed forwards while moving front and back, or they move the head excessively or with too much force. Neck pain may even result from the effort. Usually the upper back and neck do not move with ease and the coordination with the lower spine and rib cage does not occur spontaneously. In this case, an option is to stand at the side of the client and softly take the head into the two hands. The first and second finger of one hand are spread out, touch the base of the skull, and are able to lift the head slightly while it moves forward. The fingers of the other hand are flat and touch the front of the head. They can give a slight pressure to the head when moving backwards. In any case, first let the subject move a couple of times back and forth while holding the head and observing the pattern of motion of the head during this movement. Then ask the subject if they can follow you and guide the movement with your hands. While doing that, observe primarily whether the head goes up and down during the movement and then try to keep the head more or less horizontal.

DISCUSSION: A PERSONAL PERSPECTIVE

It is hoped that the practical section helps to show that an indirect approach is both feasible and effective. It follows the motto that 'a detour is often the quickest way to go'. This applies in particular when there are obstructions on the way.

In the 1970s I worked part-time in a cardiac rehabilitation unit where I introduced breathing and relaxation therapy, using biofeedback. We conducted a clinical trial comparing an experimental group (following physical exercise plus relaxation and breathing) and a control group (physical exercise only). The outcome showed a clear additional benefit (van Dixhoorn & van Duivenvoorden 1999) that has led to the inclusion of relaxation classes in the Dutch guidelines for cardiac rehabilitation. Cardiac patients in general practise valiantly what they are taught. This frequently involves the direct technique of exhaling audibly which patients found both pleasant and relaxing. However, when end-tidal CO_2 was measured, in the pilot phase of the clinical trial, it was found that many practised too long and too strong and actually hyperventilated. This was not experienced unpleasantly but was nevertheless undesirable, making the system more vulnerable. We therefore shortened the number of consecutive practice cycles from around 15 to 5, emphasized that this form of breathing was not a model for normal or optimal

breathing, and that the main purpose was to stop audible exhalation, while breathing normally and observing whether any changes were noticeable.

In the trial we measured the respiration pattern repeatedly (by covert observation) and found a decrease in respiration rate in the experimental group, but no change in the control group. The change was modest: from 15–16 cycles per minute (cpm) to 11–12 cpm, without changes in end-tidal CO_2. The slower rate was mainly due to lengthening of the exhalation pause, which is very responsive to stress (Umezawa 1992). Thus, we did not impose a respiratory pattern, but hoped we had achieved a decrease in tension which was reflected in the lower rate. Two years later, a small group of subjects was measured. Again, the experimental group was breathing slower (Fig. 7.1a.3). Two subjects were clearly 'practising' breathing during measurement, at a respiration rate of 6–7 cpm. Since we were interested in changes in natural, spontaneous breathing, they were excluded from the analysis.

On the occasion of this follow-up measurement I practised MARM for the first time (see Ch. 6.5) to assess breathing movement. It showed that the experimental group had a more costo-abdominal breathing pattern than the control group. My conclusion was not only that the spontaneous breathing pattern had changed, but also that they were sitting more at ease and less ready to get up, to which respiration responded. In other words, they were more relaxed. This strengthened my idea that a small but stable change in pattern is more relevant than a large, momentary change.

A combination of direct and indirect regulation appeared to be important: a direct technique was necessary to show that breathing regulation could be feasible and effective.

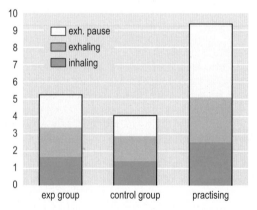

Figure 7.1a.3 Time components for experimental and control group, at 2 years follow-up, in seconds. The difference in exhalation pause time between experimental and control group is statistically significant (p < 0.01). Two subjects who practised breathing are shown but were excluded from the analysis.

This was taught mainly on an individual basis, using manual techniques as well. The indirect techniques were important to divert attention from breathing and to prevent continuous practice during the day, while at the same time promoting a change in the determinants of breathing. Stiffness of the chest appears to be almost always present and mobilizing the thorax, improving coordination with the spine, is crucial. We have no published data of our own, but indirect techniques were shown to be effective with lung cancer patients (Bredin et al 1999). The focus in that study was not to modify breathing, but to increase awareness of the factors that influence breathing and the sense of dyspnoea.

In the 1970s, the hyperventilation syndrome became a popular topic and became the main reason professionals attended my classes for breathing instructions. Because of the anxiety and panic of hyperventilation patients, the indirect approach appeared to be useful. The ability to neutrally observe natural respiratory responses to posture and mental state was valuable and needed particular emphasis. Many indirect techniques were developed to make this possible. When this was successful, treatment response was positive. However, when the experience of easy and less effortful breathing did not occur or was not convincing enough for patients to let go of the fear, psychological treatment or medication appeared to be necessary. In a recent paper, we showed that breathing therapy resulted in a clear reduction of dyspnoea complaints in stressed patients, which was mediated by reduction of upper thoracic breathing pattern (Courtney et al 2011).

REFERENCES

Bernardi, L., Sleight, P., Bandinelli, G., et al., 2001. Effect of rosary prayer and yoga mantras on autonomic cardiovascular rhythms: comparative study. BMJ 323 (7327), 1446–1449.

Bredin, M., Corner, J., Krishnasamy, M., et al, 1999. Multicentre randomised controlled trial of nursing intervention for breathlessness in patients with lung cancer. BMJ 318, 901–904.

Brosschot, J. F., Verkuil, B., Thayer, J. F., 2010. Conscious and unconscious perseverative cognition: is a large part of prolonged physiological activity due to unconscious stress? J Psychosom Res 69-4, 407–416.

Conrad, A., Muller, A., Doberenz, S., et al., 2007. Psychophysiological effects of breathing instructions for stress management. Appl. Psychophysiol. Biofeedback 32, 89–98.

Courtney, R., van Dixhoorn, J.J., Anthonissen, E., et al, 2011. Medically unexplained dyspnea: partly moderated by dysfunctional (thoracic dominant) breathing pattern. J Asthma 48, 259–265.

van Dixhoorn, J.J., 2010. Manual for Breathing Therapy. Centrum AOT, Amersfoort, The Netherlands.

van Dixhoorn, J.J., van Duivenvoorden, H.J., 1999. Effect of relaxation therapy on cardiac events after myocardial infarction: a 5-year follow-up study. J Cardiopulm Rehabil 19, 178–185.

van Dixhoorn, J., 1997. Functional breathing is 'wholebody' breathing. Biological Psychology 46, 89–90.

van Dixhoorn, J., 2007. Whole-Body breathing: a systems perspective on respiratory retraining. In: Lehrer, P.M., Woolfolk, R.L., Sime, W.E. (Eds.), Principles and practice of stress management. Guilford Press, New York, pp. 291–332.

Donaldson, G.C., 1992. The chaotic behaviour of resting human respiration. Respiratory Physiology, 88, 313–321.

Jacobson, E., 1938. Progressive relaxation. University of Chicago Press, Chicago.

Jeter, A.M., Kim, H.C., Simon, E., et al., 2012. Hypoventilation training for asthma: a case illustration. Appl. Psychophysiol.Biofeedback 37, 63–72.

Rosenkranz, M.A., Davidson, R.J., 2009. Affective neural circuitry and mind-body influences in asthma. Neuroimage., 47, 972–980.

Terai, K., Umezawa, A., 2004. Effects of respiratory self-control on psychophysiological relaxation using biofeedback involving the partial pressure of end-tidal carbon dioxide. Japanese Society of Biofeedback Research 30, 31–37.

Tobin, M.J., Chadha, T.S., Jenouri, G., et al, 1983. Breathing patterns. I: normal subjects. Chest 84-2, 202–205.

Umezawa, A., 1992. Effects of stress on post expiration pause time and minute ventilation volume. In: Shirakura, K., Saito, I., Tsutsui, S. (Eds.), Current biofeedback research in Japan. Shinkoh Igaku Shuppan, Tokyo, Japan, pp. 125–132.

Chapter | 7.1b|

Dynamic Neuromuscular Stabilization: treatment methods

Pavel Kolar, Alena Kobesova, Petra Valouchova, Petr Bitnar

See Chapter 2.1 for details of developmental kinesiology, and Dynamic Neuromuscular Stabilization (DNS) on which the methods described in this chapter are based. See also Chapter 6.1 for assessment approaches based on DNS.

INTRODUCTION

Physiological breathing is a prerequisite for physiological stabilization of the spine and vice versa. Posture closely influences breathing (Chiodini & Thach 1993, Grönkvist

et al 2002, Johansson & Stömberg 2000, Kirkpatrick et al 2010). This relationship forms the postural-respiratory function of the diaphragm. Understanding the correlation between lung function and postural activity of the diaphragm is essential for treatment outcomes (Kolar et al 2012), which is a notion that is in agreement with our clinical experience. Physical therapy focused on techniques influencing only a respiratory pattern is not sufficient for the improvement of respiratory parameters. Physical therapy treatment needs to include techniques related to the postural activity of the diaphragm. Forced expiration and the huffing technique are two airway clearance techniques that respect this functional relationship.

In patients suffering with an airflow obstruction, i.e. cystic fibrosis (CF) or chronic obstructive pulmonary disease (COPD), we advocate to combine airway clearance techniques such as the active cycle of breathing (ACBT) with chest physical therapy. Multiple therapeutic goals are established for such patients:

1. Airway clearance and assisted cough
2. Improvement of respiratory pattern by making it more efficient, which leads to normalization of ventilation parameters
3. Decreased chest rigidity
4. Increased physical fitness and exercise tolerance
5. Ultimate increase in the patient's health-related quality of life.

Autogenic drainage (AD) is a modified breathing pattern that starts with a slow, fluent, deep and prolonged inspiration and is followed by an inspiratory pause. This is followed by a volitionally controlled, very slow and long expiration, which completes the cycle. AD helps to loosen, collect and evacuate the mucus. At the end of an AD cycle, the individual is instructed to huff to expectorate the mucus. Huffing is an active, rapid but long expectoration as if breathing onto a mirror to cover it with moisture. AD and huffing are designed to replace inefficient, shallow cough. Such modified tidal breathing along with huffing is quite effective in airway mucus clearance and can be practised in almost any position, most commonly in sitting. However, the principles of optimal trunk stabilization and the proper alignment between the chest and the pelvis as described above need to be respected. The inspiration wave should reach as far as the patient's groin; the chest and the abdominal wall must expand proportionally in all directions (see Ch. 6.1, Fig. 6.1.4A,B); the chest must be maintained in a neutral position and the spine remain straight. The patient is asked to relax their shoulders, avoid activation of the accessory respiratory muscles, and utilize mainly the diaphragm and the intercostal muscles.

Different devices have been used to increase the effect of traditional thoracic therapy. Positive expiratory pressure (PEP) system breathing implements an active, muscle-assisted expiration with modified speed. PEP assists in increasing the intra-bronchial pressure during breathing against a predetermined resistance and significantly increases the diaphragm's activity. PEP from 10–100 cm H_2O is delivered by a facemask. It improves mucus clearance by increasing gas pressure behind secretions through collateral ventilation and by preventing airway collapse during expiration (McCool & Rossen 2006). No differences in pulmonary parameters between physiotherapy and PEP have been shown in patients with COPD or CF (McCool & Rossen 2006). Since 1985, the multidisciplinary approach of care for patients with CF at the University Hospital Motol in Prague has included comprehensive rehabilitation and showed good effectiveness of combined chest physiotherapy based on the principles of developmental kinesiology and airway clearance techniques. Such combined rehabilitation facilitated improved prognosis and quality of life in patients with CF (Vávrová et al 1999). Similarly, we can report a very positive experience with combination of individual chest physiotherapy and flutter utilization in patients with CF as well as in patients after chest surgery. Flutter is a plastic, pipe-like device with a steel ball placed in a circular, conical end. Exhaling through the device produces oscillatory overpressure in the airway, which helps to mobilize and evacuate pulmonary secretions and to prevent bronchial collapse and formation of atelectasis, a common consequence of mucus plugs. RC-Cornet® is another device producing gentle vibrations of bronchial walls. It is especially suitable for younger infants. Acapella® is a device of choice for airway clearance in patients who are immobilized, such as those being hospitalized in intensive care units. It allows for treatment of patients who are intubated and dependent on artificial ventilation. If a proper device is selected for a particular patient, it is well tolerated and effective. In summary, we advocate to combine individual chest physical therapy that respects genetically determined programmes and employs proper routine of respiratory-postural

function with airway clearance techniques. The goal is to increase health-related quality of life, decrease rates of pulmonary disease exacerbations, reduce hospitalizations and treat any musculoskeletal pain related to abnormal pattern of respiratory-postural function.

Regardless of the chosen type of respiratory physiotherapy, we suggest approaching posture at the same time.

TREATMENT TECHNIQUES TO OPTIMIZE A POSTURAL RESPIRATORY PATTERN

The following should be the focus when influencing the breathing pattern and trunk stabilization:

1. Influencing hypomobility and dynamics of the thoracic wall
2. Influencing spine straightening
3. Practising postural stabilization of the spine by utilizing Vojta's reflex locomotion
4. Practising postural breathing pattern and stabilization function of the diaphragm (intra-abdominal pressure control)
5. Practising postural stabilization of the spine in the positions related to developmental sequences – in modified positions and versions.

Influencing hypomobility and dynamics of the thoracic wall

The alignment and mobility of the thoracic wall are among the most important prerequisites for physiological breathing pattern and trunk stabilization. With the thoracic spine erect, the cranial ('inspiratory') position of the thoracic wall should be released and independent movement of the thorax should be achieved (movement of the rib cage independently of the thoracic spine). This is usually initiated by releasing the thoracic fasciae, especially in the area of the lower intercostal spaces, so that the subsequent training of correct activation of the diaphragm allows for thoracic wall expansion, especially between the lower ribs. Any resistance within the abdominal cavity is released by visceral techniques. Increased soft tissue resistance within the abdominal cavity limits the internal organ mobility and prevents sufficient descent of the diaphragm during breathing or postural loading. Also, it is usually necessary to mobilize the costovertebral joints and release the upper thoracic and scapular stabilizers (scalenes, sternocleidomastoids, pectoral muscles, upper trapezius) to achieve a neutral thoracic wall alignment and activate abdominal musculature. See Chapters 7.2 and 7.3 for complementary mobilization approaches.

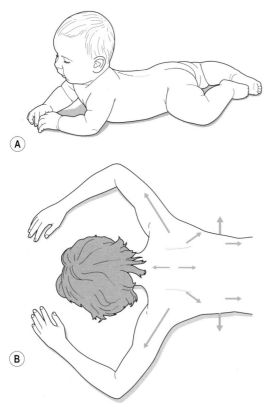

Figure 7.1b.1 Optimal sagittal stabilization in prone. **A** A healthy 4-month-old infant supports himself on the medial epicondyles and the symphysis. The spine is upright; extension and rotation are possible in all segments, including the mid-thoracic spine. **B** Assessment and training of proportional, segmental spine straightening: weight bearing on the medial epicondyles and the symphysis, spinal elongation, neutral position of the scapulae (avoid scapular retraction!), neutral chest position and symmetrical abdominal wall expansion. Practise segmental extension and rotation in mid-thoracic spine – segment by segment, one at a time. Maintain correct posture and breathe into the groin and the laterodorsal abdominal areas.

Influencing spine straightening

Practising spine straightening is another prerequisite for physiological spinal stabilization (Kolar 2006). Most often, the thoracic spine in patients with stabilization dysfunction moves as a rigid unit. Treatment includes traction mobilization techniques, active practice of thoracic spine straightening and segmental movement into extension and rotation. To accomplish this, correct scapular stabilization is important. This can be accomplished in prone with support on elbows (upper extremity (UE) closed kinetic chain). In this position, which corresponds to 4 months of physiological development (Fig. 7.1b.1A), practising thoracic spine extension and selective segmental extension is optimal (Fig. 7.1b.1B).

See also discussion of 'breathing wave' in Chapter 6.2 and Figure 6.2.11.

Activation of an optimal respiratory stabilization pattern through reflex locomotion

In the initial phase of education, reflex stimulation is used to achieve well-balanced activation of muscle synergy between the muscles of the abdominal brace (diaphragm, abdominal and pelvic floor muscles) and the back musculature (Kolar 2006, Vojta 2004, Vojta & Peters 2001). During stimulation of the thoracic zone in Phase I of reflex rolling, the diaphragm contracts through a direct and transferred stretch of the diaphragm's insertions. This contraction acts on the thorax through the ribs while the intra-abdominal pressure increases simultaneously. This is similar in reflex crawling, during which the first reaction of the stimulated zones elicits deepening of lower costal breathing and abdominal wall expansion in all directions. Individual components required for physiological stabilization are integrated within this reflexively stimulated model. These include automatic alignment of the thorax into a neutral position, spinal straightening, postural diaphragmatic breathing with expansion of the lower thoracic region, eccentric stabilization function of the abdominal muscles, centrated support function of the extremities based on positions, symmetrical facilitation of the deep and superficial muscles, etc. The goal of reflex stimulation is to elicit an optimal stabilization muscle synergy and to facilitate an experience during activation that encourages somato-aesthetic perception which can later be implemented into exercises with volitional control.

Similarly to DNS, Vojta's concept of reflex locomotion is based on developmental kinesiology. The quality of postural respiratory function evoked by reflex locomotion corresponds with an optimal quality of this pattern observed in a healthy 4–5-month-old infant. Both reflex locomotion and normal development demonstrate a pattern of physiological spinal stabilization. This is not an artificial model of an optimal stabilization outcome; it is a genetically determined, natural pattern. If the stimulation is carried out correctly, the proportional muscle coordination (as described above) is evoked automatically, the chest and pelvis are aligned correctly, with the chest being placed just above the pelvis, the pelvis and the chest axis is parallel while the whole spine is upright. Optimal coordination among the stabilizers, i.e. the concentric activity of the diaphragm and the pelvic floor and the eccentric activity of other stabilizers, occurs and, at the same time, optimal diaphragmatic breathing is triggered. An optimally developing infant, properly carrying out reflex stimulation, as well as elite athletes when aiming for the best sport performance, all demonstrate an optimal postural respiratory stereotype.

It is a stereotype that allows for maximum strength while being protective by avoiding any segmental/joint overload.

Practising a postural breathing pattern and the stabilization function of the diaphragm

The inclusion of the diaphragm into breathing and the simultaneous stabilization function without excessive or compensatory participation of the accessory breathing muscles are the goals. To accomplish this, the thorax needs to be positioned caudally and the spine should be straight. The patient is verbally and manually guided to inhale into the lower intercostal spaces and into the abdomen so that the abdominal wall expands in all directions (anterior, lateral and posterior) (see Ch. 6.1, Fig 6.1.4A,B). The umbilicus should not move cranially (an undesirable muscle pull in a cranial direction). The correct breathing pattern should be practised in supine and in sitting positions (Kolar 2006).

This is followed by practising the diaphragm's dual respiratory–stabilization function. The training is performed in various positions. During this exercise, the patient learns to include the diaphragm, whose function we are normally not aware of, during stabilization.

Practising postural stabilization of the spine in the positions related to developmental sequences – modified positions and versions

The starting position is supine with the hips and knees flexed to 90 degrees (developmental position at 4 months) (Fig 7.1b.2A).

Respiratory pattern correction. In the given position, the thorax is manually positioned into neutral alignment during respiration. Lateral movement of the thoracic wall during inspiration is facilitated by a firm manual contact and the patient consciously inhales laterally and caudally towards the pelvis without the thorax moving cranially. Expansion of the abdominal wall in all directions, including the area of the lower abdomen above the groin, is palpated.

Postural activation of the diaphragm – practice of intra-abdominal pressure control. In the same position, the abdominal wall above the groin is palpated using both thumbs (Fig 7.1b.2B). The patient is asked to briefly hold their breath after expiration and to push the examiner's thumbs diagonally down and to the sides. The patient maintains this increased intra-abdominal pressure for several breathing cycles. The same response of the abdominal wall is assessed by palpation of the posterior aspect of the abdominal wall under ribs 11 and 12. As

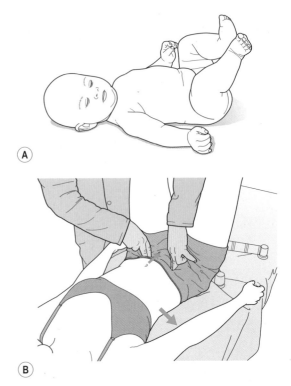

Figure 7.1b.2 Optimal sagittal stabilization in supine. **A** A healthy 4-month-old infant can lift and hold their legs above the mat; the upper gluteal sections are weight bearing, the entire spine is upright, the head is supported at the nuchal line; the lumbar spine fixes to the mat via an increased intra-abdominal pressure, the hips are functionally centrated (90° flexion, slight external rotation) – i.e. an ideal balance between the external/internal rotators, flexors/ extensors and abductors/adductors occurs; proportional, cylindrical activation of the abdominal wall and a neutral chest position. **B** The same principles are followed during the assessment and treatment of a patient in supine. Avoid back arching. This posture increases intra-abdominal pressure, and thus stabilizes the lumbar spine from the front. If this position is too difficult, the patient's lower extremities should be initially supported during practice and the support gradually removed with progression.

soon as the patient masters this coordination of the diaphragm and the abdominal wall, the demands on the control of intra-abdominal pressure are increased by incorporating upper or lower extremity movement against resistance.

The same technique is used during practice of a respiratory postural pattern in other developmental positions, such as in prone with a differentiated position of the extremities (5 months), in side-sitting (8 months), in quadruped (9 months), in a tripod position (10 months), etc. (Kolar 2006, Kolar & Kobesova 2010).

CONCLUSION

The diaphragm and its functional anatomical development play a fundamental role in breathing and in postural and sphincter functions. Disturbed CNS development and control affect movement and breathing patterns and impact visceral function. It may also lead to structural deformities. An optimal alignment of the rib cage corresponds to the position of the pelvis, with the centrum tendineum in a horizontal plane. Posture is a prerequisite for movement. The musculature of the trunk serves as a support base for upper and lower limb movement, where intra-abdominal pressure regulation contributes to spinal stabilization and ensures optimal respiratory function while also influencing visceral function. The diaphragm activates prior to movement – reactive stabilization is automatic and without volitional control. Non-physiological loading leads to reactive changes including morphological alterations due to imbalance in internal muscle forces acting on the spine during postural stabilization. Breathing assessment provides an important and sensitive evaluation of postural function and can be utilized in several positions of increasing postural difficulty.

ACKNOWLEDGMENTS

We would like to thank Ida Norgaard, DC MSc and Vanda Andel, DPT for invaluable help in preparing this manuscript. This manuscript was supported by the foundation Movement without Help, Prague, Czech Republic and by Prague School of Rehabilitation.

REFERENCES

Chiodini, B.A., Thach, B.T., 1993. Impaired ventilation in infants sleeping facedown: potential significance for sudden infant death syndrome. J Pediatr. 123 (5), 686–692.

Grönkvist, M., Bergsten, E., Gustafsson, P.M., 2002. Effects of body posture and tidal volume on inter- and intraregional ventilation distribution in healthy men. J Appl Physiol. 92 (2), 634–642.

Johansson, A., Strömberg, T., 2000. Influence of tidal volume and thoraco-abdominal separation on the respiratory induced variation of the photoplethysmogram. J Clin Monit Comput.16 (8), 575–581.

Kirkpatrick, A.W., Pelosi, P., De Waele, J.J., et al., 2010. Clinical review: Intra-abdominal hypertension: does it influence the physiology of prone ventilation? Crit Care. 14 (4), 232.

Kolar, P., 2006. Facilitation of agonist-antagonist co-activation by reflex stimulation methods. In: Liebenson, C. (Ed.), Rehabilitation of the spine – a practitioner's manual, second ed. Lippincott Williams & Wilkins, Philadelphia, 2006: pp. 531–565.

Kolar, P., Kobesova, A., 2010. Postural – locomotion function in the diagnosis and treatment of movement disorders. Clinical Chiropractic 13 (1), 58–68.

Kolar, P., Sulc, J., Kyncl, M., et al., 2012. Postural function of the diaphragm in persons with and without chronic low back pain. J Orthop Sports Phys Ther. 42 (4), 352–362.

McCool, F.D., Rosen, M.J., 2006. Nonpharmacologic airway clearance therapies: ACCP evidence-based clinical practice guidelines. Chest 129 (1 Suppl), 250S–259S.

Vávrová, V., Zemková, D., Bartosová, J., et al., 1999. Cystic fibrosis–a disease of adolescents and adults? Cas Lek Cesk. 1;138 (21), 654–659. [Article in Czech]

Vojta, V., 2004. Die zerebralen Bewegungsstörungen im Säuglingsalter: Frühdiagnose und Frühtherapie. Thieme.

Vojta, V., Peters, A., 2001. Das Vojta – Princip. Springer Verlag, Berlin.

Chapter | 7.2 |

Osteopathic treatment of thoracic and respiratory dysfunction

Leon Chaitow

Osteopathic manipulative treatment (OMT) has been used in treatment of a range of respiratory conditions for many years (Gosling & Williams 2004). For example, it has been used in cases involving: whooping cough (Kurschner 1958); hospitalized children with respiratory infections (Kline 1965); asthma (Rowane & Rowane 1999); pneumonia (Hruby & Hoffman (2007) and chronic obstructive pulmonary disease (Howell et al 1975).

In these examples it is not suggested that osteopathic attention replaced standard medical protocols, but supplemented this, with demonstrable benefit to patients.

As Hruby & Hoffman (2007) point out, OMT procedures encourage biomechanical improvements, including optimal rib cage and thoracoabdominal diaphragm motion that results in improved respiratory mechanics, as well as arterial, venous and lymphatic circulation.

Normalizing muscular and joint restrictions

The OMT methods outlined below for normalizing muscular and joint restrictions are largely soft tissue focused and are based on the type of assessment methodology outlined in Chapter 6.2. Within OMT there is a place for high velocity, low amplitude (HVLA) thrust techniques, however, these are not described in this text (see Gibbons & Tehan 2000). Alternatives to HVLA thrust approaches include muscle energy techniques (MET), positional release techniques (PRT), and mobilization methods, as described below.

These manual approaches would be combined with breathing pattern advice and exercises for home application as described in Chapter 9.

MUSCLE ENERGY TECHNIQUE (MET) PROCEDURES

A selection of MET treatment methods aimed at normalizing thoracic, spinal, rib and short postural muscle dysfunctions are described below. First, the basic 'rules' of osteopathic MET are outlined.

MET methodology

When the term 'restriction barrier' is used in relation to soft tissue structures, it is meant to indicate the first signs of resistance (as palpated by sense of 'bind', or sense of effort required to move the area, or by visual or other palpable evidence) and not the greatest pain-free range of movement obtainable.

In all treatment descriptions involving MET it is assumed that references to 'acute' and 'chronic' indicate variations in methodology which these terms call for. 'Acute' applications start at the barrier, while 'chronic' protocols commence just short of the barrier. Acute is defined as recent onset (under 3 weeks) following strain or trauma, or acutely painful (Moore 1980) – and 'acute' protocols are always used for treatment of joint restrictions – with no stretching subsequent to isometric contractions.

After an isometric contraction, the tissues are taken to the new barrier in an acute setting, and through the barrier into light stretch, in a chronic setting. In treating fragile and/or pain-ridden individuals with MET, the acute mode is always adopted – i.e. no stretching is employed! Assistance from the patient is valuable when movement is made to, or through, a barrier, if the patient can be educated to gently cooperate by not using excessive effort.

In most MET treatment guidelines the method described involves the isometric contraction of the agonist(s), the muscle(s) that most obviously requires stretching.

Mechanisms

Explanations of the mechanisms whereby MET achieves its effects have modified over the years. In the past the effects (such as reduced tone) were considered to result from *post isometric relaxation* (PIR), that followed loading of the Golgi tendon organs (Lewit 2006), in contrast to when antagonists of target tissues are involved in the isometric contraction, when *reciprocal inhibition* (RI) was regarded as the mechanism. These explanations are no longer considered sufficient to explain MET's effects (Fryer 2013, Magnusson et al 1996), with a variety of supplementary explanations emerging – summed up under a banner heading of 'increased tolerance to stretch' (Bement et al 2011, Degenhardt 2007, Schleip et al 2012). For a detailed analysis of current MET concepts see Fryer (2013), in Chaitow (2013).

Respiratory and visual synkinesis

Breathing cooperation may be used as part of the methodology of MET (Lewit 2006). A patient who is cooperative and capable of following instructions can be asked to inhale at the same time that an isometric contraction is slowly performed against resistance. The breath is held for 5 to 7 seconds, and slowly released as the effort ceases. A further inhalation and exhalation is then performed, together with the instruction to 'let go completely.' As relaxation occurs, the new barrier is engaged, or the barrier is passed as the muscle is stretched.

Eye movements are sometimes advocated during contractions and stretches, particularly by Lewit (2006), in treating muscles such as the scalenes and sternomastoid.

Additional MET variations

- Eccentric isotonic contractions, performed slowly, achieve the double benefit of both toning the weaker muscles and also releasing tone in the antagonists (Norris 2000, Parmar et al 2011).
- Pulsed muscle energy technique (pulsed MET – see below), based on Ruddy's work, can be substituted for any of the methods described in the text below for treating shortened soft tissue structures, or increasing range of motion in joints (Ruddy 1962).

Ruddy's 'pulsed MET'

When using pulsed MET the dysfunctional tissue or joint is held at its restriction barrier, at which time the patient, *against firm resistance* offered by the practitioner, introduces a series of rapid *very small contraction efforts*, usually towards the barrier. The barest initiation of effort is called for, with 'no wobble and no bounce'. This approach involves contractions that are 'short, rapid and rhythmic, gradually' increasing the amplitude and degree of resistance, thus 'conditioning the proprioceptive system by rapid movements' (Ruddy 1962). After a 10-second sequence of contractions, the patient relaxes and the tissues (or joint) are taken to a new barrier, and the process is repeated. Lewit (2009) has described use of this approach in relation to both scalene release and 1st rib mobilization (see below).

MET of selected accessory and obligatory respiratory muscles

Lewit & Simons (1984) have noted that:

- MET applied to the suboccipital muscles will also relax the sternocleidomastoid muscles
- MET treatment of the thoracolumbar muscles induces relaxation of iliopsoas, and vice versa
- MET treatment of the sternocleidomastoid and scalene muscles relaxes the pectorals.

MET treatment of a selection of the following muscles is described below: iliopsoas, quadratus lumborum, pectoralis major, upper trapezius, scalenes, sternocleidomastoid. The author of this chapter has found it clinically useful to encourage optimal mobility and flexibility of these muscles, and the associated joints – particularly in the early stages of breathing rehabilitation.

NOTE: See Chapter 6.2 for assessment methods.

MET treatment of psoas (Fig. 7.2.1)

The patient is in the supine test position – described in Chapter 6.2 – lying with the buttocks at the very end of

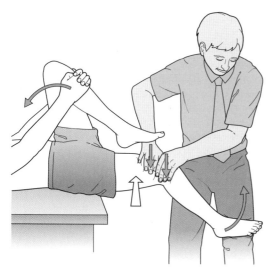

Figure 7.2.1 Position for treatment of psoas. *With permission from Chaitow 2013, Fig. 5.10A.*

the table, with the non-treated leg fully flexed at the hip and knee, and either held in that position by the patient, or by the practitioner.

The leg on the affected side should hang freely, with the medio-plantar aspect resting on the practitioner's knee or shin.

The practitioner stands sideways on to the patient, at the foot of the table, with both hands holding the thigh of the extended leg, in order to completely resist an attempt by the patient to lightly externally rotate the leg and to simultaneously flex the hip for 5 to 7 seconds. This combination of forces precisely focuses the contraction effort into psoas.

After the isometric contraction the thigh should, on an exhalation, either be taken to the new restriction barrier, without force (if acute), or through that barrier with painless pressure on the anterior aspect of the thigh (if chronic). This is held for up to 30 seconds.

MET for shortness in quadratus lumborum (QL) (Fig. 7.2.2)

The patient lies supine, positioned in a light side-bend, away from the side to be treated ('banana-shaped'). The practitioner stands on the side opposite, and slides his cephalad hand under the patient's shoulders to grasp the treated-side axilla. The patient places the arm of the side to be treated behind her neck, and grasps the practitioner's cephalad arm at the elbow, making the contact more secure. The patient's treated-side elbow should, at this stage, be pointing superiorly (see Fig. 7.2.2). If possible, the patient's non-treated-side hand should be interlocked with the practitioner's cephalad hand.

The practitioner's caudad hand is placed on the anterior superior iliac spine, on the side to be treated, and the patient is instructed to very lightly side-bend towards that side, producing an isometric contraction in QL.

After 5 to 7 seconds the patient relaxes completely, *and on an inhalation* (QL fires on exhalation) is asked to side-bend towards the non-treated side, as the practitioner assists the side-bending action of the patient, effectively stretching QL. The stretch is held for up to 30 seconds. Repeat as necessary.

MET treatment of pectoralis major (Fig. 7.2.3)

The supine patient's arm is abducted in a direction that produces the most marked evidence of pectoral shortness, assessed by palpation and visual evidence of the fibres involved.

- The more elevated the arm (i.e. the closer to the head) the more abdominal the attachments will be that are being treated
- With the arm placed more laterally, clavicular fibres will be more involved.

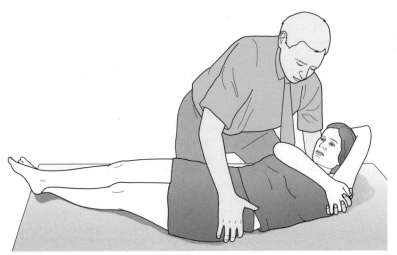

Figure 7.2.2 MET treatment of quadratus lumborum.

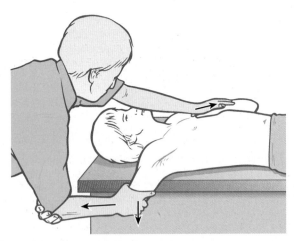

Figure 7.2.3 MET treatment of pectoralis major. *With permission from Chaitow 2013, Fig. 5.29B.*

The patient should be close to the side of the table, so that the abducted arm can be brought below the horizontal during stretching, if appropriate. The long axis of the patient's upper arm should be in line with the fibres being treated. The practitioner grasps the patient's flexed upper arm, proximal to the elbow, while the patient cups the practitioner's elbow and maintains this contact throughout the procedure. The other hand stabilizes the attachment site (i.e. is in touch with ribs, sternum and/or clavicle) during the contraction and the stretch. Placement of the patient's hand over the attachment (with practitioner's hand superimposed) acts as a 'cushion', as well as preventing inappropriate physical contact. See Figure 7.2.3.

The patient introduces a small degree of adduction and/or elevation, against resistance, for 5 to 7 seconds, using less than 25% of available strength. After the contraction, a stretch is introduced, to or through the new barrier. The arm is distracted from the thoracic or clavicular attachment, as well as being taken below the horizontal. The thoracic attachment must be constantly stabilized to prevent any movement. The stretch is held for up to 30 seconds.

MET treatment of shortened upper trapezius (Fig. 7.2.4A–C)

The patient lies supine, with head/neck side-flexed away from the side to be treated. The practitioner stabilizes the shoulder with one hand, while cupping the ear/mastoid area of the same side of the head with the other.

In order to engage the various fibres of upper trapezius, the neck needs to be held in three different positions of rotation, coupled with side-bending as described below:

1. Full side-flexion and full rotation *away from* the side being treated, involves the posterior fibres of upper trapezius (Fig.7.2.4A)
2. Full side-flexion and half-rotation *away from* the side being treated, involves the more medial fibres of upper trapezius (Fig.7.2.4B)
3. Full side-flexion away from, and rotation *towards* the side being treated, involves the posterior fibres of upper trapezius (Fig.7.2.4C).

NOTE: The MET description below should be applied with the head/neck in all three positions described/illustrated, in order to access all fibres efficiently.

Treatment details

Using a small degree of effort (under 20% of available strength), the patient attempts to take the stabilized

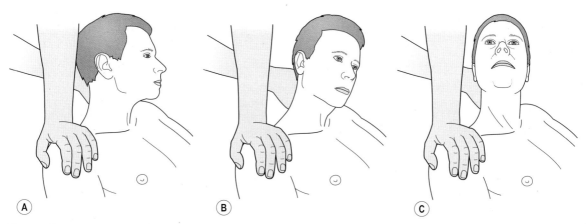

Figure 7.2.4 MET treatment of upper trapezius, showing different head positions in treatment respectively of (**A**) posterior aspects, (**B**) medial aspects and (**C**) anterior aspects of the muscle. *With permission from Chaitow 2013, Fig. 5.35.*

shoulder toward the ear (a shrug movement) and the ear toward the shoulder. This introduces a contraction of the muscle from both ends. No pain should be felt.

After a 5–7-second contraction, and complete relaxation of effort, the practitioner gently eases the head/neck into an increased degree of side-flexion and rotation, before – *with the patient's assistance* – easing the shoulder away from the ear while stabilizing the head, so achieving a light degree of stretch. This is held for up to 30 seconds.

MET treatment of short scalenes

(Fig. 7.2.5A–C)

The patient lies with a thin cushion under the shoulders to enable the neck to rest in slight extension on the treatment table surface. The head/neck is supported by the practitioner, in a neutral (i.e. not extended) position and turned away from the side to be treated.

There are three positions of rotation required in scalene treatment, with three hand placements on the thorax:

1. Full rotation produces involvement of the more posterior fibres of the scalenes on the side from which the turn is being made. The contact hand rests on the patient's hand, which lies on the upper ribs, inferior to the lateral aspect of the clavicle, acting as a 'cushion' for the practitioner to push against when introducing stretch (Fig. 7.2.5A).
2. A half rotation recruits the middle fibres. The contact hand rests on the patient's hand, which lies on the upper ribs, inferior to the mid-point of the clavicle (Fig. 7.2.5B).
3. A position of only slight turn involves the more anterior fibres. The contact hand rests on the

patient's hand, which lies on the upper portion of the sternum (Fig. 7.2.5C).

The patient is instructed to inhale and hold the breath, and to attempt to lift the forehead a fraction while turning the head toward the side being treated. Resistance from the practitioner's hand prevents both movements ('lift and turn your face').

NOTE: The effort, and therefore the counter-pressure, should be modest and painless at all times.

After a 7-second contraction, the head is eased into slight extension, with care being taken to stabilize and support the neck during the stretching phase that follows. As the patient fully exhales, the practitioner's contact hand, covering the patient's hand, lightly pushes obliquely, caudally, to follow the ribs into their exhalation position. The rib cage is held in that end-of-range position during the stretch phase of up to 30 seconds.

Visual synkinesis: a degree of eye movement can assist scalene treatment. If the patient looks downwards, towards the feet and the affected side, during the isometric contraction, this will induce a degree of contraction in the muscles. During the resting phase, when stretch is being introduced, the patient looks away from the treated side with eyes focused upward, towards the top of the head, enhancing the stretch of the muscle (Lewit 2006).

CAUTION: It is important to avoid unsafe degrees of neck extension during any phase of this treatment: *15° is suggested as the upper limit, or less in patients over 45 years of age.*

MET treatment of shortened sternocleidomastoid (Fig. 7.2.5A)

The patient is supine, in the same position as that described for treatment of the posterior aspects of scalenes (Fig. 7.2.5A) with a thin cushion/folded towel under the shoulders.

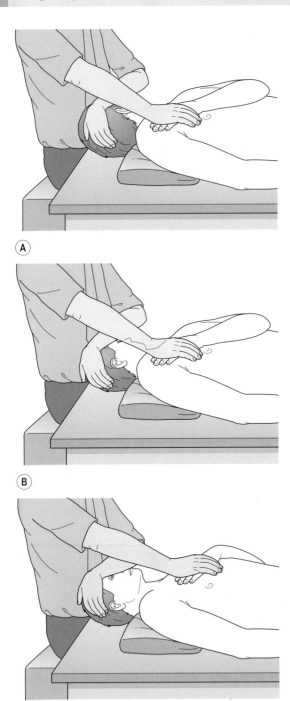

(A)

(B)

(C)

Figure 7.2.5A–C MET treatment of scalenes showing different head positions, and hand positions, associated with involving different aspects of the scalene. *With permission from Chaitow 2013, Fig. 5.37.*

Whereas in scalene treatment the instruction to the patient is to 'lift and turn' the rotated head/neck against resistance, in treating sternocleidomastoid the instruction is simply to 'slightly lift the head'. When the head is raised there is no need to apply resistance, as gravity effectively does this.

After 5–7 seconds of isometric contraction, the patient is asked to release the effort and to allow the head/neck to return to a resting position involving *a small degree* of extension, 10–15° at most.

The practitioner applies oblique pressure/stretch to the sternum, with his hand resting on the patient's 'cushioning' hand (resting on the sternum), easing the sternum away from the head toward the feet. The practitioner's other hand restrains the tendency the head will have to follow this stretch, by stabilizing it at the mastoid area. The stretch should be maintained for up to 30 seconds to achieve release/stretch of hypertonic and fibrotic structures. Repeat as necessary.

CAUTION: *Under no circumstances apply pressure* to stretch the head/neck while it is in this vulnerable position of slight extension.

MET for joint restrictions

Treatment of joint restrictions using MET involves engaging the barrier of resistance followed by the MET procedure which requires the patient to introduce a resisted isometric contraction to, or away from, the barrier, after which the new barrier is engaged. No forceful movement through the restriction barrier is used: it either retreats or it does not. As a general rule, soft tissue normalization should be encouraged prior to any joint mobilization.

A selection of MET and other methods for treatment of joint restrictions are described in this chapter. A much wider range of MET (and other) methods can be found in osteopathic and other texts, including DeStefano (2010), Ward (1997), Lewit (2009) and Chaitow (2013).

Evaluating and treating thoracic spinal restrictions using MET (Seffinger & Hruby 2007)
(Figs 7.2.6A and B)

1. The spinal segments of the seated patient should be positioned at their physiological barrier – either in one plane – for example rotation; or specific in three planes, for example involving flexion–extension, side-bending and rotation. Particular attention should be given to areas of the thoracic spine that are less flexible than normal (see Ch.6.2 for details of the slump test and breathing wave), where rib mobility may be noted as restricted, as noted in assessments described in Chapters 6.1, 6.2, 6.3 and 6.5.

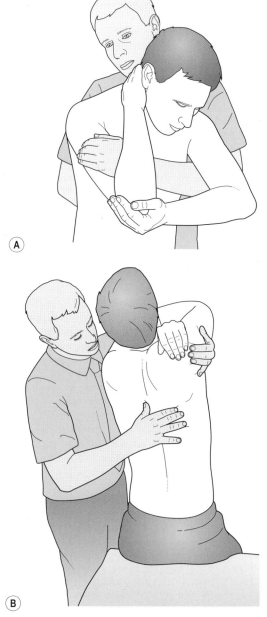

(A)

(B)

Figure 7.2.6A,B The spinal segments requiring mobilization via MET application are taken to their easy end of range, at which time an isometric contraction is requested, as described in the text. After release of the effort the joints are repositioned at their new end of range, without force.

2. The patient should then lightly contract muscles *in one direction only* – for example, translation towards, or away from, the barrier – while the practitioner totally resists any movement. The isometric contraction should be held for about 3 to 5 seconds.

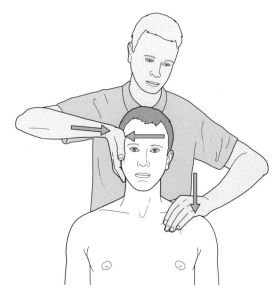

Figure 7.2.7 Pulsed MET for 1st (and 2nd) ribs on the left.

3. The amount of effort employed should be light, involving an instruction such as 'using only 25% of your strength, push towards the left.'

4. Following the isometric effort, the patient is asked to relax for 2 seconds or so, after which the practitioner re-engages the spine at its new motion barrier(s).

This process is repeated until free movement is achieved or until no further gain is apparent following a contraction.

General principles of MET for rib dysfunction

Before using MET on rib restrictions identified in tests, such as those summarized in Chapters 6.2 and 6.5, appropriate attention should be given to the attaching and overlying musculature.

MET treatment for restricted (elevated or depressed) 1st rib (Fig. 7.2.7)

The patient is seated with the practitioner standing behind. For a left side elevated 1st rib the practitioner holds the patient's left shoulder area with fingertips flexed to make contact with the superior surface of the 1st rib. The other hand stabilizes the right side of the patient's head. The patient is asked to lightly press the side of his head against that hand, in a series of rhythmic contractions, as described for pulsed MET above (see Figure 7.2.7). The objective is to encourage 10 to 20 mini-contractions (primarily of the scalenes) in 10 to 15 seconds – with no discomfort, and no objective movement. This is best achieved if the practitioner's resisting hands are firmly engaged against the points of contact. This procedure should release restricted 1st and 2nd ribs (Lewit 2009).

MET treatment for restricted 2nd to 10th ribs

For elevated ribs (restricted in inhalation position) (Fig. 7.2.8)

Clinical experience suggests that the most inferior of a group of elevated ribs should be identified and treated first. The patient is supine and the practitioner stands at the head of the table, slightly to the left, with the right hand between the scapulae, so that the right forearm supports the patient's upper thoracic region as well as the neck and head (see Fig. 7.2.8). The left hand is placed so that the thumb or thenar eminence rests on the superior aspect of the costochondral junction of the designated rib, close to the midclavicular line (for upper ribs). For ribs 7–10 the contact would be more lateral, closer to the midaxillary line, directing the rib caudally.

The upper thoracic and cervical spine is eased into flexion, as well as side-flexion towards the treated side, until motion is sensed at the site of the rib stabilization. The patient is asked to inhale fully and 'hold your breath' (isometric contraction of intercostals as well as scalenes), and to attempt to lightly return the back and head to the table (isometric contraction of levator scapulae and paraspinal muscles), against the practitioner's firm resistance.

On release and full exhalation, and with the thumb or thenar eminence holding the rib towards its caudad position, an increased degree of flexion and side-flexion is introduced. Rib motion is then reassessed.

For depressed ribs (restricted in exhalation position) (Fig. 7.2.9A&B)

Clinical experience suggests that the most superior of a group of depressed ribs should be identified and treated first.

Method 1: The patient is supine and the practitioner stands contralaterally and places his table-side arm across the patient's trunk, sliding his hand under the patient's torso, with slightly hooked fingertips engaging the costal angle of the designated rib. The patient's head or arm is suitably placed so that an isometric contraction will engage the muscle(s) most influential to the key rib (see examples below).

The patient is asked to inhale and to hold the breath, and to move the head or arm as appropriate (see below), against practitioner resistance for 5–7 seconds. On complete relaxation, the fingers draw the rib inferiorly to take out available slack, and the process is repeated following reassessment of rib movement.

The example shown in Figure 7.2.9A involves the patient introducing a flexion and rotation movement (to the left) of the head and neck – against the resistance of the practitioner's left forearm; while at the same time attempting to flex the extended shoulder, restrained by the practitioner's hand on the elbow. These isometric efforts coincide with a held breath, resulting in simultaneous isometric contractions of scalenes, pectoralis major and the intercostals.

On release of the breath, and the isometric efforts, the practitioner draws the rib inferiorly, in order to normalize its potential for subsequent free movement.

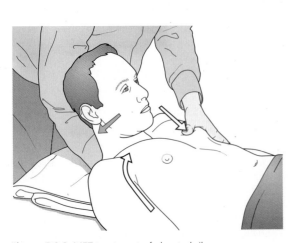

Figure 7.2.8 MET treatment of elevated ribs.

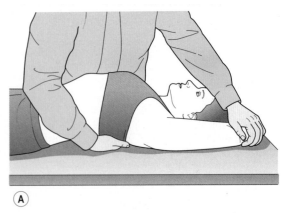

(A)

Figure 7.2.9A Treatment of depressed ribs on the left, with (in this example) rib 4 being the most superior of the affected group. The patient's left shoulder is extended, with her left hand above, or resting on her forehead.

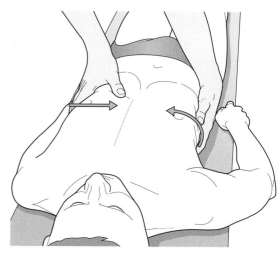

Figure 7.2.10 Mobilization of the lower rib cage using MET. *With permission from Ward 1997.*

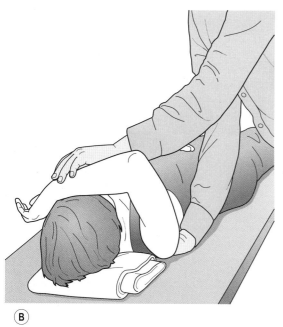

(B)

Figure 7.2.9B The patient attempts to flex the shoulder against practitioner resistance, while simultaneously inhaling and holding the breath, and also lifting and turning the head to the right. The resulting isometric contractions of the intercostal muscles, pectoralis major and the scalenes (among others) should allow easier movement of the restricted ribs, on cessation of all efforts by the patient. Following this relaxation of effort, and on the next inhalation, the practitioner introduces light fingertip traction on the rib that is depressed (i.e. restricted in its exhalation position).

Method 2: Figure 7.2.9B shows treatment of depressed ribs on the right, treated with the practitioner standing ipsilaterally. In all other ways the methodology is the same as in Method 1 above.

Lower thoracic cage release (diaphragm attachments) using MET

The patient is supine, and the practitioner stands at waist level, facing cephalad, with his hands over the middle and lower thoracic structures, fingers along the rib shafts. Treating the structure being palpated as a cylinder, the hands test its preference to rotate around its central axis, one way and then the other.

Once the direction of greatest rotational restriction has been established, side-flexion one way and the other is evaluated. Which directions of rotation and side-flexion offer the greatest resistance? The lower thorax is taken into this combined position of restriction. See Figure 7.2.10.

At this time the patient is asked to inhale and hold the breath, and to 'bear down' slightly (Valsalva manoeuvre), so introducing an isometric contraction of the diaphragm and intercostal muscles.

On release and complete exhalation and relaxation, the diaphragm should be found to function more normally and there should be a relaxation of associated soft tissues, together with more symmetrical rotation and side-flexion potential of the previously restricted structures.

CAUTION: Avoid the Valsalva manoeuvre if the patient is hypertensive or has glaucoma.

POSITIONAL RELEASE TECHNIQUES

Strain/counterstrain

Various therapeutic modalities involve the positioning of an area, or the whole body, in such a way as to evoke a physiological response that helps to resolve musculoskeletal dysfunction. The means by which the beneficial changes occur seems to involve a combination of neurological and circulatory changes which come about when a distressed area is placed in its most comfortable, most 'easy', most pain-free position (Wong 2012, Chaitow 2007).

Common basis

All positional release techniques (PRT) methods move the patient, or the affected tissues, away from resistance barriers and toward positions of ease – 'tissue comfort'. The shorthand terms used for these two extremes are 'bind' and 'ease'.

Strain–counterstrain or SCS (Jones 1981), involves monitoring the reported pain level in a tender point (any area of unusual sensitivity to which digital pressure is applied) while the area is carefully repositioned until the level of reported pain reduces from an initial level of '10', to '3' or less. This ease position is then held for up to 90 seconds, during which time (it is hypothesized), spindle resetting and circulatory changes take place to beneficially modify the status of the tissues involved, calming neural reactivity. If the tender area is an active trigger point, then the positional release process commonly deactivates it or reduces trigger point referral activity significantly (Wong 2012). See below for integrated neuromuscular inhibition technique (INIT) discussion.

Method

SCS methodology suggests maintaining pressure on a tender point, as a position is achieved in which:

1. There is no additional pain in whatever area is symptomatic, and
2. Pain in the monitored point reduces by at least 70%
3. The ease position is held for up to 90 seconds.

Strain/counterstrain (SCS) guidelines

(Wong 2012, Chaitow 2007)

The SCS guidelines are based on clinical experience and should be kept in mind when treating pain and dysfunction, especially where the patient is fatigued, sensitive and/or distressed:

- Never treat more than five 'tender' points at any one session, and treat fewer than this in sensitive individuals to avoid adaptation overload.
- Forewarn patients that, just as in any other form of bodywork, a period of physiological adaptation is inevitable, and that there will therefore be a 'reaction' on the day(s) following even this extremely light form of treatment. Soreness and stiffness are therefore to be anticipated.
- If there are multiple tender points, select those most proximal and most medial for primary attention (i.e. those closest to the head and the centre of the body, rather than distal and lateral pain points), and of these, select those that are most painful for initial attention/treatment.
- For tender points/areas on the anterior surface of the body, ease is usually found by flexion, side-bending and rotation towards the palpated point, followed by fine-tuning to reduce sensitivity by at least 70%.
- For tender points on the posterior surface of the body, extension, side-bending and rotation should usually be away from the palpated point, followed by fine-tuning to reduce sensitivity by 70%.

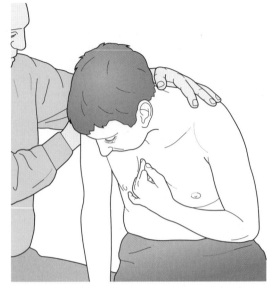

Figure 7.2.11 Practitioner instructing patient in intercostal self-treatment, using strain–counterstrain methodology.

NOTE: These guidelines can usefully and safely be taught to patients to self-treat intercostal discomfort (see Fig. 7.2.11), and/or can be used clinically in the context of enhancing thoracic mobility.

Strain/counterstrain for interspace dysfunction

Tender points used as monitors for treatment of dysfunction involving the intercostal tissues lie between the insertions of the contiguous ribs into the cartilages of the sternum. Dysfunction and discomfort in the intercostals seems to relate to non-specific stress of the thorax, sometimes following trauma, or a recent stressful coughing or asthmatic episode. Ribs may be over-approximated, and the pain reported when associated tender points are palpated may be severe. Painful tender points are common in these tissues in people with asthma, those with chronic bronchitis, and in patients with upper-chest breathing/hyperventilation breathing pattern disorders.

With the patient seated, treatment of intercostal dysfunction tender points are monitored by the practitioner, or by the patient. Once an area of tenderness is located it should be compressed sufficiently to produce a mild level of discomfort. The patient is asked to ascribe a value of '10' to the perceived pain.

NOTE: The patient is not asked to grade the level of pain, as in VAS test – but is told that, for the purpose of this treatment method, the mild pain being noted should have a value of 10.

Flexion is then introduced, with some slight rotation towards the side of dysfunction. As this takes place the reported level of discomfort should reduce markedly, until pain reduces by at least 70%. This is the 'ease' position. If fine-tuning is adequate (minor adjustments of the degree of flexion, with some side-flexion or rotation added if this helps reduce the reported pain score), the palpation-induced pain will ease. This position should be maintained for at least 90 seconds.

The methodology of positional release variations can be more fully explored in a number of texts, including Jones (1981), D'Ambrogio & Roth (1997), and Chaitow (2007).

DEACTIVATING MYOFASCIAL TRIGGER POINTS

The trigger point phenomenon, together with assessment methods, are discussed in Chapter 6.2. This chapter suggests a protocol in which a combination of modalities is used in an integrated sequence to deactivate active trigger points. An alternative approach would be to use the trigger point as a marker, so that the degree of sensitivity noted on pressure is seen to reduce as rehabilitation processes (such as postural or breathing re-education) reduce the stress on the tissues housing it (Hou et al 2002).

Variations

- Inhibitory soft tissue techniques including neuromuscular therapy/massage (Hong et al 1993)
- Chilling techniques (cold spray, ice) (Simons et al 1998)
- Acupuncture, injection (procaine, xylocaine) (Hong 1994)
- Positional release methods (D'Ambrogio & Roth 1997)
- Muscle energy (stretch) techniques (Kuchera 1997, Chaitow & DeLany 2008)
- Myofascial release methods
- Combination sequences such as INIT (see below) (Chaitow 1994, Chaitow 2011)
- Correction of associated somatic dysfunction, possibly involving manipulation and/or mobilization methods
- Education and correction of contributory and perpetuating factors including posture, diet, stress, habits of use, etc, as described throughout this book (Bradley 1999, Chaitow et al 2002)
- Self-help strategies (see Ch. 9).

CAUTION: Direct pressure should be avoided, or performed with great care:

1. If tissues are inflamed, or are in the remodelling phase, following trauma

2. In cases of malignancy
3. Close to blood vessels and nerves
4. Close to attachment sites (to avoid provoking enthesitis)
5. If pain (local or referred) is excessive.

Simons et al (1998) have suggested that in treatment of trigger points, these should receive ischaemic compression ('sustained digital pressure') for a period of between 20 seconds and 1 minute. The pressure should be gradually increased as the trigger point's sensitivity (referred sensation, as well as the local discomfort) reduces, and the tension of the tissues housing the trigger ('taut band') eases. Stretching techniques should be applied following the compression.

Fernandez de Las Penas (2006) reports that:

Ischemic compression technique and transverse friction massage are equally effective in reducing tenderness in myofascial trigger points.

The mechanisms involved may include 'neurological overload', the release of endogenous morphine-like products (endorphins, endocannabinoids, enkephalins), as well as 'flushing' of tissues with fresh oxygenated blood, following compression (McPartland & Simons 2006).

Integrated neuromuscular inhibition technique (Chaitow 1994, Chaitow & DeLany 2008, Nagrale 2010) (Fig. 7.2.12)

Having identified an active trigger point the integrated neuromuscular inhibition technique (INIT) involves a sequence commencing with application of ischaemic compression (avoided if the patient is too sensitive), followed by the introduction of positional release (see above) to ease sensitivity by at least 70%.

After the tissues have been held in 'ease' for up to 90 seconds, the patient introduces an isometric contraction into the tissues surrounding the trigger point for 7–10 seconds, after which these local tissues are stretched.

Enhancing respiratory function with adjunctive osteopathic manipulative methods

The methods outlined below are non-specific, and have a long and useful history of application in osteopathic medicine, some dating back to the early 20th century (Sleszynski & Kelso 1993, Hruby & Goodridge 1997, Hruby & Hoffman 2007).

1. Thoracic lymphatic pump technique

Lymphatic pump techniques are indicated for conditions in which enhancement of thoracic range of motion and increased expiratory efficacy is desirable, particularly in cases of chronic obstructive pulmonary disease, upper and lower respiratory infections and for postsurgical reduction of respiratory volume.

Sleszynski & Kelso (1993) demonstrated that when lymphatic pump technique was administered on the first day postoperatively in patients who had undergone cholecystectomy, there was a more rapid recovery and a quicker return towards preoperative values for FVC and FEV_1 than in patients treated with incentive spirometry. D'Alonzo & Krachman (1997) report that this technique:

> *increases vital capacity, the mobility of the rib cage, improves diaphragmatic function, clears airway secretions and possibly enhances immune function.*

This method is designed to augment pressure gradients between thoracic and abdominal regions. Variations include methods which are rhythmic and those which are continuous. Contraindications include fractures, osteoporosis, dislocations, or malignancy of the lymphatic system. Caution is advised in patients with reduced cough reflex.

Method

The patient is supine (with no food, gum or loose dentures in the mouth).

The practitioner stands at the head of the table with his hands on the patient's thoracic wall so that the thenar eminences cover the pectoral muscles just distal to the clavicle, with fingers spread towards the sides of the trunk. In this way the heels of the hands rest over ribs 2–4 (Fig. 7.2.13). A rhythmic pumping action of the thorax is introduced by means of the practitioner lightly flexing and extending the elbows, with the forearms, wrists and hands fixed, at a rate of approximately two per second. The patient is instructed to breathe normally during the process, which should continue for 2–5 minutes.

2. Rib raising

The objective is to free restrictions in rib cage motion which impact on normal respiratory effort and retard venous blood and lymph movement.

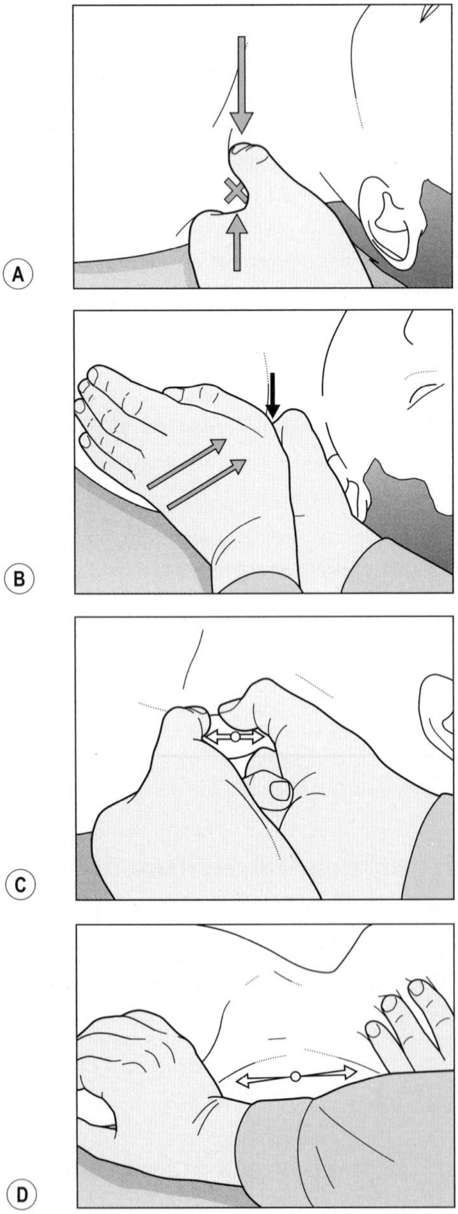

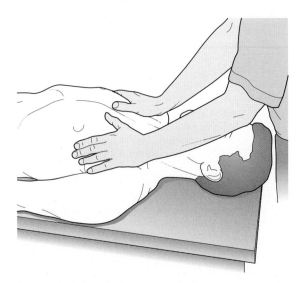

Figure 7.2.13 Lymphatic pump method.

A
B
C
D

Figure 7.2.12 INIT sequence applied to upper trapezius trigger point.

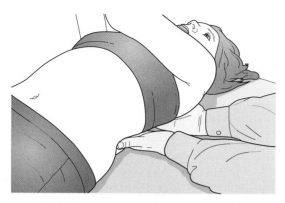

Figure 7.2.14 Rib raising method for thoracic mobilization.

The patient lies supine, with the practitioner sitting facing the patient on the side of rib restriction. The practitioner reaches underneath the patient with both arms to contact the rib angles medially with the finger pads. The contact between the practitioner's knuckles and the table serve as a fulcrum.

The practitioner applies an anterolateral traction on the contacted rib angles by flexing the wrists in order to mobilize the ribs. When a restrictive barrier is sensed the patient's ribs are returned towards neutral (Fig. 7.2.14).

This action is repeated rhythmically until an increased range of motion is sensed.

Rowane & Rowane (1999) noted the benefits to breathing function of this approach in treatment of asthma.

CONCLUSION (Box 7.2.1)

Breathing retraining requires a combination of elements:

- Understanding the processes – a cognitive, intellectual awareness of the mechanisms and issues involved (Lum 1987)
- Retraining exercises including aspects that operate subcortically, allowing replacement of currently habituated patterns with more appropriate ones
- Biomechanical structural modifications that remove obstacles to desirable and necessary functional changes (Lewit 2006)
- Time for these elements to merge and become incorporated into moment-to-moment use patterns.

Fundamental to breathing rehabilitation is a need for the individual to understand – even if in basic terms – the association between how breathing is carried out, and health in general and symptoms in particular.

Apart from appropriate biomechanical mobilization and stabilization strategies, as touched on in this chapter, breathing rehabilitation requires attention to etiological and maintaining factors that might include: ensuring adequate exercise (see Chs 1 and 2.2, as well as 7.3); an

> **Box 7.2.1 An osteopathic rehabilitation protocol**
>
> Treatment and retraining commonly involves weekly sessions for the first month to 6 weeks, followed by treatment sessions every 3 to 4 weeks, to approximately 6 months.
> - Mobilization of the thoracic spine and rib articulations, as well as pelvic joints if required
> - Focus on relaxation of structural links between the diaphragm and pelvis and lower extremity: abdominal and other thoracic fascia and musculature, including psoas, quadratus lumborum etc
> - Attention to hypertonicity in accessory breathing muscles: upper trapezii, levator scapulae, scalenes, sternocleidomastoid, pectorals, latissimus dorsi, paraspinal muscles – together with deactivation of associated trigger points
> - Attention to the diaphragm area: intercostals, sternum, abdominal attachments, costal margin
> - An educational component should be included at each treatment session
> - Retraining: pursed-lip breathing, encouraging normal thoracic movements on inhalation, together with inhibition of any tendency for paradoxical breathing, e.g. shoulders rising on inhalation; introduction of specific relaxation methods, stress management, home exercises
> - Regular review and modification as needed.
>
> General: attention to other body influences – ergonomics, posture, diet, sleep, exercise, habits of use in domestic, work and leisure situations and activities etc
>
> Possibly: hydrotherapy, tai chi, yoga, Pilates, massage, acupuncture etc

optimal dietary pattern, particularly avoidance of hypoglycaemic episodes (Steel et al 1989) (and see Ch. 4); management of biopsychosocial issues, possibly calling for stress management and/or psychotherapeutic attention (see Chs 5, 6.3, 6.4 and 7.4).

In addition, individualized breathing rehabilitation exercises are suggested that might include:

- Regular application of pursed-lip breathing exercises, with focus on exhalation and establishing a ratio in which exhalation is consistently longer than inhalation (Hochstetter 2005).
- Use of stabilization of accessory respiratory muscle methods during inhalation (as described in Chapter 9, Brugger/shoulder stabilization) (Lewit 2006).
- Time – for application of regularly practised optimal breathing patterns (morning and evening for example), to become habitual.

In addition to the (largely) osteopathic strategies described above, alternative breathing rehabilitation strategies are described in chapters: 7.1a, indirect approaches; 7.1b, Dynamic Neuromuscular Stabilization methods; 7.3, physiotherapy; 7.4, psychotherapy; 7.5, in association with speech dysfunction; 7.6, in association with athletes; 7.7, combined with use of capnography. These descriptions do not necessarily contradict each other, but offer variations that allow individualization.

A variety of other complementary methods of breathing rehabilitation are detailed in chapters 8.1, somatocognitive approaches; 8.2, Buteyko method; 8.3, Feldenkrais®; 8.4, Pilates; 8.5, Tai Chi and 8.6, Yoga. Self-help methods for home use are described in Chapter 9.

Whichever of the variety of essential and complementary methods are employed – based on patient need and preference, rather than because of adherence to any rigid protocol–breathing rehabilitation is likely to be more effectively achieved when combined with mobilization of the structures most directly involved in the act of respiration. This should include both soft tissue and articular features – the spine, ribs, fascia and muscles.

The methods described in this chapter should be seen as a small sample of a wide range of modalities, methods, techniques and protocols that may be employed in this way.

The ultimate selection of the methods discussed relates to the particular bias, experience and preferences of the author, but most basically on the individual needs of the person involved.

REFERENCES

Bement, M., et al., 2011. Pain perception after isometric exercise in women with fibromyalgia. Arch Phys Med Rehabil 92, 89–95.

Bradley, D., 1999. In: Gilbert, C. (Ed.), Breathing retraining advice from three therapists. Journal of Bodywork and Movement Therapies 3, pp. 159–167.

Chaitow, L., 1994. Integrated neuromuscular inhibition technique. British Journal of Osteopathy 13, 17–20.

Chaitow, L., Bradley, D., Gilbert, C., 2002. Multidisciplinary approaches to breathing pattern disorders. Churchill Livingstone, Edinburgh.

Chaitow, L., 2007. Positional release techniques, third ed. Churchill Livingstone, Edinburgh.

Chaitow, L., 2011. Modern neuromuscular techniques, third ed. Churchill Livingstone, Edinburgh.

Chaitow, L., 2013. Muscle energy techniques, fourth ed. Churchill Livingstone, Edinburgh.

Chaitow, L., DeLany, J., 2008. Clinical applications of neuromuscular techniques. Vol 1, second ed. The upper body. Churchill Livingstone, Edinburgh.

D'Alonzo, G., Krachman, S., 1997. Respiratory system. In: Ward, R. (Ed.), Foundations for osteopathic medicine. Williams and Wilkins, Baltimore.

D'Ambrogio, K., Roth, G., 1997. Positional release therapy. Mosby, St Louis.

Degenhardt, B., 2007. Role of osteopathic manipulative treatment in altering pain biomarkers: a pilot study. J American Osteopathic Association 107, 387–394.

DeStefano, L.A. (Ed.), 2010. Greenman's principles of manual medicine, fourth ed. Lippincott Williams & Wilkins, Baltimore.

Fernandez de Las Penas, C., 2006. The immediate effect of ischemic compression technique and transverse friction massage on tenderness of active and latent myofascial trigger points: a pilot study. Journal of Bodywork and Movement Therapies 10 (1), 3–9.

Fryer, G., 2013. Muscle energy: research evidence. In: Chaitow, L. (Ed.), Muscle Energy Techniques, fourth ed. Elsevier, Edinburgh.

Gibbons, P., Tehan, P., 2000. Manipulation of the spine, thorax and pelvis. Churchill Livingstone, Edinburgh.

Gosling, C., Williams, K., 2004. Comparison of effects of thoracic manipulation and rib raising on lung function [abstract]. Journal of Osteopathic Medicine. 7, 103.

Hochstetter, J., 2005. An investigation into the immediate impact of breathlessness management on the breathless patient: randomised controlled trial. Physiotherapy. 91, 178–185.

Hong, C.-Z., 1994. Considerations and recommendations regarding myofascial trigger point injection. Journal of Musculoskeletal Pain 2 (1), 29–59.

Hong, C.-Z., Chen, Y.-C., Pon, C., et al., 1993. Immediate effects of various physical medicine modalities on pain threshold of an active myofascial trigger point. Journal of Musculoskeletal Pain 1 (2).

Hou, C.-R., Tsai, L.-C., Cheng, K.-F., et al., 2002. Immediate effects of various physical therapeutic modalities on cervical myofascial pain and trigger-point sensitivity. Arch Phys Au5 Med Rehabil 83 (10), 1406–1414.

Howell, R., Allen, R., Kapper, R., 1975. Influence of OMT in management of patients with chronic obstructive lung disease. Journal of the American Osteopathic Association 74, 757–760.

Hruby, R., Goodridge, J., 1997. Thoracic region and rib cage. In: Ward, R. (Ed.), Foundations of osteopathic medicine. Williams and Wilkins, Baltimore.

Hruby, R.J., Hoffman, K.N., 2007. Avian influenza: an osteopathic component to treatment. Osteopathic Medicine and Primary Care 2007, 1, 10.

Jones, L., 1981. Strain and counterstrain. Academy of Applied Osteopathy, Colorado Springs.

Kline, C., 1965. Osteopathic manipulative therapy, antibiotics and supportive therapy in respiratory infections in children. Journal of the American Osteopathic Association 65, 278–281.

Kuchera, M., 1997. Travell and Simons myofascial trigger points. In: Ward, R. (Ed.), Foundations for osteopathic medicine. Williams and Wilkins, Baltimore.

Kurschner, O.A., 1958. Comparative clinical investigation of chloramphenicol and OMT of whooping cough. Journal of the

American Osteopathic Association 57, 559–561.

Lewit, K., 2009. Manipulative therapy: musculoskeletal medicine. Churchill Livingstone, Edinburgh.

Lewit, K., 2006. Manipulative therapy in rehabilitation of the locomotor system, fourth ed. Butterworths, London.

Lewit, K., Simons, D., 1984. Myofascial pain: relief by postisometric relaxation. Archives of Physical Medicine and Rehabilitation 65, 452–456.

Lum, L., 1987. Hyperventilation syndromes in medicine and psychiatry: a review. J. R Soc Med. 80, 229–231.

Magnusson, S., Simonsen, E.B., Aagaard, P., et al., 1996. Mechanical and physiological responses to stretching with and without pre-isometric contraction in human skeletal muscle. Archives of Phys. Med. & Rehab. 77, 373–377.

McPartland, J.M., Simons, D.G., 2006. Myofascial trigger points: translating molecular theory into manual therapy. J. Man. Manip. Ther. 14, 232–239.

Moore, M., 1980. Electromyographic investigation manual of muscle stretching techniques. Medical Science and Sports Exercise 12, 322–329.

Nagrale, A., 2010. Efficacy of an integrated neuromuscular inhibition technique on upper trapezius trigger points in subjects with non-specific neck pain: a randomized controlled trial. Journal of Manual and Manipulative Therapy 18 (1), 38–44.

Norris, C., 2000. Back stability. Human Kinetics, Leeds.

Parmar, S., Shyam, A., Sabnis, S., et al., 2011. Effect of isolytic contraction and passive manual stretching on pain and knee range of motion after hip surgery. Hong Kong Physiotherapy Journal 29, 25–30.

Rowane, W., Rowane, M., 1999. An osteopathic approach to asthma. Journal of the American Osteopathic Association 99 (5), 259–264.

Ruddy, T., 1962. Osteopathic rapid rhythmic resistive technic. Academy of Applied Osteopathy Yearbook, Carmel, California, pp. 23–31.

Seffinger, M., Hruby, R., 2007. Evidence-based manual medicine. Elsevier, Philadelphia.

Schleip, R., Duerselen, L., Vleeming, A., et al., 2012. Strain hardening of fascia: static stretching of dense fibrous connective tissues can induce a temporary stiffness increase accompanied by enhanced matrix hydration. JBMT 16 (1), 94–100.

Simons, D., Travell, J., Simons, L., 1998. Myofascial pain and dysfunction: the trigger point manual. Vol. 1: Upper half of body, second ed. Williams and Wilkins, Baltimore.

Sleszynski, S., Kelso, A., 1993. Comparison of thoracic manipulation with incentive spirometry in the prevention of post-operative atelectasis. Journal of the American Osteopathic Association 93, 834–845.

Steel, J., et al., 1989. Hyperventilation or hypoglycaemia? Diabetic Medicine 6 (9), 820–821.

Ward, R. (Ed.), 1997. Foundations for osteopathic medicine. Williams and Wilkins, Baltimore.

Wong, K., 2012. Strain counterstrain: current concepts and clinical evidence. Christopher Manual Therapy 17, 2–8.

Chapter | **7.3** |

Physiotherapy in rehabilitation of breathing pattern disorders

Dinah Bradley

The following BradCliff® physiotherapy approach helps establish priorities and step-by-step planning in the treatment and management of hyperventilation syndrome/breathing pattern disorders (HVS/BPDs) (Box 7.3.1).

After collating all the assessment findings (Ch. 6.3) with priorities established, an individual treatment plan can be drawn up. Find out what your patient's expectations are as well as their commitment to schedule time for retraining and recommended lifestyle changes (e.g. reduce caffeine intake). A pact with clear, measurable, attainable goals should be drawn up, to be referred back to in subsequent treatments, to chart progress.

BREATHING RETRAINING

Four basic principles in restoring normal energy-efficient and physiologically balanced breathing are:

1. Awareness of faulty breathing patterns
2. Relaxation of the jaw, upper chest, shoulders and accessory muscles
3. Abdominal/low-chest nose breathing pattern re-education
4. Awareness of normal breathing rates and rhythms, both at rest and during speech and activity.

1. The patient is half-lying (Fig. 7.3.1; chest-check test). Ask the patient to place one relaxed hand over their navel, and the other on the upper chest and clavicle. The patient is asked to take a 'deep' breath. The chances are they will take a 'big' breath instead, through the mouth, hyperinflating the upper chest first with little or no low-chest involvement – or even drawing in the stomach at the peak of inspiration. Using their own hands as guides, patients can appreciate the difference between forceful 'big' and softer 'deep' breathing. They can

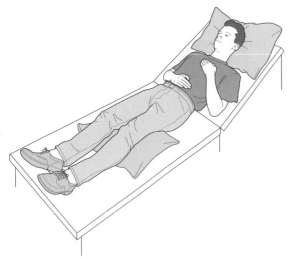

Figure 7.3.1 Half-lying; chest-check test. *From Bradley 2012.*

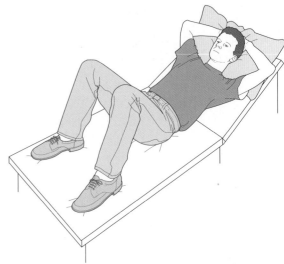

Figure 7.3.2 Beach pose. *From Bradley 2012.*

also feel the movement of their upper chest – or 'reverse breathing' – pattern, along with little or no diaphragmatic excursion/abdominal movement. Switch from mouth to nose breathing so the patient can feel the difference in both resistance and patterning.

CAUTION: It is a good idea to issue a warning at this stage that being aware of breathing is both unnatural and uncomfortable, and to be prepared for transient feelings of discomfort and 'air hunger' (Pitman 1996).

2. Once patients can identify their faulty patterns, the second step is for them to learn how to relax their upper chest and accessory muscles. A simple way of helping achieve this is to have them clasp their hands on top of their head (beach pose, Fig. 7.3.2). This helps put the upper chest muscles into 'neutral' and patients can usually immediately feel their diaphragm recruited into action. The diaphragm descends as they breathe in and their stomach gently expands, then relaxes back as they exhale.

Bending the knees helps loosen tight abdominal muscles and slowly rolling both knees together, from side to side, helps switch off tension.

Patients often describe feelings of 'air hunger' as they try to relax/release their shoulders and upper chest. (Rechecking SpO₂ saturations will help convince doubtful patients they are not hypoxic.) Swallowing and *concentrating on the out-breath* usually helps the patient to overcome this discomfort (Innocenti 1988). As progress is made the patient is encouraged to practise with their arms down and legs extended and loose, shoulders relaxed. Some patients respond well to placing a 1 kg wheatbag on their upper chest, helping focus on apical stillness and relaxation, and switching off trigger-happy accessory and facial muscles.

3. Having felt abdominal breathing while in the beach pose, concentration can be switched to low-chest breathing with quiet in-breaths dissolving into out-breaths without pause, until the end of the out-breath is reached. Habitual 'reverse breathers' will have been doing the exact opposite. Pausing instead at the top of the inhalation (tense) driven by their upper-thoracic breathing patterns, they lose the natural relaxed pause or neutral point at the end of exhalation.

A 1 or 2 kg wheatbag (depending on the size of the patient) placed over the navel provides an excellent and inexpensive biofeedback mechanism. The patient can feel, see and control the rise, fall and relaxation of the abdominal wall by focusing on the weight. Patients often remark how strange it feels at first, and how intensely they have to concentrate, followed by how exquisitely relaxing it feels when they 'get it'.

4. Restoring an energy-efficient, abdominal, nose-breathing pattern, with a *relaxed pause at the end of the exhale* often restores normal breathing rates at the same time. Sometimes counting out loud while timing helps at the beginning, with verbal coaching from the therapist. It is important that the patient be encouraged to relearn the *feeling* of 'low slow nose breathing'. Mentally repeating the phrases, 'When in doubt, breathe out' and 'Lips together, jaw relaxed, breathing low and slow' helps cement the normal rate and pattern back in place.

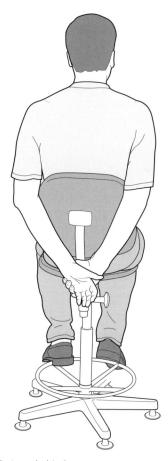

Figure 7.3.3 Arms behind. *From Bradley 2012.*

After practising while lying down, the patient may then be checked while sitting. Clasping hands together behind the chair (Fig. 7.3.3; arms behind) helps relax upper-chest muscles (a modification of hands on head). The patient is asked to 'breathe into their belt' and relax the stomach wall. As progress is made, the patient is encouraged to sit with the arms forward, hands resting on thighs, and continue energy-efficient nose breathing.

After covering these points the patient is asked to duplicate practice at home and:

- To commit to, and schedule, two 10-minute sessions each day, in lying, to switch off postural reflexes and experience relaxed stillness as a restorative process. It must be emphasized that the breathing retraining/relaxation/'time out' regimen is a three-way assault on the problem, and far from 'lying around doing nothing' is helping reset and restore energy-efficient quiet breathing.
- To adopt the beach pose in bed for 2 minutes, 'low slow nose' breathing on waking, and for 2 minutes before 'relaxing' to sleep at night.

- During the day, whether sitting or standing, on the hour every hour, the following 'stop, drop, flop' manouevre can be practised:
  STOP: chest check
  DROP: drop and soften shoulders
  FLOP: relax/go loose all over.

Timers (Hough 2001), or coloured stickers (Clifton-Smith & Bartley 2006) as visual cues give non-verbal reminders to 'stop, drop, flop'. (The patient is advised to place a dot on the rear vision mirror of their car, TV, computer, refrigerator and phone.)

The patient should be reminded that breathing retraining may feel very uncomfortable at first, and to be prepared for this. Feelings of 'air hunger' are an expected and normal reaction to resetting breathing rates and volumes (Pitman 1996).

Changing any behaviour takes time and a realistic estimate is, with *consistent practice*, between 6 and 8 weeks before habitual 'low and slow' breathing becomes re-established.

Patients need to be reminded to forget about their breathing in between times, as it is both unnatural and uncomfortable to be aware of breathing all the time. Short effective practice is the best option.

Follow-up

A follow-up appointment should be scheduled within a week to review retraining, in order to sort out any difficulties encountered and re-evaluate. The patient should be checked in lying, sitting and standing positions.

During this session, a 'sniff' test should be performed in sitting to check diaphragm action.

Sniff test seated (Box 7.3.2)

This tests bilateral diaphragm function and is useful in checking dominance of upper or lower chest patterns. Placing the hand against the patient's upper abdominal wall three fingers below the xiphoid process, ask the patient to take a quick sniff in. A firm outward movement of the abdominal wall should be felt, showing both hemidiaphragms are working.

Entrenched upper-chest breathers invariably 'sniff' into their dominant upper-chest pattern, with no diaphragmatic excursion at all, or even indrawing of their abdominal wall. Most are easily able to 'lead with the diaphragm' when shown. Trying with hands on head will help those who find it difficult. It is useful at this follow-up session to check this, to reinforce that in breathing retraining it takes time to re-establish the diaphragm as the dominant pattern.

The sniff test should be repeated at subsequent sessions to monitor progress.

Box 7.3.1 **BradCliff® Angle Check**

Patients who have hypertonic abdominal muscles, either from mental stress or overdoing 'abs' training, or both, may have a reduced xyphocostal angle, restricting normal diaphragm movement. Figures 7.3.4 to 7.3.7 show the progression of an elite 'over-abbed' Olympic athlete. A normal angle ranges between 75–90° (Nijmegen score of 38/64 at assessment). No other interventions other than breathing retraining, and the relaxation response, were given. Retesting at 10 weeks showed a Nijmegen score reduction to 14/64 and his BradCliff® angle was restored to a normal range, allowing greater diaphragm movement and power. He also won a bronze medal at the 2012 London Olympics.

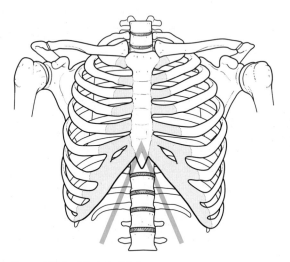

Figure 7.3.4   Week 1, 38 degrees.

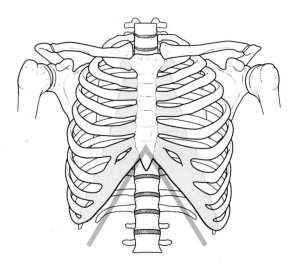

Figure 7.3.5   Week 2, 57 degrees.

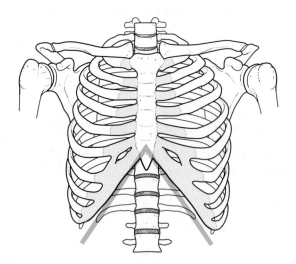

Figure 7.3.6   Week 5, 70 degrees.

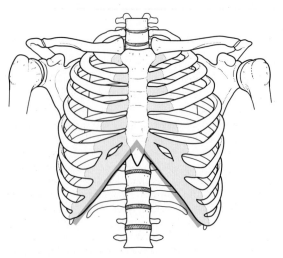

Figure 7.3.7 Week 10, 76 degrees.

Box 7.3.2 **'Sniff' test**

Unilateral paralysis can be detected in sitting by a sniff, which causes the paralysed side to rise and the unaffected diaphragm to descend.

Causes include phrenic nerve injury from surgery, trauma or carcinoma of the bronchus; neurological, including herpes zoster or poliomyelitis; or infection such as tuberculosis or pneumonia.

Bilateral diaphragm weakness or paralysis

Paradoxical indrawing of the abdominal wall is best checked in supine. Patients with, for example, multiple sclerosis, postviral infections, exacerbations of COPD (Kumar & Clarke 1998) may demonstrate weakness.

Box 7.3.3 **Rescue breathing techniques**

Rescue breathing techniques for risk situations which are likely to trigger symptoms (such as laughing, crying, high-intensity exercise, prolonged speech, humid or hot conditions, flying) include:
- Short breath-holds (to allow CO_2 levels to rise) followed by low-chest/low-volume breathing. Great care must be taken to teach patients to breath-hold only to the point of slight discomfort and to avoid deep respirations on letting go (Pitman 1996).
- Rest positions – i.e. arms forward, resting on a table or desk, to reduce upper-chest effort and concentrate on nose/abdominal breathing.
- Hands on head, or thumbs forward, hands on hips helps with breathlessness during exercise.
- Breathing into hands cupped over the nose and mouth for 10–15 seconds to rapidly raise CO_2 levels, helps patients effectively identify and separate symptoms from triggers.
- Use of a fan, with the sensation of moving air over the trigeminal nerve outlet on each side of the face, helps deepen and calm respiration.

Standing

For patients to feel abdominal breathing in standing, have them clasp their hands behind their back to reduce upper-chest involvement. Alternatively, have them clasp hands on top of the head to establish low-chest breathing.

Awareness of this, and being able to breathe abdominally in standing with arms relaxed at the sides, should be noted.

Reinforce the need to schedule time to practise breathing retraining effectively and regularly between treatment sessions.

Subsequent treatment sessions, once abdominal nose breathing is restored, can include breathing and speech, exercise, or other problem areas the patient may have integrating energy-efficient breathing into daily life, sleeping and awake (see below). Box 7.3.3 describes some techniques which can be used in situations in which symptoms are likely to be triggered.

Common coexisting problems

Asthma and chronic obstructive pulmonary disease (COPD)

Children and adults who have asthma usually experience chaotic breathing patterns during an attack (Thomas et al 2009). This is a normal response to cope with fatigue as the work of breathing increases, alternating between upper-chest/accessory and diaphragmatic/abdominal effort. Using rest positions and the 'stop, flop, drop' manoeuvre helps reduce distress while waiting for asthma medications to work (Bradley 2012). Re-establishing abdominal nose breathing patterns and normalized CO_2 levels are top priorities once the attack is over. Inspiratory muscle training (IMT) has been shown to be of benefit in abdominal/diaphragmatic pattern strengthening and in reducing exertional dyspnoea in mild to moderate asthma (McConnell

1998). Patients with COPD benefit from breathing pattern assessments, as they may experience disproportionate breathlessness in relation to their level of lung impairment (Howell 1990). This may be in part due to anxiety and/or depression over symptoms, as well as associated upper chest/mouth/increased respiratory rates. IMT has also been found to be useful in combating the sensation of breathlessness (Lisboa 1997). For those with chronic productive cough, use of oscillatory devices helps with chest clearance. A review by Hristara-Papadopoulou and colleagues (2008) examines the various brands and options.

Chronic rhino sinusitis (CRS)

Chronic mouth breathing is a constant companion of CRS, triggering chronic biomechanical and breathing pattern dysfunction. Regular saline nasal rinses, and eucalyptus steam inhalations have been shown to ease sinus congestion and restore nasal breathing (Papsin & McTavish 2003). A review of low intensity pulsed ultrasound therapy (which has a vibratory rather than heating effect), has been shown to enhance the effectiveness of antibiotic therapies by vibration of the bacteria-laden biofilms lining the sinus cavities (Bartley & Young 2008). This widespread condition (affecting 14% of the US population) is also commonly found in people with HVS/BPDs. Assisting in restoring nasal breathing is a top priority in any breathing retraining programme.

Chronic pain

Chronic pain is invariably accompanied by chronic hyperventilation, which is a perfectly reasonable reaction to it. Abdominal or pelvic pain frequently involves splinting of the abdominal muscles leading to upper-chest breathing patterns, while pain sited elsewhere may simply increase resting respiratory rates (Glynn 1981).

Promoting low tidal volume nose/abdominal breathing and relaxation are valuable additions to the patient's repertoire of pain management skills, and aids in the decrease of hyper-arousal associated with intractable pain.

Hormonal influences

Women between menarche and menopause are affected by progesterone level changes during their menstrual cycle. A respiratory stimulant, its influence in the postovulatory phase may drive $PaCO_2$ levels down as far as 25% below normal (Damas-Mora et al 1980), and lower during pregnancy (Novy & Edwards 1967). Patients with premenstrual syndrome (PMS) benefit from awareness of breathing rate changes and breathing retraining to prevent excessive CO_2 depletion and consequent HVS symptoms. Perimenopausal and menopausal hormone levels may fluctuate dramatically and women unable or unwilling to take hormone replacement therapies (HRT) have benefited from breathing retraining to reduce hot flushes and improve sleep (Freedman & Woodward 1992).

SELF-CONFIDENCE

Psychosocial measurement is an important part of assessment in chronic disorders including HVS/BPDs. Structured recording of the patient's own view of their emotional and social health and how improvements from physiotherapy interventions have helped in these areas have equal validity, along with traditional biophysical outcome measures (Chesson 1998). There are many useful scales to record these findings. One simply administered example is the Hospital Anxiety and Depression (HAD) scale (Zigmond & Snaith 1983).

This simple type of scale is recommended in those patients who express persistent anxiety or depression as their most disabling symptoms. As with the Nijmegen Questionnaire and the RoBE scale, it makes a useful educative tool as well. Referral on to and co-treatment with a psychologist or psychotherapist would be recommended as an additional option for patients with positive scores, if they wish.

Physiotherapists tend to underestimate their value as good listeners. Literally being able to get fears, frustrations and anxieties off their chests, and being able to put frightening symptoms into a physiological context can be a turning point for many patients. Chronic hyperventilation, whether a primary disorder or secondary to other physical or mental health problems, is of itself a major stress. Equipping patients with physical coping skills to deal with this is an essential ingredient in rebuilding self-reliance and confidence.

TOTAL BODY RELAXATION

Patients may have been struggling for weeks, months, even years with worrying symptoms and consequent tension brought on by breathing pattern disturbances. Ensuring patients have an understanding of the stress response is the first step. This physically based defence mechanism preparing the body for 'fight or flight' is mediated through the sympathetic branch of the autonomic nervous system (ANS). While this response is a major part of the human defence system–life-saving in some instances–the sequel to prolonged bouts of hyperarousal (Nixon 1986) is exhausting, and detrimental to health (Selye 1956).

Those in the grip of ongoing or unresolved fear or mental tension, however, may experience anxiety and/or panic episodes, which in turn may lead to avoidance behaviours/phobias (Gilbert 1999). This group of patients tend to be hypervigilant, deriving as much stress from having to control their 'fight or flight' reactions as from experiencing the initiating stressors themselves. The notion of 'letting go' is tantamount to losing control, and might at first heighten anxiety levels. Anxiety sufferers are often the first to agree that they have been dominated by their thoughts (busy brain), with poor body awareness.

A plausible explanation of these reactions helps the patient understand the process and possible initial discomforts of releasing tension.

The next step is understanding the relaxation response (Benson & Klipper 2000) where the patient learns how to identify and switch off anxiety or stress responses (mediated by the parasympathetic branch of the autonomic nervous system).

Just as the stress response is greatly influenced by fear, pain or negative thinking and emotions, so the reverse is found in eliciting the relaxation response (Fig. 7.3.8). Patients learn how to switch off negative thinking and physical tension with regular practice of 'calm stillness of mind and body'.

Mastering low volume, low chest 'minimalist' breathing is an integral part of this. Understanding both sides of the stress/relaxation equation helps equip the patient with powerful self-help skills along with awareness of the effects of CO_2 depletion from overbreathing, onset of symptoms, and consequent systems derangements (Box 7.3.4).

The third step is scheduling regular daily practice:

- Teaching a variety of mental and physical relaxation techniques helps address both physical and mental

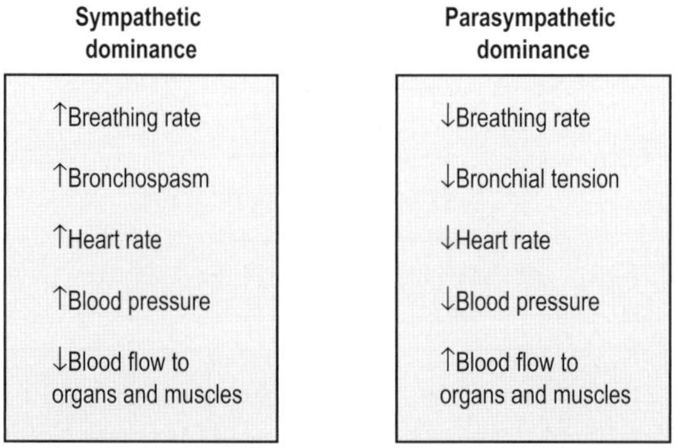

Sympathetic dominance	Parasympathetic dominance
↑Breathing rate	↓Breathing rate
↑Bronchospasm	↓Bronchial tension
↑Heart rate	↓Heart rate
↑Blood pressure	↓Blood pressure
↓Blood flow to organs and muscles	↑Blood flow to organs and muscles

Figure 7.3.8 Simplified ANS chart, indicating effects of stress/relaxation.

Box 7.3.4 **Panic attacks**

- Identifying triggers and using 'rescue breathing' techniques (Box 7.3.3) helps patients alter their perception of fear of losing control, to being 'in the driving seat'
- A discussion on the phrases 'out of control', 'under control', and 'in control' is useful
- The majority of panickers agree they spend most of their time swinging between the first two
- Learning physical coping skills and understanding the physiological consequences of overbreathing can be immensely empowering in remaining 'in control' in high risk circumstances, not 'out of' or 'under control'
- A telephone/text/email back-up service by the therapist may be offered to help panic patients regain confidence in self-managing their symptoms
- See notes on panic influences and cycles in Chapter 4.

---

approaches to stress. Variety also helps prevent boredom.

- Lying comfortably supported by pillows, with anti-gravity reflexes switched off, the patient can initially concentrate on the relaxed pause at the end of each exhalation before practising, for instance, progressive muscle relaxation (Mitchell 1987).
- Biofeedback machines, where available, make a useful therapeutic adjunct, especially when treating adolescents, notoriously resistant to relaxation.
- Hot packs, massage, acupressure or gentle stretches may be a beneficial prelude to practice.
- Prone lying is an alternative for those who at first feel vulnerable relaxing while lying on their backs. Gentle thoracic mobilizations may be added.

- Survivors of torture or abuse need specialist care. Required reading is Alexandra Hough's well-documented paper on this topic (Hough 1992).
- Progress to teaching relaxation in sitting once a positive outcome has been achieved in lying. Mini-relaxes using 'stop, drop, flop' as a guide may then be used hourly by patients – at work, in the car at traffic lights, on a bus, train or aircraft.
- A discussion about ergonomics at work should be included in this session, to review postures and breathing patterns on the job, with perhaps a worksite visit, liaising with the patient's occupational safety and health officer.
- It is important to ensure that patients understand that relaxation only helps eliminate the symptoms, not the causes of stress; examination of achievable lifestyle changes is encouraged.

SPEECH

Coordinating breathing and speaking is a common problem in HVS/BPDs where speech interferes with the background rhythm of breathing (Timmons & Ley 1994). Restoring respiratory confidence during speech is an important part of the treatment programme. Patients may fall into one, or a combination of the following groups:

1. Patients with chronic breathing pattern problems whose jobs require them to use their voices: teachers, courtroom lawyers, actors, singers, call centre and sales people for instance. They relate difficulties with breath control and vocal tone. Secondary loss of confidence and 'performance anxiety' are common additions to their repertoire of symptoms.
2. Mouth breathers with chronic sinus problems or postnasal drip with coexisting problems of cough, throat dryness and soreness.
3. Patients suffering anxiety, stress or depressive disorders, with concurrent increased sympathetic arousal, upper thoracic tension and sighing respirations often report excessive jaw and throat tightness or pain. This group often speak in a monotone. Help with voicing problems may require the additional help of a skilled counsellor.
4. Patients with a history of hiatus hernia, or gastro-esophageal reflux disease (GERD) frequently complain of irritated throat, chronic throat clearing, shoulder tension and vocal fold impairment. In response to gut discomfort, upper-chest breathing becomes the norm. Abdominal bracing leads to ineffective breath control while speaking – commonly petering out before the end of a sentence is reached (it is important to check medication compliance).

Common to all groups is reduced diaphragmatic strength/usage.

Assess speaking and breath control in sitting and standing, once an abdominal pattern is re-established, perhaps at the second or third session. The most common problems are:

- Hyperinflating the upper chest when starting to speak
- Forgetting to pause for breath during speech
- Speaking to the very end of the out breath, followed by a gasping inhalation.

Having the patient read from a simple text, or recite the alphabet out loud if they have reading difficulties, is an effective way of identifying problems and correcting them. Steps include:

- Relaxed breath out before speaking
- Breathe in softly through the nose to start
- Light, low-chest mouth-breaths between sentences
- Speak slowly.

IMT can benefit those who find mouth/diaphragm breathing difficult.

Any continuing voice/speech problems should be referred on to a speech pathologist or speech therapist. See Chapter 7.5 for voice/vocal fold problems.

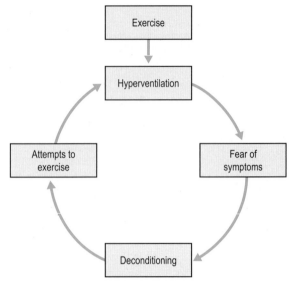

Figure 7.3.9 Deconditioning cycle.

EXERCISE

The ability to exercise depends on the capacity of the cardiovascular and respiratory systems to increase delivery of oxygen to the tissues and remove excess carbon dioxide and metabolites. Although the normal oxygen cost of breathing at rest is less than 2% of resting oxygen consumption, up to 30% of total oxygen consumption may be used to move and aerate the lungs and chest wall during episodes of hyperventilation (Koeppen & Stanton 2006). For patients who are habitually using more oxygen than usual to move air *at rest* (hyperventilating), the oxygen cost of apical breathing itself may limit their exercise capability.

A mechanical problem often coexists with this set of events. Chronic upper-chest breathers hyperinflate with exercise and reach the bony limits of their chest wall rapidly, and misinterpret the feeling of constriction as breathlessness or misattribute symptoms to more sinister causes. (Chest wall pain due to overstretching of intercostal structures, the sequel to habitual upper-chest breathing, is a prime example of the patient thinking of heart attacks rather than musculoskeletal injury.)

Fear of effort becomes established, often triggered by unpleasant symptoms of breathlessness and fatigue. The latter may be central fatigue, with generalized feelings of low energy/unwellness, mediated in part by a shift of the acid-base balance (pH) toward alkalosis (Grossman & Wientjes 1989). Protection of pH is maintained by excretion of alkalis such as bicarbonate via the kidneys. Potassium and phosphates are also depleted (Magarian 1982), which causes muscle fatigue.

Lactic acid build-up in the skeletal muscles from compromised metabolic efficiency leads to aching and stiffness. Breathlessness in reaction to unbuffered acids reaching the central circulation triggers further hyperventilation (Lewis 1954).

Peripheral fatigue, where the venous system fails adequately to clear the accumulated waste products of metabolism from muscles during exercise, adds to the misery. The 'vicious circle' is complete. These patients then have the secondary problem of loss of condition (Fig. 7.3.9).

Physical fitness is described in Altug and Miller's (1990) *Teacher's Guide for Fitness for Living* as:

> *the body's ability to meet the normal demands of everyday life – work and recreation – with ease and with enough margin to adequately cope with emergencies.*

Patients who have been struggling with disordered breathing patterns and physiological sequelae often admit to falling far below this ideal. Some patients have fallen so far below they experience symptoms usually associated with heavy exercise while doing quite light activities.

CAUTION: The level of exercise a patient may undertake requires careful judgment with consideration as to age, nutritional status, exhaustion levels and sleep patterns. See Figure 7.3.10.

A useful rule of thumb is to discourage fatigued patients from resuming aerobic exercise until balanced breathing and improved sleep patterns (adequate rest and restoration of homeostasis) are re-established.

Fitness recommendations have changed emphasis from an exercise training/fitness to a physical activity/health

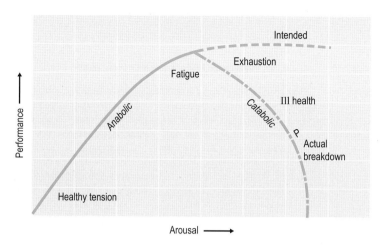

Figure 7.3.10 The human function curve. Performance relates to coping ability and efficiency. Arousal relates to effort and, at the higher levels, to struggle. 'P' represents the 'catastrophic cliff edge' of instability where little further arousal is required to precipitate a breakdown. *Dr Peter Nixon.*

model which uniquely incorporates *moderate* intensity and *intermittent* physical activity (Warburton 2006). This is a more attractive prospect for most people – especially the drastically unfit, or those in sedentary jobs. Accumulated exercise times *gradually* increase towards a total of 30 minutes' brisk activity a day, 6–7 days a week, which can be broken into 10-minute segments. Activity may be varied.

As little as 2 minutes three times a day may be a suitable starting point for the very unfit, or those suffering exhaustion, once proper breathing has become familiar. IMT has been shown to benefit those with limited exercise capacity because of obesity (Edwards et al 2012) and may 'provide a useful priming or preparatory strategy prior to entry in a physical training programme for overweight and obese adults.'

Nutrition: Box 7.3.5 makes some recommendations on nutrition and exercise.

Establishing an exercise programme

A supervised session covering breathing with activity begins with a review of expected changes to breathing during exercise:

- Increases in breathing rates and tidal volumes in tandem with increased oxygen consumption (normal)
- Loss of the rest phase at the end of exhalation (normal)
- Upper-chest involvement during effort (normal)
- Switching from nose to mouth breathing at extremes of effort keeping in mind that the very unfit will reach those extremes rapidly (normal)
- Breathlessness is not harmful, merely a signal to slow down or stop, recover, check breathing before continuing ('stop, drop, flop').

Box 7.3.5 Nutrition

- Good nutrition is an important aspect of fitness; many patients admit that their diet as well as their fitness levels are equally less than adequate.
- Fluctuating blood glucose levels may trigger symptoms in patients with high-carbohydrate diets which produce rapid rises followed by sharp falls to fasting levels – or below (Timmons & Ley 1994).
- Patients are recommended to eat a breakfast which includes protein and to avoid going without food for more than 3 hours (Hough 2001).
- This fits in with a mid-morning and afternoon protein snack as well as the usual three meals a day.
- This is particularly relevant to patients who experience panic attacks or seizures which have been shown to be more likely to strike when blood glucose levels are low (Timmons & Ley 1994).
- Referral to a dietician may be warranted.

Walking or climbing stairs is an easy way to observe breathing rates/patterns and pulse rates in response to exercise. Using an oximeter to check SpO_2 saturations:

- Demonstrates normal values to anxious or sceptical patients
- May signal undiagnosed cardiopulmonary disease if oxygen desaturation accompanies breathlessness in falls below normal minimum levels (95%) during exercise. Further investigations would be indicated.

Once confident about breathing with exercise, patients can self-manage with individualized graduated programmes if required, or resume regular gym or sports activities. The advantages regular enjoyable exercise brings are:

- Aerobic benefits (cardiovascular efficiency)
- Improved digestion/bowel function
- Improved sleeping patterns/relaxation responses
- Release of opiopeptoids into the bloodstream (e.g. mood and sleep enhancer, serotonin).
- Improvement/maintenance of bone density (important to those on long-term courses of steroids and to postmenopausal women).

REST AND SLEEP

A common and debilitating symptom experienced by patients with breathing pattern disorders is erratic sleep patterns/vivid dreaming. Recovery and repair for optimum physical and mental health depends on restful sleep and relaxed rest. Being deprived of this causes a great deal of stress, anxiety and exhaustion to already overloaded body systems. Sleep regulating centres (SRCs) in the brainstem process information from different parts of the body – joint, organ and muscle receptors – as well as from higher cortical levels, to either:

- induce sleep (lowered levels of stimulation to the SRC)
- encourage wakefulness/alertness (high SRC stimulation).

A calm mind as well as a relaxed body are prerequisites to restorative sleep.

Sleep involves two entirely different cycles in which significant changes to the respiratory system occur:

1. *Slow wave or quiet sleep.* This is deep and restful, characterized by reductions in peripheral vascular tone, blood pressure and respiratory and metabolic rates. CO_2 levels increase as hypercapnic responses are attenuated. Some dreaming may occur but these dreams are seldom remembered. This is considered the physical restoration phase.
2. *Rapid eye movement (REM) sleep.* Approximately every 90 minutes slow wave sleep changes to REM sleep which lasts between 5 and 30 minutes. Also called paradoxical sleep, because the brain is quite active during this phase, this sleep is thought to be linked to mood and emotional adaptions. Slight increases in heart and metabolic rates and blood pressure, irregular breathing and reduction in tidal volumes occur; despite reduced muscle tone, including muscles of the upper airways, intercostals and accessory muscles (which dissociate from diaphragmatic activity (Hough 2001), muscle twitching and rapid eye movements can be observed. Dreams during this cycle are often remembered, at least in part (Koeppen & Stanton 2006). REM sleep

may be absent in those suffering extreme tiredness, but returns after adequate rest/sleep.

A vicious cycle is established

People with chronic breathing pattern disorders who have low-level or fluctuating CO_2 levels by day commonly report startled waking at night, with rapid breathing. Having managed to fall asleep, CO_2 levels start to rise (reduced minute volumes) to higher than accustomed daily levels (Bootzin & Perlis 1992). This stimulates the respiratory centres to increase respiratory drives in order to reduce CO_2 to habitual daytime levels. Vivid dreams or nightmares are often experienced at this time, along with a pounding heart. Sleep itself becomes feared (Box 7.3.6).

Re-establishing normal sleep patterns

- Breathing retraining: restoring low-volume, low chest breathing patterns during waking hours helps re-establish higher CO_2 tolerance by the respiratory centres

---

Box 7.3.6 Sleep disturbances

This cycle may not exist in isolation. A sleep history assessment will determine other common causes of sleep disturbance such as:

- physical problems (e.g. chronic pain)
- drugs (whether prescribed or recreational) which are CNS stimulants (e.g. bronchodilators, caffeine, amphetamines, nicotine)
- environmental factors (e.g. crowded conditions, noise, pollution)
- behavioural reasons (e.g. boredom, daytime sleeping)
- psychiatric problems (e.g. clinical or reactive depression)
- social problems (e.g. unemployment, relationship problems, grief)
- upset diurnal rhythms (e.g. shift work)
- snoring bed partner
- sleep disorders such as obstructive sleep apnoea
- addictions (e.g. alcoholism, drug dependence including hypnotics).

Noting these and finding relevant specialist agencies to address the underlying problem, where necessary, must be the first priority before dealing with the coexisting insomnia.

- Prior to sleep, or when sleep is broken, breathing awareness with total body relaxation helps reduce hyperarousal and promotes sleep
- Discussion about sleep rituals/preparation
- Commitment to an individualized sleep plan for 2–6 weeks.

Sleep hygiene checklist

Discuss how and why to:

- Instigate calming pre-sleep rituals to reduce hyperarousal (relaxing music, warm bath, avoidance of mental stimulants, e.g. TV news, late night videos/cinema/theatre, debates/arguments)
- Reduce/stop dietary stimulants, e.g. replace coffee, chocolate, strong tea with decaffeinated, herbal teas or warm milk
- Check soft drinks and over-the-counter (OTC) pain medication labels for caffeine levels
- Do not exceed the 300 mg recommended daily limit of caffeine (the equivalent of three cups of coffee)
- Ban daytime naps (disturbs diurnal/circadian rhythms)
- Avoid late evening spicy or heavy meals
- Restrict late evening alcohol consumption (reduces upper airway muscle tone, triggering snoring/poor sleep architecture)
- Avoid late exercise/gym sessions (stimulating)
- Reduce stress levels (good and bad) in the bedroom – ban telephones, electronica, eating and drinking, or writing in bed – to reinforce bed as a place to sleep
- Making love is an exception. Deep post-orgasmic relaxation, however, only lasts 4–5 minutes: if sleep is not reached in that time, it is of no added benefit. Anxieties about sex may require specialist help.
- Keep evening fluid intake to a minimum to avoid bladder frequency.

These simple considerations, if adhered to, help restore restful and replenishing sleep.

Sleep retraining

Drug therapies may be required in some circumstances, such as:

- Severe chronic disabling insomnia causing extreme distress
- Transient sleep problems associated with shift work or jet lag
- Sleep disturbance related to emotional upheaval or serious illness.

Toward independence

CREATING AN INDIVIDUAL PROGRAMME

Having completed the detective work, and covered where necessary the areas listed above, putting together an acceptable programme for the patient to follow is the next step.

While the assessment session requires a lot of talk and inquiry, following sessions would be more action-based, with breathing retraining, education and relaxation taking up the majority of time. As progress is made (and recorded), other specific topics, as judged applicable, may be covered.

Weekly physiotherapy sessions will be needed until patients have stabilized and feel more confident in self-management skills. Appointments may then be spaced out with half-hour check-ups or telephone/email/text communications only required.

Recording objective markers at 2-monthly intervals – such as re-doing the Nijmegen Questionnaire or RoBE scale, rechecking thoracic trigger point pain levels, mobility and balance, sleep changes, days off work/school – provides positive feedback to patients as well as outcome measures for data collection for future research.

REFERENCES

Altug, Z., Miller, M., 1990. The natural exercise prescription. Clinical Management 9(3).

Bartley, J., Young, D., 2008. Ultrasound as a treatment for chronic rhinosinusitis. Medical hypothesis. Elsevier Science Direct.

Benson, H., Klipper, M., 2000. The Relaxation Response. Harper Collins, New York.

Bootzin, R., Perlis, M., 1992. Non pharmacological treatments of insomnia. Journal of Clinical Psychology 53 (6) (suppl).

Bradley, D., 2012. Hyperventilation syndrome/breathing pattern disorders. Random House, New Zealand.

Chesson, R., 1998. Psychosocial aspects of measurement. Physiotherapy 84 (9), 435–438.

Clifton-Smith, T. Bartley, J., 2006. Breathing Matters. Random House, New Zealand, pp. 101.

Damas-Mora, J., Davies, L., Taylor, W., et al., 1980. Menstrual respiratory changes and symptoms. British Journal of Psychiatry 136, 492–497.

Edwards, A.M., Maguire, G.P., Graham, D., et al., 2012. Clinical study: four weeks of inspiratory muscle training improves self-paced walking performance in overweight and obese adults: a randomised controlled trial. Journal of Obesity Volume 2012 (2012), doi:10.1155/2012/918202.

Freedman, R.R., Woodward, S., 1992. Behavioural treatment of menopausal hot flushes: evaluation by ambulatory monitoring. American Journal of Obstetrics and Gynecology 167, 436–439.

Gilbert, C., 1999. Breathing and the cardiovascular system. Journal of Bodywork and Movement Therapies 3 (4), 215–224.

Glynn, C.J., Lloyd, J.W., Folkhard, S., 1981. Ventilatory response to intractable pain. Pain 11 (2), 201–211.

Grossman, P., Wientjes, C., 1989. Respiratory disorders: asthma and hyperventilation syndrome. In: Turpin, G. (Ed.), Handbook of clinical psychophysiology. Wiley, New York, pp. 519–554.

Hough, A., 1992. Physiotherapy for survivors of torture. Physiotherapy 78 (5), 323–328.

Hough, A., 2001. Physiotherapy in respiratory care, third ed. Nelson Thornes, UK.

Howell, J.B.L., 1990. Behavioural breathlessness. Thorax 45, 287–292.

Hristara-Papadopoulou, A., Tsanaka, J., Diomou, G., et al., 2008. Current devices of respiratory physiotherapy. Hippokratia 12 (4), 211–220.

Innocenti, D.M., 1998. Hyperventilation. In: Pryor, J., Webber, B., (Eds.), Physiotherapy for respiratory and cardiac problems. Churchill Livingstone, Edinburgh, pp. 449–461.

Koeppen, B.M., Stanton, B.A., (Eds.), 2006. Berne & Levy Physiology, sixth ed. Mosby, Philadelphia.

Kumar, P., Clarke, M., 1998. Clinical medicine, fourth ed. W B Saunders, Edinburgh, pp. 826.

Lewis, B.I., 1954. Chronic hyperventilation syndrome. JAMA 151, 1204–1208.

Lisboa, C., 1997. Inspiratory muscle training in chronic airflow limitation: effect on exercise performance. Eur Resp J. 10, 1266–1274.

McConnell, A., 1998. Inspiratory muscle training improves lung function and reduces exertional dyspnoea in mild/moderate asthmatics. Proceeding of the Medical Research Society. Clinical Science 95, 4P.

Magarian, G.J., 1982. Hyperventilation syndromes: infrequently recognised common expressions of anxiety and stress. Medicine 62, 219–236.

Mitchell, L., 1987. Simple relaxation. John Murray, London.

Nixon, P.G.F., 1986. Exhaustion: cardiac rehabilitation's starting point. Physiotherapy 72 (5), 129–139.

Novy, M.J., Edwards, M.J., 1967. Respiratory problems in pregnancy. American Journal of Obstetrics and Gynecology (Dec 1), 1024–1045.

Papsin, B., McTavish, A., 2003. Saline nasal irrigation: its role as an adjunct treatment. Canadian Family Physician 49, 168–173.

Pitman, A., 1996. Physiotherapy for hyperventilation video. Physiotherapy for Hyperventilation Group, c/o Anne Pitman, Physiotherapy Department. The London Clinic, 20 Devonshire Place, London, UK.

Selye, H., 1956. The stress of life. McGraw Hill, New York.

Thomas, M., McKinley, M.K., Mellor, S., et al., 2009. Breathing exercises for asthma: a randomised controlled trial. Thorax 64(1), 55–61.

Timmons, B.H., Ley, R., 1994. Behavioural and psychological approaches to breathing disorders. Plenum, London.

Warburton, D.E.R., Nicol, C.W., Bredin, S.S.D., 2006. Health benefits of physical activity: the evidence. CMAJ March 14, 2006 vol. 174 no. 6 doi: 10.1503/cmaj.051351.

Zigmond, A.S., Snaith, R.P., 1983. The Hospital Anxiety and Depression Scale. Acta Psychiatrica Scandinavica 67, 361–370.

Psychological training and treatment of breathing problems

Chris Gilbert

This chapter focuses on interventions with a psychological component, including emotional factors, habit change, self-regulation, cognitive psychotherapy and dealing with panic. As long as mental intent is engaged, learning to improve breathing is in part a psychological process. This is especially true when a dysfunctional breathing pattern is based on disordered thinking and feeling. Identifying and changing such things is a bigger order than having steadier breathing, but is not always necessary. Proceeding as if the breathing alone needs to be changed may be sufficient. Because of the bidirectional relationship of body and mind, physical or behavioural changes generally also have an impact on the emotional state. In this view, one person can come for help with the breathing pattern and end up feeling more psychologically stable, while another comes in for psychotherapy and ends up having more stable breathing.

A person with respiratory symptoms interprets those symptoms in a certain way, and this affects what kind of practitioner to consult: physician, nutritionist, acupuncturist, osteopath, chiropractor, psychotherapist or physical therapist. Each person's choice thus displays a biased belief about the source of the symptoms. Each of these disciplines (and others besides) has a valid approach to breathing problems, and each discipline can offer some relief through its particular approach to the same set of symptoms – especially if the beliefs of the practitioner match the beliefs of the patient.

Trying to guide or retrain someone's breathing usually involves teaching brief exercises that simulate natural relaxed breathing. With repeated practice and self-correction, the conscious intervention may become less conscious and more habitual. Several books describe methods for retraining breathing along these lines, and they reflect careful observation and practice (Bradley 2012). This chapter offers a few general guidelines, with attention to the psychology of controlling the breath. More details are available in Chaitow et al (2002).

Changing one's breathing is not the same as improving a tennis serve or ski technique; breathing is a continuous, fully automatic process that does not require conscious supervision. Also, since breathing is so essential, there are multiple controls and safeguards to ensure its operation. Teaching someone to interfere in this process is in a way presumptuous; with full attention we can commandeer the breathing mechanism temporarily, but as soon as the mind wanders elsewhere, automatic control returns.

Yet improvement in breathing pattern is quite possible. The interaction between voluntary and involuntary can be addressed with respect for the deep, protective systems which try to ensure adequate air exchange in spite of conflicting messages from various areas of the brain. Problems which disrupt breathing may derive from emotional sources, from injuries, poor posture or habits acquired through compensation for some other factor, as detailed in preceding chapters. Assuming there is no structural or medical impediment to restoring normal breathing, the challenge is to allow the body to breathe on its own, in line with the metabolic needs of the moment and without excessive input from higher centres.

If a chronic or intermittent emotional state is contributing to the breathing problem, it would seem that both would have to be changed together. Yet if we accept that the mind is affected by the breathing as well as the reverse, the separation becomes artificial, an expression of an assumed mind–body dichotomy. We can describe interaction, mutual influence, reciprocity and synchrony until the distinction starts to seem like an artifact of language and ultimately pointless. Our English language enforces the mind/body distinction, but biological reality predates language.

Most of the inappropriate breathing changes which create problems happen without conscious intent. An individual does not usually decide to suspend breathing in order to think more clearly; breathing just stops. In this sense breathing is automatic in the way that stomach contractions are. Yet the abundant nerve connections from the cortex to the breathing centres permit us to direct our breathing very thoroughly. The most basic neural control centres in the pons and medulla receive inputs from chemoreceptors for fine-tuning of breathing variables, but they also receive input from the limbic structures (emotional input) from the reticular formation when the person is awake (general arousal, alertness), and from the cerebral cortex via corticospinal neurons for full voluntary control. It is this last pathway that can be practised, or 'exercised', in order to strengthen its dominance over breathing patterns.

SELF-MASTERY

When we ask a patient to breathe in a certain way we are encouraging mastery of a system which may be a source of great fear and worry. Many patients are initially uneasy about trying to alter their breathing; such attempts may trigger gasps or sighs, or else an apparent refusal to tamper with a biological process which they perceive as threatening. This alienation from a natural body function amounts to a withdrawal of responsibility, leaving the breathing process to be driven by emotional states. This alone constitutes a strong rationale for 'breathing exercises' – what is being strengthened is voluntary control, intentionally modifying or reversing influences from emotional centres.

To learn to interrupt out-of-control breathing, finding an entry point for conscious intent is helpful. This requires extending the conscious mind into a new and sometimes frightening realm. Breathing may be the body function holding the most menace because it is associated with possible suffocation and death. For some individuals, breathing is particularly linked to emotions and may be a major route of emotional expression, representing something far more than simple air exchange. If so, requesting conscious regulation of this process is close to requesting conscious regulation of anger, grief, or feelings of abandonment – a much larger order. So kindness and patience is helpful with patients who balk at regulating the breath or have special difficulty with the task.

HYPERVENTILATION

In the case of habitual hyperventilation, reducing breathing volume calls for introducing pauses somewhere, reducing depth of the inhalation, reducing overall breathing rate, or slowing the exhalation so that the volume of air flow per unit time is reduced. Some of these are more difficult than others even with attention fully focused on the goal. When asked to pause at the end of an exhale, for example, many people simply cannot. They will partially comply, but will draw a slight amount of air in, either knowingly or unknowingly. When asked to exhale slowly, there may be little reversals, 'sneak breaths' on the way out. And if asked to not sigh so much (a common problem in chronic hyperventilation), often the reverse happens instead: more sighing, as if thinking of the possibility stimulates more of it.

Pausing the breath

Breath-holding, voluntary apnoea, is a simple place to begin. The breath can be stopped either with the throat open or with the throat closed. Pressing the back of the tongue against the soft palate seals the air passage and blocks all air movement. Breath-holding with the throat open is usually harder as it requires suspending all breathing-related movement, but it seems to more effectively extend conscious control.

In any case, stopping the breath is within everyone's repertoire. It is of course advisable when swimming underwater, and is also part of the 'freezing' reflex. Interrupting breathing to produce sound is part of vocalization. We can also exhale forcefully, as when blowing out a flame. These are both manipulations of the breath for a specific purpose. But meddling with the mechanism in the abstract often feels threatening to those who most need to do it. Interrupting breathing may evoke latent fears; those who want access to air at all times may ostensibly comply when asked to pause, but will still pull a little extra air. It can be detected either with a strain gauge or by close observation. Short breath-holding time is one indicator of a tendency to hyperventilate, and may indicate excessive air hunger or fear of build-up of CO_2 – the so-called 'suffocation alarm' (see Preter & Klein 2008). Some patients cannot exceed 10 seconds of breath-holding at first; 30 seconds is reasonable; and 45 should be within reach (see Ch. 8.2). Using a pulse oximeter can display to the patient reassuring evidence that the O_2 saturation does not drop very much during breath-holding.

Interjecting a pause is the wedge, or 'foot in the door' of conscious control of breathing. It is useful to practise pausing with the throat both open and closed, to feel the difference. Once that is mastered, the next step is a pause at the end of the exhalation. This differs from a post-inhalation pause and is usually harder. The object is to allow a complete exhalation to 'happen', simply by releasing all breathing muscles and letting movement subside, then resting just a moment before the next inhalation.

In favour of the post-exhalation instead of post-inhalation pause, keeping the lungs filled creates tension and strain in the muscles of inhalation. Pausing after the inhalation creates temporary hyperinflation, which works against relaxation and proper emptying of the lungs. Pausing after inhalation does not seem to occur naturally except when accompanying a state of suspense. Pausing after the exhalation is more relaxing, since the breathing system reduces volume by slowing frequency, reducing depth, and lengthening the post-exhalation pause. Attention can be directed toward the sinking down of the chest, the deflating of the abdomen, the release of used air, and the quietness that ensues when all motion stops.

For individuals anxious about breathing, their uneasiness is being confronted by asking them to do what they usually avoid. Learning to tolerate a brief pause develops tolerance of CO_2 build-up, but this can provoke major fear if the person has had attacks of hyperventilation-linked panic. So it is important to go slowly, but also to convey that voluntary breathing control is worth learning. One must assume that an optimal breathing pattern is accessible if only the conscious mind can be got out of the way.

Alleviating acute hyperventilation

If a person is visibly hyperventilating and it can be determined that the state is not due to organic factors but is being maintained by anxiety, this is an emotional emergency and not a medical emergency. This condition is frequently encountered by emergency personnel, especially when chest discomfort is involved. A minor tranquillizer will terminate such episodes within a few minutes, but leaves the person with the conclusion that the solution to subsequent attacks lies in another pill.

The state of panicky hyperventilation can also be considered a state of heightened suggestibility. Brief hyperventilation is often used as the final 'push' to enter a hypnotic state, and many hypnotists routinely ask for deep breathing to facilitate entering a trance (Baykushev 1969). Cerebral hypoxia compromises orientation and perception of reality. The emotional distress adds further to the need and willingness to be helped, and so anyone with a suggestion of authority or special knowledge is in a good position to give directions at such times.

Direct instruction works well here. For example: 'I can see you're very nervous and you're breathing pretty heavily. Would you like me to help you? You need to get control of your breathing, because it's a big part of the problem. Do you feel you're not getting enough air?' (*consider response*) 'You're getting plenty of air. You're breathing enough for three people! But the way you're breathing prevents your body from absorbing it. If you breathe more slowly, you'll start to absorb more oxygen. Let me help you. Watch my hand. Breathe with my hand.'

Then begin pacing the person's breathing with your hand, rising for inhalation, falling for exhalation, like a conductor, following the existing rhythm at first and then starting to lead it: in other words, following, pacing, and finally leading. Following the person's breathing in the beginning imposes no requirement to change anything, but provides an external reflection of the breathing pattern. As the person's attention is fixated on the moving hand, the internally-directed drive is somewhat interrupted.

'False equilibrium' and adaptation to imbalance

If an overbreathing pattern is fairly persistent it will feel familiar or even normal, regardless of the symptoms generated. This is partly due to the body's adaptation to the lower CO_2 levels, which includes reduction of bicarbonate buffer. The result is that achieving 'normal' breathing briefly will be opposed by the adaptation, which expects abnormal breathing to continue. Reducing breathing volume will raise CO_2 toward normal, but may initiate a feeling of not getting enough air. Also, the patient may be used to hyperinflation, so that reduced volume and a full, relaxed exhalation do not feel right. Finally, if mouth breathing has become a habit, the extra resistance of nose breathing will feel odd at first.

This adaptation to an imbalanced situation can be explained to the patient with reassurance that the physiology will adjust in time to an improved, lower level of breathing. Presenting printed norms showing where CO_2 and oxygen saturation should be, can be convincing enough to motivate acceptance and home practice.

USING A CAPNOMETER

(A full description of clinical capnometry is covered in Chapter 6.6, so only a few comments will be offered here).

Checking for presence of hyperventilation

Since both the depth of inhalation and the rate of breathing combine to determine total air flow, it is difficult to decide by observation alone whether an individual is actually hyperventilating at a given moment. The florid cases are obvious, with rapid breathing and heaving chest. But if the overbreathing is more subtle, sampling the exhalations for a minute or two with a capnometer – especially while the patient is being distracted – adds more weight to a decision about whether the patient is truly hyperventilating. With a capnometer, a single sample of $ETCO_2$ can be obtained in less than 30 seconds, but this reading does not necessarily imply anything beyond that moment. It may represent a habitual style, a transient state or anxiety about the measurement process itself. If it is high, it could be because the presence of opiate medication is suppressing respiration. Within a certain range, $PaCO_2$ fluctuates continuously and is more labile in some people than others. A single deep breath can push the next breath's CO_2 content temporarily below 35 mmHg, while suspending breathing for 30 seconds may result in the next exhalation reading over 45.

With capnometry, a series of end-tidal readings is easily obtained, but the information is only a beginning. If certain symptoms are being reported (light-headedness, chest discomfort, confusion, etc.) and the $PETCO_2$ is low as well, then making this connection can be very helpful. If the end-tidal CO_2 is initially low (<35 mmHg), slow breathing may be requested directly, and with luck the capnometer will reflect a rise in CO_2 toward normal. This gives the patient a sense of potential control, but requires full attention to the task of breathing less. Thinking of other things, creating a calm mental state, may be sufficient to normalize the breathing without focusing on it directly. Speaking softly to the patient about the seashore, mountains or some other pleasant and relaxing experience will usually induce a calm state which reduces breathing volume temporarily, with a corresponding rise in CO_2. The implication of this should be clear to the patient. Assigning home practice, perhaps a prepared audio recording in the therapist's voice, or listening to peaceful music, can provide a temporary 'scaffolding' for the more autonomous skill development.

Demonstrating the effects of emotional recall

The work of Ashley Conway (see Ch. 5) as well as Dudley (1969) and others has demonstrated the 'thinness' of the interface between emotions and breathing in some people. If the respiratory system is acting out each emotional state that runs through the mind and is forever preparing for some new imaginary threat or recalling alarming events, then physiological stability will be significantly compromised. Using the capnometer (as well as other

methods for monitoring breathing) helps to magnify and sharpen patients' awareness of their breathing responses to various emotional states. This information is of course useful to the therapist also, not only to confirm that the breathing reacts strongly to induced emotion, but also to identify more precisely which topics and emotions affect the breathing. But until this information is understood by the patient it has little practical use. The capnometer can be used like any other psychophysiological monitoring instrument, in the manner of a polygraph examination, except that the goal is to detect strong emotional responses.

Relevant connections such as the ones in the case study cited in Chapter 6.4 (Box 6.4.2) are not always so clear or retrievable, but it is often enough to ask the patient to describe a recent instance of hyperventilating while being monitored with the capnometer. Normally this request elicits a detailed memory, but if the person begins to describe the incident the entire response may begin again. In this case, the patient can then see that thinking about the symptoms can recreate the symptoms, along with a lowered $ETCO_2$ as independent evidence. Seeing such evidence of the body–mind connection usually impresses the patient with how self-generated the symptoms actually are. With an adequate sense of self-efficacy, this fact can be translated into more active control.

Boxes 7.4.1 and 7.4.2 contain miscellaneous practical tips for breathing training both with and without the aid of biofeedback devices.

COGNITIVE THERAPY

An important step in changing breathing patterns with symptoms is helping the patient to deal with the rapid, fairly automatic assumptions being made about the meaning of the symptoms. Rapid heartbeat, for instance, could represent to the patient an impending heart attack. With that interpretation it is no wonder that a panic attack ensues. Mild dyspnoea resulting perhaps from a tense diaphragm could be interpreted as impending suffocation, light-headedness as about to lose consciousness, tingling fingers as an approaching stroke, and so on. Helping the patient to reinterpret these 'symptoms' as mere sensations from the hyperventilation, coupled with a cognitive proneness to catastrophizing, provides a new angle on things.

The concept of automatic thoughts has been developed by the school of cognitive therapy (Beck 2011) and holds that such thoughts emerge from underlying assumptions about what things mean. The deepest level of belief might be 'I am at particular risk from heart attack because there is heart disease in my family.' Given that assumption, the individual will be predisposed to react to benign chest sensations, heart palpitations, or tachycardia as a confirmation of these deeply held beliefs. The automaticity of this process means that the matter is not necessarily referred

---

Box 7.4.1 **Breathing instruction tips using biofeedback devices**

1. Practise some simple task such as typing or playing a video game while breathing is being monitored with a capnometer, HRV or EMG (scalenes or upper trapezius). Set a reasonable threshold for keeping the breathing steady, abdominal, slow, etc. using an audio alarm to notify that the threshold has been exceeded. This method splits the attention between the task and maintaining the intended breathing control; it facilitates habit formation.

2. To prolong exhalation as a way to slow breathing rate: use a strain gauge, thermistor at the nostril or capnometer to display exhalation. This trains slow release of breathing muscles, building conscious control.

3. Practise desensitization to a memory or scenario associated with emotional tension, using breathing as a gauge (HRV, EMG in the neck/shoulder area, or $ETCO_2$). The goal is to maintain relaxed breathing while dwelling on something disturbing. This tends to hasten desensitization to the topic and develop 'psychophysiological indifference'.

4. Improve discrimination and inner awareness of breathing quality by 'weaning' from feedback and requesting the 'best guess' about whatever is being monitored: breathing rate, muscle, $ETCO_2$ or HRV. Closing the eyes and either producing a requested level or guessing at the reading builds interoception and is usually an engaging challenge.

Box 7.4.2 **Breathing instruction tips without biofeedback**

1. Have the patient place small adhesive labels in the home, automobile, or work environment as reminders to check breathing. Printed 'BREATHE' labels can be placed strategically where the person wants to be reminded to maintain relaxed breathing.

2. Use computer software or smartphone apps dedicated to pacing breathing: these display a rhythmic change in something which guides the breathing practice at a rate that can be adjusted as desired. (For example, the E-Z Air Plus programme available from http://www.bfe.org/breathpacer.htm (Accessed June 2013)).

3. Enlist someone close to the patient to observe breathing as the patient goes about daily activities; observe style of breathing, rate, regularity, pauses, nose vs mouth, and give feedback to the patient.

4. Practise breathing control while recalling a distressing experience or imagining a stressful scene. Do brief intervals separated by relaxation rests. This strengthens control over both the breathing and the emotional response.

5. If frequent sighing is a problem, encourage gradual change in the habit not by trying to prevent the sigh, but making it shallower (reduce sigh volume). This is similar to allowing a 'forbidden' food but having only a small portion.

---

to the conscious mind for decision; it has already been decided. The conscious mind becomes occupied instead with the next step, such as deciding where the closest hospital is. This anxiety will feed back into the physiological system which is producing the symptom, sustaining the state or provoking it to even greater levels of alarm.

It can be revealing to question the patient about the assumed meaning of symptoms related to hyperventilation. Teaching control of breathing without explanation may seem to be sufficient, but even if the chest or neurological symptoms abate, the patient may covertly decide that a heart attack has simply been postponed. Intervening at a higher level – challenging the assumption that the sensations signal approaching disaster – can interrupt a disruptive and very persistent vicious cycle. Salkovskis et al (1996) represents this clinical approach, implying that breathing retraining can often be bypassed when the implicit meaning of the hyperventilation symptoms is uncovered, challenged and changed.

Cognitive therapy works with thinking errors, but tends to stay at the conscious level of mental life. Emotional interference with breathing can be quite complex; the state of confusion and disorientation resulting from hyperventilation can be punishing, but for some people it may be rewarding if it helps to temporarily escape decision or responsibility. The act of hyperventilating can create temporary depression, agoraphobia and fear of death; the symptoms may lead to misdiagnosis of schizophrenia, hysteria, conduct disorders and hypochondria. It can aggravate pre-existing psychiatric disorders. Fensterheim (1994) reviewed these matters, and stresses the prevalence of fear of death in people who hyperventilate. This can include a general feeling of doom or imminent death, the fear of death or loss of a significant person, and fear of fatal medical illness.

Panic disorder

Panic attacks are not strictly a breathing pattern problem, but there is often a strong relationship in that low resting CO_2 due to overbreathing is common in panic disorder (Meuret et al 2008). Whether the breathing aberration is a cause, an effect or a corollary of panic has been debated for years. Not all those with panic disorder suffer from hyperventilation; some have no detectable disruption in breathing and no complaints about it.

Many practitioners teach breathing control as a therapy for panic attacks, countering hyperventilation. The most recent method developed involves home practice with portable capnometers and recorded instructions for paced breathing. The capnometers record and store the end-tidal CO_2 records produced during practice, and these are evaluated and discussed during periodic meetings with the therapist-trainers (Meuret et al 2008, 2010). In this research, cognitive therapy for panic prevention was contrasted with breathing instruction; the two approaches to panic treatment were applied to separate but equivalent patient groups. The results showed equivalency of the two therapies; training to maintain pCO_2 in the normal range worked as well as the cognitive-behavioural approach. Both approaches showed long-term reductions in agoraphobic behaviour, perceived control and panic symptom severity (but see also Kim et al 2012).

Cardiac rehabilitation

One of the largest studies of cardiac rehabilitation including breathing-based relaxation was done in The Netherlands by Jan van Dixhoorn (van Dixhoorn et al 1989, van Dixhoorn & Duivenvoorden 1999). Survivors of recent heart attacks underwent six hours of individual instruction in a simple relaxation technique which centred on breathing, in addition to regular aerobic exercises and 'care as usual' – which a control group received without the breathing instruction.

Follow-up data were collected for 5 years afterwards; incidence of subsequent heart trouble was lower in the relaxation-plus-exercise compared with the exercise-only group. The breathing-based relaxation procedure provided a clear advantage. At follow-up, breathing and heart rate were reduced and respiratory sinus arrhythmia was stronger in the relaxation group, indicating lowered sympathetic tone. ST-segment depression diminished (meaning less evidence of myocardial ischemia) and in the following years serious cardiac incidents occurred in 37% of the exercise group, compared to 17% in the relaxation group, with fewer hospitalizations for cardiac problems. In addition, the cost of the breathing intervention was more than offset by reduced medical costs. All this resulted from 6 hours of instruction.

The way the study's author Jan van Dixhoorn (see Chapter 7.1a) taught relaxation via breathing was subtle, personal and to some extent individualized, introducing each person to their own breathing in a way designed to create detached awareness and insight. Improved body awareness rather than performance of a particular physical routine was considered central to the entire intervention, and the desired respiratory change was coupled to passive awareness and self-observation. Breathing-based relaxation was integrated into daily routines by practising in a variety of positions and situations.

Recommended rest breaks were defined as exercises in self-awareness rather than 'relaxation', which his population of cardiac patients would have considered being lazy or 'falling behind'. The goal was to train the patients to restore homeostatic balance, and the intervention simply requested a 'before and after' comparison. To do this required entering an objective state that disrupted ongoing emotional states which contribute to stress.

REFERENCES

Baykushev, S., 1969. Hyperventilation as an accelerated hypnotic induction technique. International Journal of Clinical and Experimental Hypnosis 17 (1), 20–24.

Beck, J., 2011. Cognitive behavior therapy: the basics and beyond, second ed. Guilford Press, New York.

Bradley, D., 2012. Self-help for hyperventilation syndrome: recognizing and correcting your breathing pattern disorder. Kyle Books, Canada.

Chaitow, L., Bradley, D., Gilbert, C., 2002. Multidisciplinary approaches to breathing pattern disorders. Churchill Livingstone, London (Ch. 5 & 8).

van Dixhoorn, J., Duivenvoorden, H.J., Staal, H.A., et al., 1989. Physical training and relaxation therapy in cardiac rehabilitation assessed through a composite criterion for training outcome. American Heart Journal 118 (3), 545–552.

van Dixhoorn, J., Duivenvoorden, H.J., 1999. Effect of relaxation therapy on cardiac events after myocardial infarction: a 5-year follow-up study. Journal of Cardiopulmonary Rehabilitation 19 (3), 178–185.

Dudley, D.L., 1969. Psychophysiology of respiration in health and disease. Appleton-Century-Crofts, New York.

Fensterheim, H., 1994. Hyperventilation and psychopathology: a clinical perspective. In: Timmons, B.H., Ley, R. (Eds.), Behavioral and psychological approaches to breathing disorders. Plenum, New York.

Kim, S.,Wolburg, E., Roth, W.T., 2012. Opposing breathing therapies for panic disorder: a randomized controlled trial of lowering vs raising end-tidal pCO_2. Journal of Clinical Psychiatry 73 (7), 931–939.

Meuret, A.E., Wilhelm, F.H., Ritz, T., et al., 2008. Feedback of end-tidal pCO_2 as a therapeutic approach for panic disorder. Journal of Psychiatric Research 42 (7), 560–568.

Meuret, A.E., Rosenfield, D., Seidel, A., et al., 2010. Respiratory and cognitive mediators of treatment change in panic disorder: evidence for intervention specificity. Journal of Consulting & Clinical Psychology 78 (5), 691–704.

Preter, M., Klein, D.F., 2008. Panic, suffocation false alarms, separation anxiety and endogenous opioids. Progress in Neuropsychopharmacology & Biological Psychiatry 1, 32 (3), 603–612.

Salkovskis, P.M., Clark, D.M., Gelder, M.G., 1996. Cognitive-behavior links in the persistence of panic. Behaviour Research and Therapy 34 (5/6), 453–458.

Chapter | **7.5** |

Speech and singing

Eva Au Zveglic

Dysphonia is a term that describes disorders of the voice. Previously, literature has speculated as to whether breathing disorders are the cause of a type of dysphonia, known as vocal cord dysfunction (VCD) (Greene 1984). VCD (Box 7.5.1) is the 'paradoxical adduction of the vocal cords during inspiration' (Noyes & Kemp 2007). Anxiety has been observed as a characteristic in both VCD and breathing pattern disorders (BPD). However, the absolute cause of VCD is not yet known, although similarly to BPD, treatment commonly incorporates relaxation techniques, breathing retraining and cognitive behavioural therapy.

When individuals with BPD are learning to improve their breathing control at rest, it is appropriate to coordinate this process with attention to any associated dysfunctional activities of daily living, such as phonation. Phonation is the production of sound from oscillation of the vocal folds (or 'vocal cords') and resonance of the vocal tract, both of which are essential for normal speech and singing function. Good posture and breathing control are included as part of technique training by both acting and singing teachers, as these features profoundly influence voice production, and since some types of dysphonia may be evident in this population (Noyes & Kemp 2007; Greene 1984).

The signs and symptoms of dysphonia include:

- Breathlessness during speaking or singing
- Loss of voice
- Throat discomfort
- Pain
- Hoarse voice

Box 7.5.1 **Vocal cord dysfunction**

In VCD the cords do not abduct appropriately during inspiration. This causes an obstruction to ventilation. Therefore this condition has been wrongly diagnosed as asthma in some patients (Noyes & Kemp 2007). Like breathing disorders, the cause of VCD is unknown and occurs in absence of organic disease. In the case of VCD, the intervention of a speech pathologist and/or psychologist may be helpful.

- Lump sensation in the throat
- Wheeziness
- Stridor.

Dysphonia in breathing disorders may be due to different causes and present with different signs and symptoms. In more complex cases of dysphonia, the intervention of an otolaryngologist, psychologist and/or speech pathologist is essential. Therefore a multidisciplinary approach is recommended to effectively treat these conditions (Van Houtte et al 2011). This chapter explores the possible causes of dysphonia in relation to breathing dysfunction. Basic assessment and treatments during singing and speech are also explored.

complain of an inability to speak properly. Some report that they mainly feel these symptoms during public speaking or only when singing, while others complain that it occurs all the time. Phonation tasks require good coordination of breathing with numerous muscles. In classical singing techniques, such as Appoggio (Box 7.5.2), it is believed that breathing exercises are key to effective vocal control (Miller 1996, p.23). Exercise 1 is a good example of an appoggio breathing exercise that can also be used as a more advanced exercise for breathing dysfunction. Therapists have an important role in teaching breathing control if they have a comprehensive understanding of the biomechanics and anatomy of breathing.

HOW BREATHING DISORDERS AFFECT THE VOICE

Poor breathing coordination and phonation

One of the most common signs of breathing dysfunction is breathlessness while speaking. Loud gasps of inhalation may be audible between phrases. The individual may also

Box 7.5.2   The Appoggio Technique

The Appoggio Technique is a classical Italian opera singing technique focusing on the use of good breathing control, effective muscle use and posture. The position of the sternum is used as a prompt to prevent over-activity of the upper chest and effective lung expansion on inspiration. This technique also encourages quiet inspiration during phonation.

Exercise 1 – A breathing control exercise for singers (adapted from Miller 1996)

Please note that this is an advanced exercise for singers and those who have mastered a desired breathing pattern. Do not try this if normal breathing control is difficult.

- Ensure diaphragmatic breathing by putting one hand on your upper chest and the other on your upper abdomen.
- Count mentally through each phase of inhalation, holding and exhalation.
- Inhale for 5 counts, hold your breath for 5 counts, exhale for 5 counts. Then inhale for 6 counts, hold your breath for 6 counts and exhale for 6 counts. Now inhale for 7, etc. (follow the cycles below until you reach 10 counts for each phase).
- Count at your own comfortable pace. As you improve in your control of breaths, slow down your counting pace as much as you can.

- Inhale and exhale quietly through the nose or slightly parted lips.
- Keep the jaw, neck, shoulders and chest relaxed throughout the exercise.
- The use of a metronome can be useful to maintain a moderate pace.
- Maintain a continuous pace between the three phases.
- Stop the exercise if you feel symptoms of dizziness, anxiety or shortness of breath and resume slow relaxed breaths.
- If you are unable to complete the entire exercise at first, break it up into components and progress as tolerated.
- Recite each counting cycle once and progress down the cycles in a continuous rhythm.

Inhale		Hold breath		Exhale
1 2 3 4 5	→	1 2 3 4 5	→	1 2 3 4 5
1 2 3 4 5 6	→	1 2 3 4 5 6	→	1 2 3 4 5 6
1 2 3 4 5 6 7	→	1 2 3 4 5 6 7	→	1 2 3 4 5 6 7
1 2 3 4 5 6 7 8	→	1 2 3 4 5 6 7 8	→	1 2 3 4 5 6 7 8
1 2 3 4 5 6 7 8 9	→	1 2 3 4 5 6 7 8 9	→	1 2 3 4 5 6 7 8 9
1 2 3 4 5 6 7 8 9 10	→	1 2 3 4 5 6 7 8 9 10	→	1 2 3 4 5 6 7 8 9 10

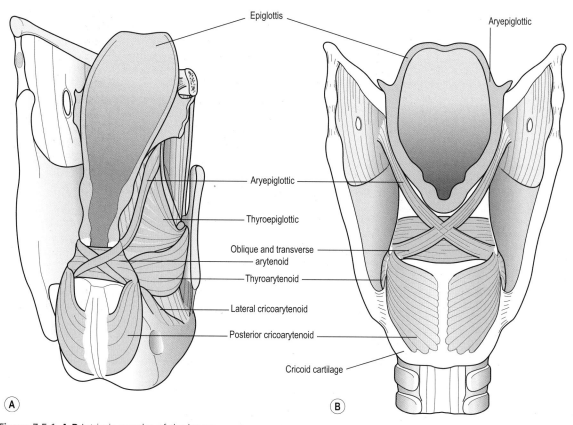

Epiglottis

Aryepiglottic

Aryepiglottic

Thyroepiglottic

Oblique and transverse arytenoid

Thyroarytenoid

Lateral cricoarytenoid

Posterior cricoarytenoid

Cricoid cartilage

(A)

(B)

Figure 7.5.1 A,B Intrinsic muscles of the larynx.

The larynx

The extrinsic muscles of the larynx influence its position while intrinsic muscles abduct (open) and adduct (close) the vocal folds for the production of voice and respiration (Fig. 7.5.1A&B). Intrinsic muscles also influence the tension of the vocal folds.

Autonomic disturbances in breathing disorders may also affect laryngeal function due to its innervation from branches of the vagus nerve. As discussed in chapter of this book (Chaitow et al 2002), the vagus nerve is part of the parasympathetic outflow of the autonomic nervous system. Branches from this nerve control the intrinsic muscles of the larynx that adduct, abduct and lengthen the vocal folds. There is evidence that vagus nerve stimulation causes voice changes (Handforth et al 1998) and vocal cord dysfunction (Zumsteg et al 2000).

Normally, the *lateral cricoarytenoid* and *interarytenoid muscles* adduct the folds during vocalization (Fig. 7.5.2). During expiration, they also partially adduct to allow some air to still remain in the lungs to prevent alveoli closure.

Conversely, the vocal folds are abducted during inspiration by the *posterior cricoarytenoid* muscle to allow air to enter the lungs (Figs 7.5.3 & 7.5.1B).

Posture and hypertonicity

Poor posture and muscle hypertonicity in breathing dysfunction (Ch. 4, Chaitow et al 2002) affects the position of the larynx. Laryngeal position is influenced by the pull of surrounding muscles (Shipp 1987). As the larynx is attached to the hyoid bone, the suprahyoid muscles that elevate the hyoid bone will also elevate the larynx (Fig. 7.5.4). Hence, if the suprahyoid muscles are continuously hypertonic, the larynx will be elevated at rest (Van Houtte et al 2011). Therefore this position has been associated with dysphonia (Mathieson et al 2009).

Usually the larynx is automatically elevated during swallowing. Elevation of the larynx is also a way of stiffening the vocal cords to reach higher pitches in singing but this is not the best way to alter pitch. A lower vertical position of the larynx is more desirable and pitch change should be achieved by using the intrinsic cricothyroid muscle

205

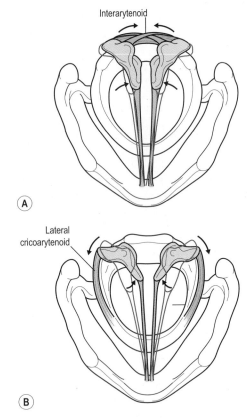

Figure 7.5.2 **A,B** Vocal cord adduction.

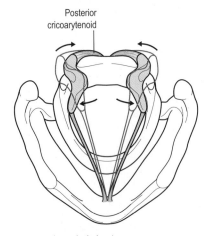

Figure 7.5.3 Vocal cord abduction.

(Fig. 7.5.1A) to tilt the thyroid over the cricoid (Iwarsson & Sundberg 1998).

To reach higher pitches the thyroid tilts more forward over the cricoid to lengthen the vocal folds (Fig. 7.5.5). This tilt is restricted if the tissues surrounding the larynx are tight, or if the neck position is altered. For example, compare how your laryngeal prominence (Adam's apple) moves when you sing in a neutral neck position, compared with when your neck is in full extension. You should feel that it is more difficult for your laryngeal prominence to move downwards when your neck is extended.

The diaphragm

Reduced diaphragm effectiveness in breathing disorders results in a reduction of inspiratory volume. The greater the volume, the greater the recoil of the lungs for generating pressure below the glottis (subglottal pressure) during voice production (Leanderson & Sundberg 1988). When lung recoil is reduced, the abdominal muscles will activate to help generate subglottal pressure. Functional residual capacity (FRC) is the volume of air that remains in the lungs at the end of passive expiration due to this recoil. Therefore when phonation starts at a lung volume below FRC, more abdominal muscle activity is necessary. This pressure causes a steady flow of air that rapidly opens and closes the vocal folds to produce sound waves. Larger lung volumes correspond to greater pressures needed for louder sounds or higher pitches. Hence in breathing dysfunction, when inspiratory volumes are low and abdominal muscles are weak, less pressure occurs to oscillate the folds. Consequently the individual will strain the voice with compensatory muscles.

Diaphragmatic contraction on inspiration also improves the vertical position of the larynx (Iwarsson & Sundberg 1998). When the diaphragm contracts caudally, a downward tracheobronchial pull occurs causing the attached larynx to assume a more vertical position (Shipp 1987). This is important for good vocal resonance due to the length of the vocal tract which shortens when the larynx is elevated. In breathing dysfunction, upper chest breathing occurs rather than diaphragmatic, reducing vertical laryngeal positioning.

The abdominal and pelvic floor muscles

Finally, (as mentioned in Chapter 4 of Chaitow et al, 2002), weakness of the deep internal abdominal muscles (DAM) and pelvic floor muscles (PFM) may be evident. DAM refers to the transversus abdominis (TA) and internal oblique muscles. The co-activation of both muscles is necessary when greater subglottal pressures are needed during production of higher pitches or greater sound amplitude. These muscles also activate when the individual phonates below FRC (Leanderson & Sundberg 1988).

Co-activation of the PFM and DAM achieves greater subglottic pressures by pushing the diaphragm upwards (Talasz et al 2010). Figure 7.5.6C demonstrates how this works. The pelvic floor contracts eccentrically during inspiration and concentrically with greater force during expiration (Hodges et al 2007). When the DAM and PFM are weak, the external anterolateral (i.e external obliques and rectus abdominis) muscles compensate and less pressure occurs cephalically (Fig. 7.5.6B). Therefore to produce greater pressure and airflow towards the vocal folds, the individual strains the muscles around the neck, potentially leading to a 'lump' or 'soreness' in the throat during loud speech or singing.

TAKING A HISTORY

Phonation problems are bound to vary between patients. Therefore taking a detailed history is necessary to identify the specific causes and maintaining factors of the problem. It is helpful to differentiate between symptoms that appear to be directly related to breathing dysfunction and those that relate to pre-existing conditions/pathologies. For example, a singer with vocal fold nodules will have throat pain, hoarseness and limited vocal range in the absence of a breathing disorder.

In some patients, vocal problems occur during speech but not during singing. Therefore the patient should be asked to carefully describe details related to the onset, and provocation, of their symptoms. Some singers may only experience difficulties during challenging phrases in their singing. Examples of specific questions include:

- What precisely is experienced when vocal problems occur?
- Is there a feeling of a lump in the throat?
- Is there voice loss or a change in the voice?
- Is there breathlessness during phonation?
- When do symptoms occur?

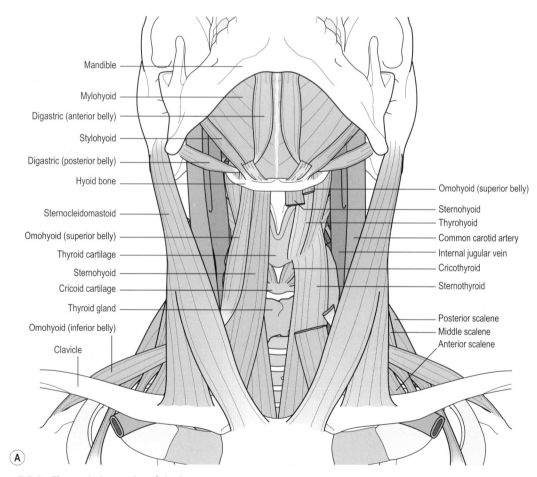

Figure 7.5.4 The extrinsic muscles of the larynx.

Continued

- Do symptoms only occur during singing or during loud speech?
- Has the voice changed since breathing problems occurred?
- Does the voice change only in certain circumstances?
- Were there vocal problems prior to the breathing disorder?

The individual's past medical history may offer clues as to what might be contributing to vocal dysfunction. For example, previous childbirth, incontinence, back injuries and abdominal surgery can weaken abdominal and pelvic floor muscles. Previous surgery around the larynx can also contribute to vocal strain problems due to post-surgical inflammation of the laryngeal area, and/or adhesions.

Psychological conditions such as depression can contribute to both breathing dysfunction and some types of dysphonia (Van Houtte et al 2011). In this circumstance, the intervention of a psychologist may be necessary. Knowledge of pre-existing conditions will indicate what treatment limitations there might be, and what disciplines to refer to.

Taking a social history includes specific questions about occupation and recreational activities that might impact on assessment and treatment. It may also indicate whether what is prescribed is likely to fit comfortably into the individual's lifestyle. Enquiry should be made as to whether speaking, acting or singing activities are work related, or are more socially oriented.

Asking about the individual's occupation may offer clues regarding emotional and psychological stress that might be contributing to breathing and vocal disorders. Additional enquiry regarding stress-management strategies may be informative.

ASSESSMENT

Observation

While taking a history, the clinician should discreetly observe the degree of coordination between breathing and speech. This candid assessment is important as the patient might alter their breathing pattern if they are conscious of being observed.

Things to observe include:

- The quality of the voice
- The ability to finish phrases and sentences
- The speed of the speech
- The audibility of the inspiration
- The use of the respiratory muscles during breaths
- The amount of upper chest or abdominal movement during respiration
- Mouth or nose breathing.

Commonly in breathing dysfunction, the individual may speak very rapidly. Breathing can also change during

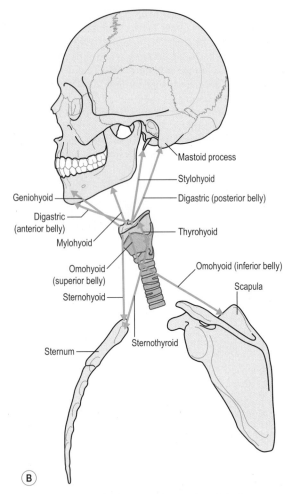

Figure 7.5.4, cont'd. The extrinsic muscles of the larynx.

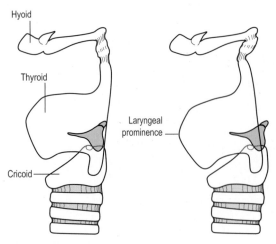

Figure 7.5.5 Cricothyroid muscle action.

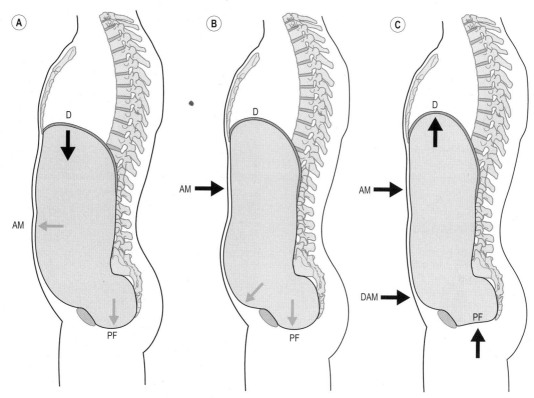

Figure 7.5.6 A–C Pelvic floor and abdominal muscles during inspiration and expiration. Arrows = direction of muscle contraction during: inspiration (**A**); expiration with weak PF and DAM (**B**); and expiration with co-activation of PF and DAM (**C**). D, diaphragm; AM, anterolateral muscles; PF, pelvic floor muscles; DAM, deep anterolateral muscles. *From Talasz et al 2010, International Urogynecology Journal.*

different phonation activities. Some singers may breathe well with the diaphragm during singing but not during normal speech. This may be due to a higher awareness of their breathing during singing but not during other activities. Therefore they may only experience symptoms during speech. In novice singers, symptoms may occur only in singing as this activity produces a greater demand on the vocal system. Hence it is important to observe the use of respiratory muscles and posture during different phonation tasks. In some patients, vocal disturbances may only occur during components of an activity. For example, a singer may only experience a 'lump in the throat' during singing at very high pitches. Observation of breathing, posture and how the patient vocalizes during these occasions is important. The clinician may see that the patient increases muscle tone of the head, neck, shoulders and chest during these times, due to anticipation anxiety. Increased tone of the suprahyoid muscles elevates the larynx instead of allowing the larynx to be in a vertical position for efficient phonation. The neck posture could also change, as there is a tendency for individuals to increase retraction and extension of the neck to reach higher pitches. Such compensatory strategies must be pointed out to the patient in order for them to correct these habits in their practise.

Muscle tone of the neck, shoulders and chest can be assessed with palpation and observation (see Chs 2.2 and 6.2). In breathing pattern disorders, increased muscle activity of the sternocleidomastoids, upper trapezius and the pectoralis muscles are visible during inspiration. Pettersen & Westgaard (2004) found that upper trapezius activity reduced thoracic expansion in inspiration.

Palpation

In order to palpate whether there is early and/or overuse of the external anterolateral abdominal muscles, the hands are placed around the midlateral abdominal area. During normal speech, minimal activity should be palpated in these areas. The recoil of the lungs and some PFM co-activated with DAM is sufficient to produce speech (Leanderson & Sundberg 1988, Hodges et al 2007).

Over-or early activity can indicate that these muscles may be weak or dysfunctional.

The patient should be asked to self-palpate the chest and abdominal areas to obtain self-awareness of their breathing during phonation. During such self-assessment, the patient places one hand over the upper sternum and one hand over the upper abdominal area (see Fig. 6.2.1) in order to ascertain whether they predominantly use the upper chest for quick inhalations between phrases, during singing or speech. Loud audible gasps of air indicate overuse of the accessory muscles and some narrowing of the vocal tract during inspiration. Overuse of chest, shoulders and neck muscles prevents good diaphragmatic excursion and reduces thoracic expansion.

Dynamic ultrasound equipment

Musculoskeletal physiotherapists have used dynamic ultrasound to assess and train TA activation in the treatment of lower back pain. Dynamic ultrasound has good inter- and intra-rater reliability for TA measurements (Koppenhaver et al 2009). This method can be used to observe abdominal muscle activity during phonation. The ultrasound head is placed just above the iliac crest of one hip, directly below the axilla. Thickening of the TA would indicate good TA activity (Fig. 7.5.7). No thickening occurs during quiet breathing and during normal speech as TA activity is minimal. However, this activation is far greater when there is an increase in loudness or during high pitches of the voice. When there is absent TA activity, the internal and external oblique muscles compensate to provide the pressure necessary to push the diaphragm upwards during forced expiration.

It is also important to assess spinal posture. A neutral spine results in better TA activity necessary for phonation (Pinto et al 2011). In the appoggio technique, the singer is asked to attain a higher sternal position to prevent too much flexion of the spine. Too much flexion reduces lung volumes. However, this prompt could also result in overcompensation by hyperextension of the spine. This results in a deviation from the desired neutral spine posture. The patient should be assessed and given exercises in different positions because spinal posture could vary in lying, sitting and standing.

TREATMENT

Breath control in phonation

Chapter 7.3 discusses breathing retraining. This is an important component of training before the therapist attempts to work on the coordination of breathing during phonation. Teaching good breathing technique during speaking may be too difficult to undertake during the first

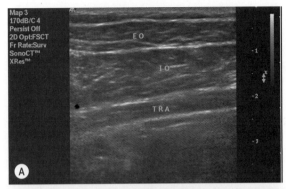

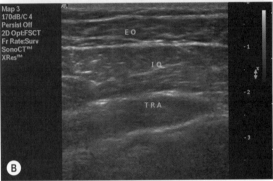

Figure 7.5.7 Dynamic ultrasound images of the abdominal muscles, (**A**) before a TA contraction; (**B**) during a TA contraction. EO, external obliques; IO, internal obliques; TRA, transversus abdominis. *Courtesy of Mr John Leddy - www .dynamicultrasound.org*

session as education and breathing exercises may be overwhelming. Some professional singers, actors and public speakers may already know how to use their diaphragm well, but still have incoordination of breathing due to the hypertonicity of their upper chest and neck muscles (Pettersen & Westgaard 2004). Other professionals may not have vocal symptoms during singing as they have better awareness of their breathing during this task but have symptoms when they are speaking. Treatment may include re-education and awareness of these overactive muscles.

Sometimes breathlessness during speech resolves as the patient improves their breathing control and specific vocal treatments may not be necessary. However, if speaking and singing does not improve, referral to a multidisciplinary team is indicated.

Motor learning theory in breathing and vocal dysfunction treatment

Motor learning involves learning a skilled task and then practising with a goal in mind until the skill is executed automatically (Schmidt & Wrisberg 2007). For example, learning to play a song on the piano initially takes a lot of thought and practise before the task is automatic and executed skilfully. This process involves both sensory feedback and motor systems and is integral in motor task learning.

Phonation is an example of a complex motor task that involves the coordination and timing of many muscles. Usually this task requires little thought in normal speech. However, in breathing disorder patients, poor habits are acquired in their motor activity of breathing and speech. Even without breathing disorders, the task of singing effectively requires good motor control and practise. Therefore motor learning can be used in the retraining of breathing coordination with speech or singing. Postural re-education, correcting respiratory muscle use, and reducing unnecessary accessory muscle activity, can be used to refine motor control in phonation.

Pettersen & Westgaard (2004) used biofeedback equipment to reduce unnecessary trapezius activity during singing. Biofeedback allowed singers to improve their motor control of these muscles through a visual medium. Therefore biofeedback, mirror reflection and palpation are all good ways of achieving sensory feedback during practise of phonation and breathing.

Many breathing pattern disorder patients may speak rapidly and have poor timing of breaths in speech. They either gasp a breath mid-sentence or speak too long before quickly sucking a breath with their upper chest. It can be useful to ask the patient to listen, look and feel their upper chest and diaphragmatic excursion during phonation to encourage awareness of the way they coordinate their breaths.

For both singing and speech, it is important that inspiration is quiet. Even traditional singing methods encourage quiet inspiration during singing (Miller 1996). It is important that the patient focuses on quiet breathing during singing or speaking as part of their motor learning.

To reduce sympathetic tone, relaxation is important to slow down the speed of speech and breathing. Before retraining vocal tasks, slow relaxed breathing is encouraged for a few minutes. If the patient finds it difficult to improve abdominal breathing in the upright position, it may be helpful to start with practise while lying down.

Simple phonation tasks such as reciting numbers or the alphabet are good to use, as they do not require a lot of complex thought. This allows the patient to concentrate on how they breathe between phrases, their posture and muscle tension. It is advisable to ask the patient to recite in their mother tongue if their first language is not English. Exercise 6 is an example of an exercise that can be used to improve motor control of breathing and phonation.

Musculoskeletal manual therapy and voice retraining

In some patients tightness of the neck and thoracic area of the body reduces the ability to use muscles effectively for breathing and phonation. For example, tightness of the external obliques reduces the 'bucket handle' rib movement in inspiration, of the 5th to 12th ribs. Passive and active stretching of the external obliques may reduce excessive tightness, potentially enhancing thoracic expansion. See the chapters in Section 7 for manual approaches to enhance respiratory, and therefore vocal function.

In one study, Mathieson et al (2009) demonstrated that massage of the suprahyoid and sternocleidomastoid muscles reduced muscle tension in patients with dysphonia. This reduction in tension improved acoustic quality and reduced vocal tension discomfort in this patient group. Referral to a clinician familiar with manual techniques will be required if there are tight connective tissues and muscles that alter the patient's posture and function.

Expiratory muscle training

Dynamic ultrasound imaging is used to train TA activation in lower back pain (Ferreira et al 2007). However, this can also train TA activation during singing and loud speech. Poor proprioceptive feedback of these muscles may be associated with their dysfunction and therefore ultrasound provides good visual feedback for TA activation (Radebold et al 2001).

If the patient lacks activation of the TA needed for loud speech and singing, it is important to aim to increase awareness of this muscle first. Thickening of the TA occurs on the ultrasound screen as the muscle contracts correctly. The ultrasound will also show over-activation of other muscles, such as the external obliques.

If the clinician does not have access to dynamic ultrasound equipment, prompts and palpation can also be used to train abdominal activity. See Exercises 2 and 3 below.

CONCLUSION

Dysphonia associated with BPD may be due to various reasons. These include:

- Poor coordination of breathing
- Diaphragmatic dysfunction
- Cognitive factors
- Autonomic disturbance
- Weak/poor activation of abdominal and pelvic floor muscles.

Similarly to BPD, dysphonia presents differently in different individuals. Therefore research into the causes of dysphonia may be difficult and this may be why evidence on this condition within the BPD population is also lacking.

Exercise 2 – Learning to contract TA

- Commence in supine with a pillow supporting behind the knees to maintain a neutral spine.
- Instruct the patient to isolate a TA contraction by contracting the lower abdominal muscles below an imaginary belt line. This imaginary line is below the umbilicus.
- Ask the patient to use three fingers to palpate approximately 3 centimetres below the umbilicus. He/she should feel a slight deep isolated contraction if the TA is activated.
- Contract for 1 second and relax.
- Now ask the patient to do this contraction with the PFM contraction at the same time.
- Hold this co-contraction for 1 second and repeat for 10 repetitions.
- If the individual cannot contract up to 10 repetitions, encourage relaxation of these muscles for 45–60 seconds. Then repeat the number of repetitions the individual can achieve. Do three sets and practise at least once a day.
- If a 5 second co-contraction is achieved easily, ask them to use this contraction while doing Exercise 4.
- Introduce Exercises 5–7 in later sessions as the individual progresses.
- Also progress to doing these exercises in sitting and standing once the individual can achieve phonation with the co-contraction easily in supine. However in these upright positions, ensure that the individual maintains the neutral spine.

Exercise 3 – Four-point kneeling

Alternatively, four-point kneeling may be a better position for contractions if the individual finds it difficult to feel the TA in supine. In this position, awareness of these muscles may increase due to the effects of gravity on the abdominal area (Richardson & Jull 1995).

If TA contraction is too difficult for the individual, ask him/her to contract the anus and vagina. For men, instruct them to contract the pelvic floor as if the muscles were lifting the testicles upwards. Hodges et al (2007) found that the TA and PFM co-activate together during expiration. Novice singers tend to contract these muscles less in singing compared with professional singers (Talasz et al 2010). Correct any over-activity of compensatory muscles, such as the external obliques, by palpating these superficially. Good use of TA and PFM are necessary to avoid vocal strain.

Once the patient can isolate contraction of these muscles, commence training these muscles during phonation. Exercises 4–7 can be used while the patient concentrates on appropriate abdominal contractions.

Exercise 4 – Expiration against resistance

- Gently inspire a normal breath through the nose. Inspiration must be quiet.
- Keep the mouth and jaw relaxed as you expire a long 'ss' sound as long as you can.
- Contract the pelvic floor and lower transversus abdominis muscles to help you exhale as long as possible.
- The 'ss' should be smooth and not vary in loudness.
- Rest before repeating the above again.
- Also practise from a large inspiratory volume.
- Rest for 45 seconds to 1 minute between 'ss' exhalations. If the individual feels dizzy, light-headed or breathless, rest for a few minutes longer until the symptoms disappear.
- Do 3 sets of 3 repetitions. Aim to do 3–4 sessions a day. Alter the number of repetitions or sets according to how fatigued or breathless the individual feels.

Exercise 5 – Bubble blowing

- Put a long thick straw into a bottle of water. Don't fill the bottle too much as water will spill over the top.
- Start after normal resting expiration (FRC).
- Blow out through the straw and expire as long as you can to make bubbles.
- Focus on using the pelvic floor and lower transversus abdominis muscles during blowing.
- Rest for 45 seconds to 1 minute between blows. If the individual feels dizzy, light-headed or breathless, rest for a few minutes longer until the symptoms disappear.
- Do 3 repetitions for 3 sets. Aim to do 3–4 sessions a day. Alter the number of repetitions or sets according to how the individual feels.

Exercise 6 – Alphabet practise

- Recite the alphabet loudly but very slowly.
- Start after normal resting expiration (FRC).
- Contract the pelvic floor as you vocalize. This should be a sustained contraction until the next inspiration.
- The inspiratory volume is equivalent to a tidal volume.
- Inspiration is slow, quiet, controlled and through the nose.
- During speech, the tongue, neck and facial muscles are relaxed.
- Recite 'A B C D [inspire] E F G H [inspire] I J K L [inspire].'
- As the patient improves, add extra letters before the next inspiration.
- E.g. 'A B C D E F [inspire] G H I J K L [inspire].'
- As breathing coordination improves, the patient can then hold their breath in place of some of the inspiratory breaths, e.g. A B C D (pause) E F G H (inspire) I J K L M (pause) N O P Q (inspire).

Exercise 7 – Singing

- Commence after normal resting expiration (FRC).
- Inspire a small breath gently through the nose.
- Ask the patient to sing 'Hmm' during a musical phrase.
- During phonation, highlight the use of the pelvic floor and lower internal abdominal muscles.
- The patient must be reminded to keep the tongue, throat, glottis, neck and chest muscles relaxed. The mouth is also closed gently.

A holistic assessment and treatment of individuals with dysphonia seems most appropriate. So far some literature recommends a multidisciplinary approach to the treatment of this condition. Therefore greater awareness of dysphonia may be necessary within other disciplines, such as physiotherapy, that do not traditionally treat this condition.

There is still a paucity of studies on the effectiveness of treatment techniques for dysphonia. There is already evidence for motor learning and abdominal muscle training in other conditions but not yet in dysphonia. With updated and more affordable imaging equipment, such as dynamic ultrasound, our knowledge of how muscles and tissues work in contribution to phonation may improve in the future.

REFERENCES

Chaitow, L., Bradley, D., Gilbert, G., 2002. Multidisciplinary approaches to breathing pattern disorders. Churchill Livingstone, Edinburgh.

Ferreira, M.L., Ferreira, P.H., Latimer, J., et al., 2007. Comparison of general exercise, motor control and manipulative therapy for chronic low back pain: a randomized trial. Pain 131, 31–37.

Greene, M.C., 1984. Functional dysphonia and the hyperventilation syndrome. Br. J. Disord. Commun 19 (3), 263–272.

Handforth, A., DeGiorgio, C.M., Schachter, S.C., et al., 1998. Vagus nerve stimulation therapy for partial onset seizures: a randomized active-control trial, Neurology 51 (1), 48–55.

Hodges, P.W., Sapsford, R., Pengel, L.H., 2007. Postural and respiratory functions of the pelvic floor muscles, Neurourol. Urodyn. 26 (3), 362–371.

Iwarsson, J., Sundberg, J., 1998. Effects of lung volume on vertical larynx position during phonation. J. Voice 12 (2), 159–165.

Koppenhaver, S.L., Hebert, J.J., Fritz, J.M., et al., 2009. Reliability of rehabilitative ultrasound imaging of the transversus abdominis and lumbar multifidus muscles. Arch. Phys. Med. Rehabil. 90 (1), 87–94.

Leanderson, R., Sundberg, J., 1988. Breathing for singing. Journal of Voice 2 (1), 1–12.

Mathieson, L., Hirani, S.P., Epstein, R., et al., 2009. Laryngeal manual therapy: a preliminary study to examine its treatment effects in the management of muscle tension dysphonia. J. Voice 23 (3), 353–366.

Miller, R., 1996. The structure of singing. Schirmer, Cengage Learning, Boston.

Noyes, B.E., Kemp, J.S., 2007. Vocal cord dysfunction in children. Paediatr. Respir. Rev. 8 (2), 155–163.

Pettersen, V., Westgaard, R.H., 2004. The association between upper trapezius activity and thorax movement in classical singing. J. Voice 18 (4), 500–512.

Pinto, R.Z., Ferreira, P.H., Franco, M.R., et al., 2011. The effect of lumbar posture on abdominal muscle thickness during an isometric leg task in people with and without non-specific low back pain. Man. Ther 16 (6), 578–584.

Radebold, A., Cholewicki, J., Polzhofer, G., et al., 2001. Impaired postural control of the lumbar spine is associated with delayed muscle response times in patients with chronic idiopathic low back pain. Biomechanics 26 (7), 724–730.

Richardson, C.A., Jull, G.A., 1995. Muscle control-pain control. What exercises would you prescribe? Manual Therapy 1 (1), 2–10.

Schmidt, R., Wrisberg, C., 2007. Motor learning and performance: a situation-based learning approach, fourth ed. Human Kinetics, Champaign.

Shipp, J., 1987. Vertical laryngeal position: research findings and application for singers. Journal of Voice 1 (3), 217–219.

Talasz, H., Kofler, M., Kalchschmid, E., et al., 2010. Breathing with the pelvic floor? Correlation of pelvic floor muscle function and expiratory flows in healthy young nulliparous women. Int. Urogynecol. J. 21 (4), 475–481.

Van Houtte, E., Van Lierde, K., Claeys, S., 2011. Pathophysiology and treatment of muscle tension dysphonia: a review of the current knowledge. J. Voice 25 (2), 202–207.

Zumsteg, D., Jenny, D., Wieser, H.G., 2000. Vocal cord adduction during vagus nerve stimulation for treatment of epilepsy. Neurology 54 (6), 1388–1389.

Chapter | **7.6** |

Breathing pattern disorders and the athlete

Tania Clifton-Smith

INTRODUCTION

'If breathing is not normalised no other movement pattern can be' (Lewit 1980).

Little attention has been paid to the breathing pattern of the athlete until recently. Historically this area of research has been dominated by sports physiologists who have focused on ventilation and the delivery of oxygen. Research is now starting to look at the muscles of respiration and even breathing patterns (Vickery 2007).

BREATHING PATTERN DISORDERS

A current working definition has been postulated within the physiotherapy literature: 'Inappropriate breathing which is persistent enough to cause symptoms, with no apparent organic cause' (Clifton-Smith & Rowley 2011). This is the favoured definition of the author as it encompasses hyperventilation and breathing pattern disorders, and can also include acute and chronic episodes. Once the pattern is established, the breathing pattern disorder becomes habituated and can exist as an entity of its own or exist alongside the trigger. For example, if an athlete has an inefficient breathing pattern when competing, this may cause premature breathlessness, or lower limb fatigue that is non-reflective of cardiovascular fitness or any organic pathology. Alternatively, if a breathing pattern disorder is evident at rest, this too may well impair performance. Therefore breathing patterns for an athlete must not only cover performance and sport, but also patterns at rest. If possible, the initial triggers or reasons for the development of the disordered pattern, whether acute or chronic in presentation, should be ascertained, as this may be helpful when considering treatment protocols.

In the literature there appear to be three main categories attributed to triggering breathing pattern disorders: biomechanical, physiological/biochemical and psychological factors (Gardner 1996). Relevant examples of how these apply to the athlete are given below.

Biomechanical

- **Increased work of breathing** with repetitive postures and some specific sports, for example the aerodynamic posture of cyclists compromises the thoracic cavity, and swimmers who exercise in a supine position not only have the positional dynamics but also the imposed hydrostatic pressure of water to work against.
- **Altered muscle recruitment patterns**. If the superficial abdominal muscles fire prior to the deep abdominal stabilizers (transversus abdominis) this can result in altered trunk stability.
- **Hyperinflation** appears to be common amongst the athlete groups who move excessive volumes of air during their sport. Often the athlete fails to return to normal volumes at rest (authors' observations); in particular this has been noted in swimmers and rowers.
- **Past injuries** such as trauma to the nose, commonly in sports such as rugby and boxing.

Physiological/biochemical

Changes to rate, pressure and volumes will have an effect on gas exchange – in particular to the athlete.

- **Pre-existing organic disorders.** Asthma, chronic sinusitis, exercise-induced bronchospasm, and vocal cord dysfunction (see Ch. 7.5).
- **Diet or drug related.** E.g use of performance-enhancing drugs
- **Altitude related.** Breathing patterns adapt to altitude to compensate for the lack of oxygen. Athletes are now using these adaptations and altitude training to help their performance.
- **Environments.** E.g cold, dry, hot or humid training locations, outdoor pollutants or allergen surges.
- **Sleep cycles.** Ultradian and circadian rhythm can be disturbed with frequent air travel.
- **Tachypnoeic shift.**[1] A change in breathing rate whilst maintaining tidal volume. During exercise this is dysfunctional as the athlete is breathing too fast and will not be able to maintain adequate ventilation.

---

[1]Tachypnoeic breathing involves an abnormally rapid rate (more than 20 breaths per minute in adults), Mosby's Medical Dictionary, 8th edition. © 2009, Elsevier.

Emotional/psychological

Performance anxiety, choking, past experiences, pain, panic disorders, depression, suppressed emotion, conditioning or learned responses or ego threat.

BIOMECHANICAL CONSIDERATIONS

The muscles of respiration are uniquely adapted for endurance, but their function can be compromised as they are involved in both respiration and postural stability. It is pertinent to the athlete that altered motor recruitment patterns can lead to increased workloads, reduced mechanical advantage, and increased ventilatory requirements.

Pressure control: biomechanics

The diaphragm is required to perform the dual role of respiration plus postural control/stabilization during movement (Hodges & Gandevia 2000). The muscles essential to static and dynamic stability are the diaphragm, transversus abdominis, multifidis and the pelvic floor muscles. Of all the abdominal muscles, transversus plays the most significant role in synchronizing pressure changes with the diaphragm for optimal respiration as well as stability and postural support (De Troyer et al 1990).

When these muscles work together in harmony, ideal intra-abdominal pressure occurs which predominantly protects the lumbar spine (Hodges & Gandevia 2000). These muscle groups, plus the accessory muscles of respiration, not only assist with optimum pressure control within the whole body and spinal support, but also contribute to motility of fluid-based systems within the body, i.e. gastrointestinal, lymphatic drainage, arterial and venous circulation (Massery 2006). Structurally, at the top of the system regulating pressure control, are the vocal folds and the surrounding musculature, in particular the intrinsic laryngeal muscles. Hence voice and vocal control is also reliant on this system. The most commonly presented disorder relevant to athletes at the top of the system is vocal cord dysfunction (VCD) (inspiratory stridor) or paradoxical VCD (PVCD). The diaphragm sits in the middle and the pelvic floor at the bottom of this system. Optimal pelvic floor function is also related to appropriate diaphragmatic activity. The diaphragm, due to its position, has often been referred to as the pressure generator.

Pressure control: muscle length tension relationship

Breathing is a rhythmical function so the diaphragm constantly contracts and relaxes. The diaphragm is at its most relaxed at the end of the exhalation phase. If the diaphragm returns to a relatively constant resting position at the end of each contraction–relaxation cycle, this will maintain respiratory load and breathing frequency. Another important factor to consider is the zone of apposition. This is the area of the diaphragm encompassing the cylindrical portion, which corresponds to the inner aspect of the lower rib cage. The transversus abdominis muscle, alongside the diaphragm, plays a large role in the prediction of this zone and pressure regulation (Urmey et al 1998). The zone of apposition relates to the resetting end-position of the diaphragm and the corresponding efficiency of movement. The smaller the zone of apposition the less force created during a cycle of respiration, and conversely the larger the zone the greater the force. For example an incomplete exhalation, as seen in hyperinflation, leaves the diaphragm in a lower, flatter position; this is a smaller zone of apposition versus that of a complete exhalation, which allows a fuller doming, and a correspondingly larger zone. This highlights the importance of full breathing cycles for maximum force and power during exercise.

If the respiratory accessory muscles, or the abdominal muscle group, shorten or are weakened, the diaphragm is unable to return to its optimal resting position, and as a result pressure generation is decreased. Pressure can therefore determine the length–tension relationship, i.e. shortened muscles create less force, the muscle length tension relationship is altered, and the work of breathing increases. Optimal pressure gives strength to an otherwise weak external structure. If the system is weakened, gas exchange inefficiencies may also occur, often leading towards arterial hypocapnia.

Muscle recruitment/motor patterns

Muscle recruitment and motor patterns are important not only to preserve intra-abdominal pressure but also in lumbo-pelvic stability and all the other biomechanical functions, such as those related to motility.

Should there be a deviation away from the optimal trunk lumbo-pelvic recruitment pattern, such as the oblique muscles firing first, then pressure, ventilation volumes, stability and ultimately the work of breathing, can be affected (Hodges & Gandevia 2000).

In a professional athlete population it has been documented that low back pain (LBP) is one of the most common reasons for missed playing time (Bahr et al 2004). On ultrasound imaging, athletes who have been identified with a breathing pattern disorder often display increased resting tone (hypertonicity) of the superficial abdominal muscles (author's observations). It is known that in people with LBP there is evidence of delayed activation of the transversus abdominis muscle and increased activity of superficial lumbo-pelvic muscles (Hodges 1999). If these muscles are over-active at rest, in particular the superficial abdominal muscles, they can act as a corset (often associated with hyperinflation of the lungs and reduction of the zone of apposition). This corseting effect

may be an attempt to increase spinal stability via increasing the intra-abdominal pressure. Hodges et al (2005) showed that the stiffness of the lumbar spine is increased when intra-abdominal pressure is elevated. However, this learned bracing will ultimately reduce stability: the transversus does not work in synchronization with the diaphragm: the zone of apposition decreases, along with the ultimate force-generating ability of the diaphragm.

It is vital clinically to not only consider the stability of the trunk, but to also consider the role of respiration and the muscles of breathing.

In the literature there are multiple exercise programmes for the deep muscles of the lumbo-pelvic region, with no or little consideration of respiratory patterns. Therapists need to look at innovative exercise programmes utilizing the whole system, such as abdominal exercises that incorporate breathing patterns in various postures. Additionally, limb movements above the head will increase postural demands for stabilization, as will utilization of the voice. Clinically, this author often designs client programmes involving Swiss ball trunk stability exercises, whilst abdominally breathing, moving arms above head height and reciting a poem, the alphabet or singing. The goal is for the diaphragm to coordinate breathing, trunk and voice control.

Alternatively, with any upper trunk dysfunction such as rotator cuff disorders, breathing patterns must also be considered. Patients with neck, shoulder and general upper torso pain commonly have faulty breathing patterns (Perri & Halford 2008). In upper chest breathing the sternocleidomastoid muscles, the scalene muscles, and the upper trapezii muscles are increased in activation (Falla 2004).

Breathing entrainment

If breathing is coordinated to the rhythm of motion, a locomotor-respiratory coupling may occur. This possibly occurs in order to achieve an economical advantage (Mahler et al 1991, Polemnia 2007). The coupling is characterized by the ability to change breathing pattern and rate, to meet changing physiological demands, for example during running, the ability to switch breath to stride ratio depending on ventilatory demands. The runner at a low speed may take one breath to two strides (1 : 2 ratio), but with a higher speed may switch to one breath every four strides (1 : 4 ratio) (Polemnia 2007). During rowing, the following patterns are proposed by Steinacker (1993):

1. One exhalation during the stroke, i.e. oar in the water and one inhalation during recovery (1 : 1).
2. With higher speeds, demand and increased ventilation, one complete breathing cycle (inhale and exhale) during recovery, one complete breathing cycle during the stroke phase (1 : 2).

In the last decade, studies have emerged regarding the possibility of breathing entrainment occurring in sport.

Entrainment has been observed in many elite professionals in their sport, whilst the concept has not been shown amongst novices in the sports (Mahler et al 1991). Such observations suggest that the elite athlete has an innate natural rhythm, or has adapted through various training regimes. It may be that with experience professional athletes learn to avoid a tachypnoeic shift at high-exercise intensities. Many coaches instruct athletes to control ratios deliberately in order to ensure that sufficient oxygen is available for movement, but there are virtually no studies on intentional control, especially under high ventilatory loads (Polemnia 2007).

Research is needed in these areas – the author's observations are that awareness of the exhalation phase can alter performance with favourable outcomes as seen by Vickery (2007).

Dynamic hyperinflation

An end result of an upper chest breathing pattern can be dynamic hyperinflation. If body mechanics and motor patterns alter, physiological changes may also occur; the body can acclimatize to this 'new' pattern in as short a time as 24 hours (Gardner 1996). Often individuals present with dynamic hyperinflation and increased resting tone of the superficial abdominal muscles, which creates a self-induced corset, so that normal breathing becomes difficult, resulting in serious physiological, mechanical, and psychological changes (see Ch. 6.4). Breath stacking, in which inhalation exceeds exhalation, over time during exercise, leads to hyperinflation, and airflow can become limited, so that oxygen reaching the alveoli is decreased, as dead space volume increases. If prolonged, adaptations of muscle fibres may occur to preserve strength and increase endurance.

PHYSIOLOGICAL CONSIDERATIONS

Hyperventilation

A lowering of CO_2 levels in the blood, causing an increase in pH, creates many physiological changes. Of particular relevance to the musculoskeletal system is the alteration of sensory and motor axons, altered oxygen (O_2) uptake via the Bohr effect, smooth muscle constriction, and lowered pain thresholds. See Chapters 1 and 3 for more on this topic.

Threshold alteration to sensory and motor axons causes depolarization or excitation of the nerve motor unit which contributes to an increased central nervous system arousal. The increase in pH improves muscle function, as seen in short duration cycle sprints (Bishop et al 2004). If prolonged, however, over-stimulation, fatigue and ultimately increased sensitization can become a problem. During hyperventilation, haemoglobin binds tightly to oxygen, reducing the release of oxygen to tissue cells (Bohr effect suppression) in particular to the periphery. Chronicity can deplete the bicarbonate buffer, resulting in immediate muscle lactate build-up at low levels of exercise (Nixon & Andrews 1996).

The discovery of smooth muscle cells in collagen which constrict when pH rises (Restini & Bendhack 2006), can potentially explain the presentation of increased muscular and fascial tension amongst individuals with breathing pattern disorders. This implies breathing disorders will play a part in fascial/connective tissue sites: ligaments, menisci and possibly spinal discs. It has also been suggested that in the hypermobile individual, the altered breathing pattern exists as a means to increase tone and stability via the effect of respiratory alkalosis on contractile smooth muscle cells (Chaitow 2004).

'Blood stealing'

The diaphragm muscle requires movement to maintain its own healthy blood supply. During the relaxation phase, blood flow to the diaphragm muscle is regulated. It has been shown that the relaxation phase is responsible for accommodating most of the changes in blood perfusion brought about by increased diaphragmatic work (Hussain & Magder 1991). Diaphragmatic blood flow is reduced during inspiration and can be completely abolished during forceful contractions. Perhaps another explanation for the stitch?

During maximal exercise blood flow to the diaphragm and inspiratory muscles represents 15% of the total oxygen cost of exercise (Wetter et al 1999), and as exercise increases, the respiratory muscles demand more and more of the total body oxygen consumption. The work of breathing during maximal exercise results in marked changes in locomotor muscle blood flow, cardiac output and both whole-body and active-limb oxygen uptake. It is believed the compromised locomotor blood flow is associated with noradrenaline (norepinephrine), suggesting enhanced sympathetic vasoconstriction (Romer & Dempsey 2006). Evidence exists of a metaboreflex, with its origin in the respiratory muscles (Sheel et al 2001). It is believed this reflex can reduce blood flow to the lower limbs, via stimulation of sympathetic nervous system vasoconstrictor neurons. The fundamental goal is the protection of oxygen delivery to the respiratory muscles, thus ensuring the ability to maintain pulmonary ventilation, proper regulation of arterial blood gases, pH, and overall homeostasis. This concept has been referred to as blood stealing – the respiratory muscles stealing blood from the lower limbs (McConnell 2011). The important point to note here is that when all systems are challenged, breathing will remain as the final driving force, in other words, 'breathing always wins' (Massery 2006). See Figure 7.6.1 highlighting the effect breathing pattern changes have on performance.

Breathing: Altered pattern/poor initiating pattern

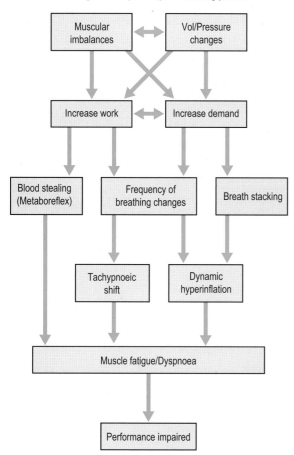

Figure 7.6.1 Breathing pattern disorders and impaired motor performance. *From Bradley & Clifton-Smith 2009.*

Take, for example, a couple of runners talking, jogging and breathing who reach a set of 200 steps; as the ventilatory demand increases so does the breathing demand. It becomes harder to converse, and as the demand further increases, breathlessness (dyspnoea) may occur. Dyspnoea alerts the system that it is under pressure; pace is eased, and regulating of the breathing pattern occurs. The goal of the system is to preserve and regulate respiration. This alarm system or warning system applies to the individual with COPD, through to elite athletes. It is a complex system, however research into breathing pattern disorders has shown the benefits that good efficient breathing patterns can play in the appropriate desensitizing of this 'alarm' (Vickery 2007).

Hypoxic training

Awareness of altitude training became evident after the 1968 Olympics in Mexico City, which has an elevation of 2240 metres (7349 ft) above sea level. Endurance athletes did poorly as opposed to sprint (anaerobic) eventers, validating theories that performance outcomes can be affected by altitude.

Historically athletes who wished to utilize the concept of altitude training would train at high altitudes. The goal and purpose was to increase erythrocyte volume and ultimately enhance sea-level maximal oxygen uptake (VO$_2$max) and endurance performance. New theories suggest other factors may be involved in the improvement of performance. Other central (such as ventilatory, haemodynamic or neural adaptation) or peripheral (such as muscle buffering capacity or economy) factors play an important role (Wilber 2011). Currently there are several altitude/hypoxic training models. For the purposes of this chapter the author will not go into details but suggests that the reader reviews the literature.

PSYCHOLOGICAL/EMOTIONAL CONSIDERATIONS

Any athlete, particularly the elite athlete, is exposed to many internal and external pressures. Performance anxiety has been shown to have close associations with breathing pattern disorders (Masaoka & Homma 1997); similar changes are seen with anticipatory anxiety. For example, fear of dyspnoea is a major factor in panic attacks and anxiety (Ley 1997). It is often the sensation of dyspnoea or muscle discomfort that will limit performance.

In the case of the athlete, it is not only anxiety surrounding potential symptoms such as breathlessness, but also anxiety surrounding the performance itself that can affect, or be affected by, a breathing pattern disorder. It is important to note, however, that the factors surrounding anxiety are too complex and interrelated to suggest that there can be a simple causal effect. The connection between psychological state and respiration is bi-directional, suggesting breathing should be examined as an independent variable affecting the psychological process. For example the use of nose, low and slow breathing during warm-up routines to maintain autonomic stability, preserve energy and maintain cortical control.

Choking under pressure is well documented in the sports literature. Jordet et al (2008) found that choking in major football (soccer) penalty shoot-outs corresponds well with a three-step model involving ego threat, emotional discomfort and self-regulation failure. Performers who self-regulate well can successfully cope with both high levels of ego-threat and discomfort; working on improving one's self-regulation is a natural way to prevent choking under pressure. Working with the breath is a powerful tool for self-regulation.

Figure 7.6.2 is a simple representation of the processes described above, as well as resulting symptomatic presentations.

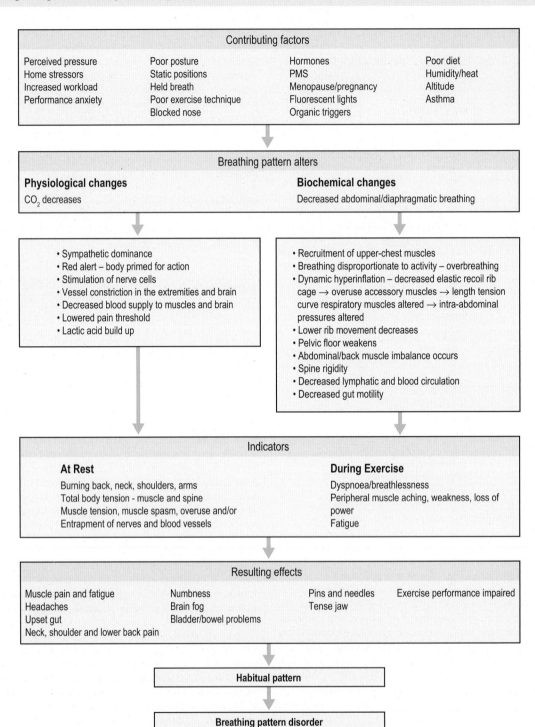

Figure 7.6.2 Breathing and the musculoskeletal connection. *From Bradley and Clifton-Smith 2005.*

GUIDELINES FOR CLINICAL IMPLEMENTATION

Full observation, assessment and treatment protocols are addressed elsewhere in the book, therefore only key points, pertinent to the athlete, are considered here.

Assessment indicators for the athlete

Athletes should be questioned on:

- The history of organic disorders, especially respiratory-related from birth. For example, childhood asthma is indicative of potential altered patterns from a young age.
- Co-existing medical conditions, in particular asthma, exercise-induced asthma/bronchospasm (EIA, EIB), gastro-esophageal reflux disease (GERD), postnasal drip (which can cause pharyngeal erythema) and sinusitis.
- Habitual coughing and throat clearing.
- Past injuries: pain/discomfort.
- Exercise history: What type of exercise? When and how, with details of training programmes and recuperation time.
- General health: coughs, cold, flu, chest infections. These are indicators of the immune system's status.
- Sleep is another important homeostatic indicator. Bed time? How many hours slept? Is sleep interrupted? And is the individual refreshed on waking?
- Relaxation: many individuals confuse downtime and real-time relaxation. Downtime includes things like watching TV, reading a book/magazine or gardening. Relaxation is a conscious practice to still the body and thought processes. Does the patient visualize and/or use the power of mental preparation (for an important presentation or sporting event)?
- Stitch pain: which side and when?

Sinclair's theory of stitch published in the 1950s is still considered valid. Sinclair felt that stitch is a diaphragmatic pain, caused by pull on the peritoneal ligaments. When exhalation occurs on heel strike the lungs empty, a heavy strain is placed on these ligaments and the diaphragm, resulting in spasm and tension – and possibly stitch pain (Sinclair 1951).

Breathlessness experienced during sport/activity

The individual should be asked what the breathlessness feels like, and when it occurs. Breathlessness during activity could relate to exercise-induced bronchospasm/asthma (EIB/EIA), or vocal cord dysfunction (VCD), or exercise-induced hyperventilation (EIH). Many athletes who present with 'breathlessness' are given a diagnosis of asthma, without further investigation, and this is not surprising, considering the statistic in the literature on asthma and athletes.

Competitive athletes appear to have a high prevalence of asthma and EIA, particularly athletes participating in winter endurance sports.

Theoretically a higher incidence of airway hyper-reactivity occurs when air is cold and dry, and when there is a high ventilatory rate, airborne allergens and other irritants' particles will worsen symptoms in the lower airways. Consequently, not only winter sports athletes, but also endurance-trained athletes may be at increased risk of developing asthma/EIB (Kippelen et al 2005).

Differential diagnosis: EIA/EIB, VCD, HVS, Swimming-Induced Pulmonary Edema (SIPE), other lung disorders or poor physical fitness.

An athlete with VCD typically identifies the neck or throat as the source of airway restriction; in EIA/EIB the chest is commonly identified as the source of tightness. Wheezing, cough, shortness of breath or chest pain are more closely associated with EIA, whereas whistling sounds (due to narrowing of the respiratory tract) and a stridor at the level of the larynx, characterized by a harsher noise like that of sawing, are indicative of VCD. VCD is the inability to inhale, and a lack of responsiveness to bronchodilators is the rule, and is more commonly seen in young female athletes. Another condition to be mindful of is SIPE, which presents in elite swimmers. Symptoms include shortness of breath, prominent cough, significant sputum production, haemoptysis and wheezing. SIPE significantly influences performance. It is not clear what predisposes to its occurrence. One theory is that pulmonary oedema occurs as a result of damage to the blood-gas barrier (BGB), as a result of the need to overcome high capillary pressures during extreme exercise (Adir et al 2004).

Objective considerations

BradCliff® Ski Jump Test (Fig. 7.6.3)

Lying in supine with knees bent

This test checks for hyperinflation/over-tensed superficial abdominal musculature in the supine position.

1. Ask for permission to palpate.
2. Run your hand along the lower rib cage from lateral to medial.
3. A flaring of the lower ribs at the costal border is indicative of hyperinflation/over-tensed superficial abdominal musculature.

BradCliff® Angle Test (Xyphocostal border) (Fig. 7.6.4)

Lying in supine

If abdominal muscles are tense and the rib cage is hyperinflated, the angle of the caudal opening is altered from

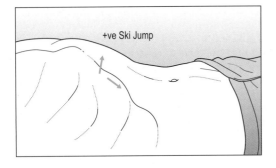

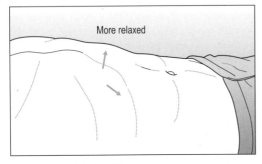

Figure 7.6.3 BradCliff® Ski Jump. *From Bradley & Clifton-Smith 2009.*

the average expected norm of approximately 90 degrees (clinical observations).

Measuring this angle before treatment, and then again after treatment, might prove useful. The angle is often reduced in patients with Breathing Pattern Disorders (BPD), coinciding with a splinted abdomen, and hyperinflation. Patients are often surprised at the difference that relaxed abdominal breathing can make to the shape of the rib cage. Conversely the angle is often greater in patients with respiratory disorders, especially Chronic Obstructive Pulmonary Disease (COPD), due to the flattening of the diaphragm.

Note that the Ski Jump and BradCliff Angle Test can be repeated within the session. These objective measures often improve significantly which helps to reconfirm the importance of breathing awareness.

Dynamic observations

It is useful to observe the locomotor respiratory pattern on a treadmill, exercising, or rowing machine depending on equipment available. To meet the increase in ventilatory demand of exercise, breathing patterns alter to allow increased volumes. Upper chest and mouth breathing are recruited to allow larger volumes of air. The point at which the pattern changes possibly corresponds with the respiratory compensation point – the onset of hyperventilation during incremental exercise that is thought to represent the body's attempt to compensate for metabolic acidosis (Meyer et al 2004).

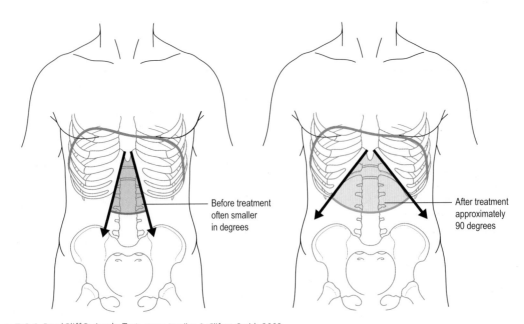

Figure 7.6.4 BradCliff® Angle Test. *From Bradley & Clifton-Smith 2009.*

TREATMENT PROTOCOLS FOR THE ATHLETE/SPORTS INDIVIDUAL

High performance individuals are aware that all factors in their lives impact on each other and each factor requires special attention if goals and aspirations are to be achieved.

The BradCliff® Method of breathing for athletes considers a four-step treatment programme. Note this is only an overview; in-depth descriptors of treatment regimes require a full assessment of an individual, followed by a personalized treatment and/or rehabilitation plan. Presentation may be due to pain, asthma or the desire to improve performance. Goals may then be to improve function via desensitization and homeostatic balance, or utilize breathing patterns to allow respiratory adaptation to enhance performance.

Breathing re-education for rest and recovery

It is important for an individual to know what calm optimal breathing at rest feels like, and to understand how the body systems work. This step endeavours to guide the individual to an optimal breathing pattern. Education of the musculoskeletal, biomechanical workings of the diaphragm and associations with other muscle groups is important, particularly to athletes. Simple physiological explanations of breathing efficiency during exercise are also likely to be beneficial.

Various postures and positions are utilized in the clinic, including at rest in supine to sitting and standing postures. Optimal breathing patterns and optimal posture go hand in hand, for example it is advisable to check in standing that posture is balanced, the abdominals are engaged but not over-active, and that gentle diaphragmatic breathing is achieved.

Prior to sport

Educate on the use of breathing skills to encourage focus and body awareness such as awareness of nose, low, slow breathing during warm-up sessions. This reinforces the normal/optimal breathing pattern established in the clinic, encouraging blood flow to the diaphragm, while helping to avoid poor breathing patterns during the warm-up phase prior to an event.

Sport specific

Energy-efficient breathing assists with all sports. Good breathing patterns at rest are essential: this ensures the individual is starting from a mechanical and physiological advantage.

Depending on the sport, specific techniques can be implemented. The paper this author cites with enthusiasm for future research is by Vickery (2007). This study examined the effect of breathing pattern retraining (BPR) on cycling performance, and on respiratory, metabolic and perceptual responses during an incremental test in competitive cyclists. The retraining comprised 10 minutes daily at rest, and awareness of a pursed-lip pattern during cycling. Pursed-lip breathing elongates the exhaled breath, through resistance, avoiding breath stacking, hyperinflation and a tachypnoeic shift. The results at 4 weeks showed enhanced endurance performance and improved incremental peak power. Vickery believed the changes to be due to altered respiratory mechanics and a reduced perception of exertion. This is significant in the world of sport and highlights the value of breathing pattern awareness and training to optimize performance.

Resistance training of the breathing muscles

Resistance to the respiratory muscles can be achieved via flow limitation or pressure loading. Flow reduction training is known as inspiratory flow resistive loading. Pressure loading can be either inspiratory or expiratory. Inspiratory pressure loading is the preferred method of resistance training, by this author, for athletes. Inspiratory muscle training (IMT) has the most scientific research, with respect to the effects on sport and performance (see http://www.powerbreathe.com/imt-clinical-trials-and-medical-research (Accessed June 2013) for research papers). The POWERbreathe and threshold devices have been shown to be the most versatile, cost-effective and time-efficient devices to use in pressure-threshold inspiratory muscle training (McConnell 2011).

Prior to use of any threshold devices the therapist should have a clear understanding of how to instruct on use, and of any contraindications. See the above references for in-depth knowledge on inspiratory muscle training.

CONCLUSION

Breathing and the muscles of respiration can be a major factor in the ultimate training and outcomes of anyone participating in sport. Athletes, and in particular the elite athlete, need to be assessed and treated with all three categories in mind: biomechanics, physiology and psychology. Biomechanics needs to consider both postural and respiratory demands.

REFERENCES

Adir, Y., Shupak, A., Gil, A., et al., 2004. Swimming-induced pulmonary edema: clinical presentation and serial lung function. Chest. 126 (2), 394–399.

Bahr, R., Andersen, S., Loken, S., et al., 2004. Low back pain among endurance athletes with and without specific back loading – a cross-sectional survey of cross-country skiers, rowers, orienteerers, and nonathletic controls. Spine 29, 449–454.

Bishop, D., Edge, J., Davis, C., et al., 2004. Induced metabolic alkalosis affects muscle metabolism and repeated-sprint ability. Med Sci Sports Exerc 36, 807–813.

Bradley, D., Clifton-Smith, T., 2005. Breathe Stretch and Move. Random House NZ.

Bradley, D., Clifton-Smith, T., 2009. BradCliff® Manual. Writers Inc. Auckland, New Zealand.

Chaitow, L., 2004. Breathing pattern disorders, motor control, and low back pain. Journal of Osteopathic Medicine 7 (1), 34–41.

Clifton-Smith, T., Rowley, J., 2011. Breathing pattern disorders and physiotherapy: inspiration for our profession. Physical Therapy Reviews 16 (1), 75–86.

De Troyer, A., Estenne, M., Ninane, V., et al., 1990. Transversus abdominis muscle function in humans. J Appl Physiol. 68 (3), 1010–1016.

Falla, D., 2004. Unraveling the complexity of muscle impairment in chronic neck pain. Man Ther 9, 125–133.

Gardner, W., 1996. The pathophysiology of hyperventilation disorders. Chest 109 (2), 516–535.

Hodges, P., 1999. Is there a role for transversus abdominis in lumbo-pelvic stability? Manual Therapy 4 (2), 74–86.

Hodges, P., Gandevia, S., 2000. Changes in intra-abdominal pressure during postural and respiratory activation of the human diaphragm. J Appl Physiol 89, 967–976.

Hodges, P.W., Eriksson, A.E., Shirley, D., et al., 2005. Intra-abdominal pressure increases stiffness of the lumbar spine. J Biomech 38 (9), 1873–1880.

Hussain, A., Magder, S., 1991. Diaphragmatic intramuscular pressure in relation to tension, shortening, and blood flow. J. Appl. Physiol. 71, 159–167.

Jordet, G., 2008. Performing under pressure: what can we learn from football penalty shoot-outs? Sport & Exercise Psychology Review 7 (2), 13.

Kippelen, P., Caillaud, C., Robert, E., et al., 2005. Effect of endurance training on lung function: a one year study. Br J Sports Med 39, 617–621.

Lewit, K., 1980. Relation of faulty respiration to posture with clinical implication. Journal of the American Osteopathic Association 79, 525–529.

Ley, R., 1997. Panic disorder and agrophobia: Fear of the fear or fear of the symptoms produced by hyperventilation? Journal of Behavior Therapy and Experimental Psychiatry 18, 305–316.

Mahler, D.A., Shuhart, C.R., Brew, E., et al., 1991. Ventilatory responses and entrainment of breathing during rowing. Med Sci Sports Exerc 23 (2), 186–192.

Massery, M., 2006. The patient with multi-system impairments affecting breathing mechanics and motor control. Cardiovascular and Pulmonary Physical Therapy Evidence and Practice, fourth ed. Mosby & Elsevier Health Sciences, St. Louis, MO (Chapter 39), pp. 695–717.

McConnell, A., 2011. Breathe strong perform better. Human Kinetics, U.S.A.

Masaoka, Y., Homma, I., 1997. Anxiety and respiratory patterns: their relationship during mental stress and physical load. International Journal of Psychophysiology 27, 153–159.

Meyer, T., Faude, O., Urhausen, A., et al., 2004. Is lactic acidosis a cause of exercise induced hyperventilation at the respiratory compensation point? British Journal of Sports Medicine 38, 622–625.

Nixon, P., Andrews, J., 1996. A study of anaerobic threshold in chronic fatigue syndrome (CFS). Biological Psychology 43 (3), 264.

Perri, M., Halford, E., 2008. Pain and faulty breathing: a pilot study. J Bodyw Mov Ther 4, 297–306.

Polemnia, G., 2007. Intentional control of motor-respiratory coordination. Journal of Sport & Exercise Psychology Jul Supplement 29, pS51.

Restini, C., Bendhack, L., 2006. Involvement of non-selective Ca2+ channels in the contraction induced by alkalinization of rat anococcygeus muscle cells. European J Pharmacology 553, 288–296.

Romer, L., Dempsey, J., 2006. Legs pay out for the cost of breathing! Physiology News 65, 25.

Sheel, A., Derchak, P., Morgan, B., et al., 2001. Fatiguing inspiratory work causes reflex reduction in resting leg blood flow in humans. J Physiol 537, 277–289.

Sinclair, J., 1951. The Side Pain of Athletes. The New Zealand Medical Journal 50 (280), 607–612.

Steinacker, J.M., 1993. Physiological aspects of training in rowing. International Journal of Sports Medicine 14 (Suppl 1), 3–10.

Urmey, W., De Troyer, A., Kelly, K., et al., 1998. Pleural pressure increases during inspiration in the zone of apposition of diaphragm to rib cage. J Appl Physiol. 65 (5), 2207–2212.

Vickery, R., 2007. The effect of breathing pattern retraining on performance in competitive cyclists. http://repositoryaut.lconz.ac.nz/handle/10292/83 (Accessed June 2013).

Wetter, T.J., Harms, C.A., Nelson, W.B., et al., 1999. Influence of respiratory muscle work on VO(2) and leg blood flow during submaximal exercise. J Appl Physiol 87, 643–651.

Wilber, R.L., 2011. Application of altitude/hypoxic training by elite athletes. J. Hum. Sport Exerc. 6, No. 2.

Chapter | **7.7** |

Capnography in treatment of BPD

Laurie McLaughlin

This chapter reviews the use of capnography as an adjunct to traditional breathing interventions as well as adding unique management strategies through monitoring respiratory indicators. The success (or lack thereof) of any therapeutic input can be determined allowing for customized treatment programmes.

Once problem areas have been isolated through the evaluation process a management plan can be developed. Capnography can be used as a test-retest or outcome measure for whatever treatment intervention is used such as those outlined in the various chapters in Section 7. It can also be used specifically for treatment providing real-time information that can be used to connect breathing style with physiology providing a powerful tool for change.

GENERAL CONCEPTS

Watch your own breathing and voice quality when speaking with the patient. People tend to entrain breathing with one another. Try to make sure they 'catch you' and you don't 'catch them'. Keep your voice calm, quiet and relaxed.

The **principles of good breathing**, as discussed in Chapters 7.2, 7.3 and elsewhere, will be reinforced during the session using capnography as added information and input. These principles can be summed up as:

Nose (as opposed to mouth breathing, see Ch. 2.3)
Low (lower chest rather than upper chest)
Slow (breathing at 8–14 breaths per minute at rest)
Let Go (passive exhale, let go of muscle tension)
Quiet (making the breath quiet helps to keep the volume in check)

I suggest that patients memorize nose, low, slow, let go, and quiet to remind them about what to check in with, when they find themselves experiencing symptoms they associate with poor breathing. Through testing, they will know which particular aspects to pay attention to (McLaughlin 2009).

Self-discovery/awareness training

Changing breathing has a great deal to do with education and self-awareness. Once people understand the importance of breath to their wellbeing, and how their current style of breathing is negatively affecting health, the process can become one of self-discovery. Seeing the capnographic feedback helps associate the feelings of good respiratory chemistry with the style of breathing that creates those feelings. Also, the sensations of poor respiratory chemistry (usually lower CO$_2$) can be associated with the style of breathing creating those sensations. These experiences are then internalized so that noticing symptoms associated with poor breathing becomes a cue to adjusting the breathing pattern. With time, people can learn to tune into ever-subtler cues. Peter Litchfield (2012) refers to this style of learning as 'inside out' where people essentially 'work it out' on their own, with the help of capnography readings and some guidance or facilitation. 'Outside in' learning uses a more direct approach, where people are told what they are doing incorrectly and given specific instruction about how to change. Clinical experience suggests that a combination of these approaches proves to be the most successful.

Case history

One young woman who had been experiencing ongoing neck pain and headaches for 18 months following a motor vehicle accident, rented a capnograph for home use to help her understand how breathing was contributing to her problem. She was asked to record her breathing, both when she was in significant pain, as well as at times when she wasn't in quite as much pain. She was also instructed to notice her breathing mechanics, upper or lower chest, rate, etc. She observed that when she was in a great deal of pain, she breathed in her upper chest, and at a faster rate. When her pain wasn't as bad, she breathed more slowly and less in her upper chest. It was then suggested that when she was in significant pain, she should check her breathing, and shift to the breathing style she used when her pain was reduced, to see if it had any effect. She was able to report a reduction in pain when breathing mechanics were changed to the style used when she was in less pain. She could have been given this information, but working it out for herself made the learning more profound. Some people, on the other hand, would prefer to be told what they are doing wrong, and how to fix it, or they may become quite frustrated, aggravating their breathing.

Wave play

Wave play is a mainstay of breathing retraining with capnography, where information is available immediately in response to whatever change is made to the breathing style. Simply watching the waveform for ETCO$_2$, respiratory rate and pattern, while experimenting with the principles of good breathing, provides rich information, facilitating connections between the inner experience and the breathing process. Experimenting with these principles can be helpful in gaining understanding as to how best to breathe in order to optimize the ETCO$_2$, rate and pattern.

Rate/ratio retraining

In the CapnoTrainer™ software there is an application called the 'Mechanics Training' screen (Fig. 7.7.1) that is helpful for both assessing and training respiratory rate. There is a 'bouncing ball' that is followed up an incline during inhalation, down the decline during exhalation and across the bottom for the pause in between breaths. A great deal of diversity and individuality in human breathing patterns has been noted including the ratio of inhalation to exhalation, although inhalation is generally thought to be of shorter duration than exhalation (Benchetrit 2000). However, equal inhalation and exhalation times have also been described (Fried 1999). To show the impact of altering the ratio, the rate of the inhalation and

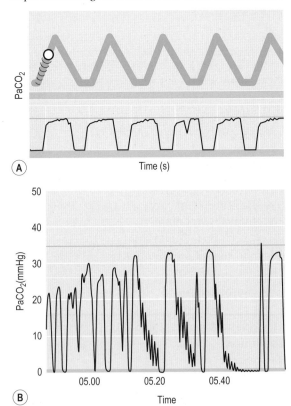

Figure 7.7.1 A The 'mechanics training' screen (heavy, blue waveform) allows the 'speed' of the bouncing ball that moves up and down the slopes of the upper waveform to be adjusted to various breathing rates. The slope of the incline (inhalation) and decline (exhalation) can be adjusted to experiment with the ratio of inhalation to exhalation. The lower (black) waveform shows the levels of the individual's ETCO$_2$, and the effects of the various rates and ratios can be monitored with the capnometer. Note that the height of the wave on the screen represents the estimated level of CO$_2$ in millimeters of mercury (mmHg). **B** This jagged line on the decline representing inhalation shows gasping which is indicative of increased inspiratory effort where the individual is reaching for their breath. This is considered a poor pattern.

the exhalation (and therefore the bouncing ball) can be adjusted on the screen, to illustrate the 'feel' of breathing at different ratios. The CO_2 values can be monitored to determine whether the individual's efforts are improving end tidal carbon dioxide ($ETCO_2$), by helping levels rise towards normal, or are making matters worse.

It is important to be able to balance rate and depth of inhalation/exhalation, no matter how fast or slow patients are breathing. The idea is for the individual to connect with the somatic experience of rate/depth so they are not held to a narrow range through habit. As patients gain skill in breathing, practising with different rates and depths while keeping the $ETCO_2$ above 35mmHg, helps with their breathing agility, providing a wider range or repertoire of breathing styles. It may be useful to request individuals to cycle through breathing rates, from low to high, initially within the normal range. Raising the rate beyond normal resting rates, such as to 20 breaths per minute, can also be helpful as there are times when a faster rate *is normal* as people are not always at rest! Reducing the rate to below 8 breaths per minute can be used to train relaxation. For example, six breaths per minute which, interestingly, saying the rosary or a yogic mantra accomplishes, is generally thought to be ideal, as it has been shown to encourage parasympathetic activity, and thereby help to balance autonomic function (Bernardi et al 2001).

In Fig. 7.7.1B, the patient was exerting a great deal of effort to 'catch' the breath. This gasping or breath spasm is seen as a choppy line on the inhalation (the down-slope). The gasp is audible particularly if the ears are blocked by earplugs or fingers. Once the individual tunes into the sound of their breath, with an emphasis on making it quiet while watching the screen, they can smooth out the waveform and improve the breathing pattern.

Negative play

Sometimes no matter what cues or 'tricks' are tried, people have difficulty making a change. One way to have them 'find it' is to have them exaggerate the fault, then lessen the exaggeration, increase it again and so on until bit by bit they can connect with that behaviour and learn to minimize it. For example, one woman seemed unable to stop breathing in her upper chest. She tried self-monitoring her upper chest and abdomen while upright and lying down among other things but despite understanding what she was trying to do she simply couldn't 'find' how to do it and was becoming frustrated. She was then asked to breathe WAY up into her chest and really lift her sternum up. Interestingly, she could figure out how to do more of it quite easily. She was then asked to do a bit less, a bit more again, back and forth while she gradually gained control. $ETCO_2$ readings were also observed, showing improvement when she was able to breathe in her lower chest, which reinforced the change. The same process can be applied for a fast respiratory rate, forced exhalation, and so forth.

Context retraining

Since breathing is context dependent, testing and retraining in the context of where the problems are, represents an important aspect of management. People can often control their breathing while in your office but will need to have the tools to do so when facing challenges in their life that trigger poor breathing.

Intentional overbreathing

Recreating the internal context of poor chemistry may be the most important teaching technique of all. Helping people recognize the sensations associated with breathing well, versus those associated with breathing poorly provides an extremely valuable learning tool. Once the patient

Case history

R described having symptoms associated with exertion. He was tested on a treadmill with an incline. As soon as the $ETCO_2$ values dropped, he reported that he was experiencing the leg cramping and shortness of breath that were concerning him. He was encouraged to pay attention to how his breathing had changed. He noticed he was breathing in his upper chest and straining to inhale after forcing an exhalation. He then focused on breathing in his lower chest as he prolonged his exhalation, while allowing the breath to come naturally, rather than straining for it. He was able to see the difference on the screen and feel his symptoms lessen. Once he made that connection he no longer had problems with exercise.

Case history

Another patient complained of lateral elbow pain in their dominant arm. Manual therapy to the upper extremity helped to some degree but she still had trouble at work where she spent a great deal of time at the computer using a mouse. She did well on the standardized tests except for the concentration test where her $ETCO_2$ dropped. She used a capnograph at her desk and was able to test her breathing when she began to have symptoms. There was a correlation with the onset of her elbow pain and lower $ETCO_2$ values. (See Fig. 7.7.2.)

As she paid attention to how her breathing changed, she realized that she elevated her shoulder girdle, braced her abdominal muscles and breathed shallowly when she had to concentrate. She now uses the alarm on her computer to sound every 20 minutes, so she can check her breathing, and no longer experiences elbow pain.

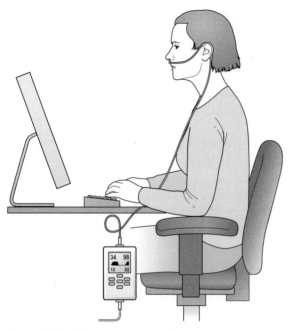

Figure 7.7.2 Using a capnometer during computer work.

can identify the type of breathing that reproduces symptoms, and even more powerfully, how to change breathing to restore good chemistry and abolish symptoms, the skills for managing breathing in the context of daily life are present.

! Intentionally lowering CO_2 is not appropriate for patients with cardiac pathology, severe asthma or a history of panic attacks. Reinforce that the patient should stop if they become uncomfortable. Have a paper bag available to rebreathe into if necessary. There are, however, risks associated with rebreathing into a paper bag if the person is hypoxic or has cardiac pathology. It is important, when using a paper bag, not to block access to fresh air, otherwise oxygen in the bag will very quickly be used up, which is dangerous to some people. Leave space around the margins of the bag for fresh air to flow in. The use of oximetry can be helpful if there is uncertainty regarding oxygen status (Callaham 1989). Ask the patient to increase breath volume initially, and gradually increase the rate if necessary, to bring the $ETCO_2$ down. Have the patient pay attention to thoughts, emotions and bodily sensations, as the numbers go lower, and to reverse the process of lowering the $ETCO_2$ by

Case history

J was assessed a few months after he started his new executive job right after completing his MBA. He had begun to experience left-sided chest pain during exertion and while stressed. This resulted in multiple trips to the Emergency Room where he was tested and cleared for cardiac pathology. Instead he was given a diagnosis of anxiety disorder, which he found quite disturbing and quite frankly unbelievable as he had always seen himself as a 'cool, coping kind of guy'. He was certain that he had a cardiac problem that was missed. Examination identified a myofascial trigger point in his left pectoralis minor that reproduced left-sided chest pain when palpated. His $ETCO_2$ was found to be 30 mmHg. Intramuscular needle stimulation helped to deactivate the trigger point but did not solve the exertional or stress related chest pain. While lying supine he was able to bring his $ETCO_2$ up to 40 mmHg fairly easily, following good breathing principles reinforced with wave play. Once he sat up, his $ETCO_2$ promptly plummeted and became worse on standing. He held himself rigidly upright in an almost military posture, projecting an image of being 'strong' and 'ready'. This was pointed out, and he worked to release his global muscles and adopt a more relaxed posture while watching the capnograph. As he relaxed and tuned into his breath he was able to bring the $ETCO_2$ numbers up to 40 mmHg. The next step was to have him connected to the capnometer while using his smartphone. The minute he

concentrated on the screen his numbers went down. He was able to see the difference, as to how his breathing had changed, and learned to change it back. The true epiphany however came while on a business trip to San Francisco. Air travel often challenges poor breathers as airplanes are pressurized to about 7000 feet. That means there is less oxygen available, which stimulates the peripheral chemoreceptors in the aorta. This increases the respiratory drive, resulting in a higher minute volume to meet oxygen requirements. People who already have a tendency to overbreathe will often respond to the increase in drive by breathing more rapidly. This produces feelings of breathlessness, establishing an overbreathing vicious cycle resulting in hypocapnia. Exertion had always been a trigger for him. Walking the San Francisco hills while sightseeing, compounded by the stress of wanting to do a stellar job, worked together to produce a full blown chest pain episode. He was fearful that he was having a fatal heart attack. He checked his breath and realized he was breathing poorly. He changed it back to the breathing he had come to associate with good breathing chemistry, and his chest pain went away. He *finally* accepted that it was indeed his breath that was responsible for his chest pain and there truly wasn't a lurking cardiac problem. It was very gratifying to witness his new-found confidence, once he felt assured that his heart was healthy and he no longer fitted the 'anxiety disorder' label.

changing the breathing volume, rate or location (back to diaphragmatic from upper chest) in order to bring the CO_2 levels back up. Once the values can be brought down and up at will, the mastering of breathing difficulties is under way. By attending to ever-subtler cues of when blood chemistry is changing as symptoms appear, by checking the breathing pattern, and when necessary reverting to breathing well, the symptoms of poor breathing can become the stimulus for improved breathing.

High performance and sport

When treating endurance athletes, capnography can be used while exercising on a bike or treadmill to isolate the anaerobic threshold (see Ch. 6.6). Wave play can help to extend the individual's time in the aerobic envelope. Carbon dioxide feedback is an excellent way for athletes to become sensitive to the signs of anaerobic metabolism. By learning these signs, the athlete can remain in the aerobic window while performing an endurance sport.

Case history

E, a health professional, had days when she experienced dyspnoea, a sense of being unable to get a satisfying breath. Some mornings she would find herself unable to go to work as she couldn't 'catch her breath'. Careful interviewing about symptom onset was an integral part of helping her to understand her problem. Questioning revealed that it did not occur upon waking and was not present until she was sitting eating breakfast, and thinking about her upcoming day. It became clear that the stress she was feeling about the day ahead changed her breathing, making her feel short of breath. Her response to this symptom involved trying even harder to achieve a satisfying breath, making her feel even worse. Once this cycle was established she did not know how to get herself out of it, resulting in some missed work days. Intentional overbreathing while connected to the capnograph reproduced her feelings of breathlessness and dyspnoea. When she replicated her typical response, her ETCO$_2$ levels went even lower. She was able to see that her strategy for managing the symptoms actually made her worse. Once she de-emphasized inhalation and focused on relaxing through exhalation, while watching the waveforms (wave play) she learned how to change her breathing for the better and stopped her sense of breathlessness. This process offered her insight to her thoughts, feelings and stressors. When she began to have feelings of breathlessness she learned to become an observer of her thoughts, facilitating good 'mental hygiene' where she opted to change her negative self-talk, to something more positive. Now, instead of falling victim to a conditioned response, she monitors her breath, allowing her to choose to breathe well.

When the individual can identify signs that suggest that the anaerobic threshold is approaching, effort/exertion can be reduced in order to prevent the threshold being crossed, allowing continued participation in the activity.

Athletes have been shown to reach exhaustion 45 seconds sooner when they overbreathe before exercising (Walsh et al 2006). This has implications for achieving best performances. Capnography can help athletes to identify faulty breathing patterns, triggered by stress for example, and to learn to change them. (See Ch. 7.6 for more on breathing and the athlete.)

Since respiratory chemistry has such an impact on oxygen delivery (Levitsky 2007, Thomson et al 1997) athletic performance can be adversely affected by poor breathing habits. A top level figure skater had trouble with leg pain while skating. The pain became pronounced in specific sections of her programme. Using mental imagery to run through her programme while connected to a capnograph, it became clear that she became hypocapnic during those painful times. When she identified the faulty breathing, and improved it, her pain diminished, helping her deliver an Olympic gold medal-winning performance. Any sport requiring focus and precision (golf, marksmanship, etc) can be enhanced when the brain is more fully perfused with oxygen, which can only occur with optimal breathing. Capnography can provide feedback to the athlete and therefore assist them in achieving their personal best.

COMMON CLINICAL PRESENTATIONS

Breathing too fast

When the respiratory rate goes above the typical 8–14 breaths per minute at rest, there is a tendency toward an increased minute volume. The amount of air passed through the lungs is in excess of that required to support the metabolic requirements at the time, resulting in hypocapnia.

Once the person is connected to the capnograph it can be useful to switch to the 'Mechanics Training' screen to match the current breathing rate, and to then request that attention be paid to that rate. The individual will often comment that it seems fast. Adjusting the screen to a slower rate that is within the 'normal' resting rate – say 12 breaths per minute – allows observation as to how that affects the CO_2 reading.

To further investigate the effect of different breathing rates on CO_2 levels, modification of the breathing rate to the low normal range, followed by raising to an even higher level than at the start, offers further challenges. Initiating another drop provides the individual a chance to experience and reflect on the feelings associated with these different rates. Tuning into the *feelings* is a valuable tool in learning self-regulation.

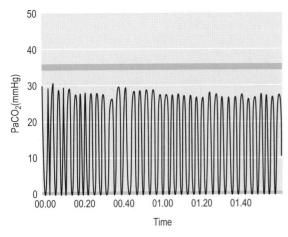

Figure 7.7.3 Rapid (20 breaths per minute) breathing rate.

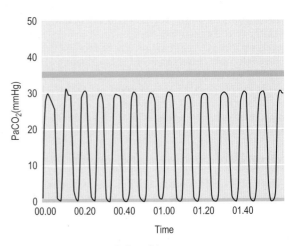

Figure 7.7.4 Hypocapnic breathing.

Case history

A university student complained of back pain and was clearly anxious (fidgeting etc.). She was unable to sit and study due both to her back pain and an inability to concentrate. She was breathing at 20 breaths per minute when sitting at rest (Fig. 7.7.3). An obvious place to start was to have her decrease her breathing rate in order to see if it had an effect on the $ETCO_2$ level. With this patient, a simple decrease in respiratory rate, along with a manual therapy and motor control approach to her back pain, allowed her to sit comfortably and to focus sufficiently to study and pass her exams. Breathing retraining was necessary as the manual therapy approach to her pain was used initially and brought only moderate success. Once the breathing intervention was added there was an abrupt improvement in her symptoms, and it was then far easier for her to activate her core muscles. Before the breathing retraining she struggled with being able to isolate the core muscles.

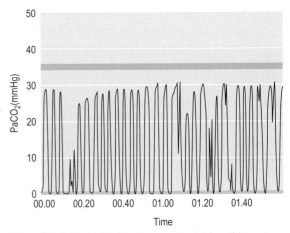

Figure 7.7.5 Rapid (18 breaths per minute) breathing rate.

Too much volume

Sometimes the respiratory rate can be within normal limits and yet the person is still hypocapnic, as in the screen image below (Fig. 7.7.4). If the rate is normal and the $ETCO_2$ is low it means that the volume is too high. This pattern is often associated with upper chest breathing.

There are many different methods that can help people to stop breathing in their upper chests, for example, monitoring the upper chest with one hand and the abdomen with the other can help bring awareness to the faulty mechanics, setting the stage for change (see HiLo test in Ch. 6.2, Fig. 6.2.1). In addition, requesting 'quiet breathing', taking in only a gentle sip of air, can be helpful. The idea of breathing 'up from the toes' can also assist individuals to maintain the focus (and locus) low, rather than in the upper chest. Using a tactile reminder such as TheraBand™ or even a towel around the lower chest can bring focus to that area and facilitate movement there. Lying supine and even raising the lower body relative to the upper body with cushions or bridging can stimulate diaphragmatic or lower chest breathing. Using negative play can also help the patient isolate the 'feel' of where they are breathing so they can 'find it' and make the appropriate change. Which particular strategy is best can be determined by watching the capnography readings or engaging in 'wave play'.

Poor rate, pattern and ETCO₂

In Fig. 7.7.5, the patient is breathing too quickly at 18 breaths per minute, with a choppy pattern and low $ETCO_2$

Case history

A patient with fibromyalgia, tested at 26 mmHg ETCO$_2$ while lying supine (Fig. 7.7.6A) – her best reading of the standardized tests (and where the low end of normal is 35 mmHg). She was enthusiastic about wanting to change her breathing and went home to practise, however she ended up decreasing her respiratory rate as well as her ETCO$_2$ values which went down when re-tested to 23 mmHg (Fig. 7.7.6B)! Her intentional manipulation of her breath had a negative effect. The patient opted to rent a capnograph for home use, to ensure that she was practising correctly. She started with normalizing her ETCO$_2$ levels, while lying supine, using wave play, counting her breath to optimize the ratio of inhalation/exhalation, followed by a brief pause, while saying 'ahhhhh' to herself as she exhaled. When she was able to get her ETCO$_2$ consistently above 35 mmHg, she moved to sitting, and went through the same process. After that she worked on standing, doing meal preparation in the kitchen and eventually walking on the treadmill. Her pain levels improved dramatically as did her functional level. She was able to participate in a Pilates exercise programme without experiencing any exacerbation of her symptoms, which had been a problem for her in past attempts at exercise.

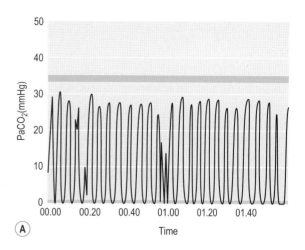

(A)

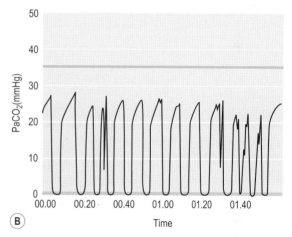

(B)

Figure 7.7.6 A Patient lying supine with low ETCO$_2$ (26 mmHg) readings together with rapid breathing rate. **B** After ineffective home practising, breathing rate and ETCO2 decreased to 23 mmHg.

(27 mmHg). With so many things to work on, it is tempting to tell the patient many things all at once, which can be confusing, leading to further distress. If this occurs, it might be useful to simplify and pick one thing to work on at first. Most overbreathing incorporates too much inhalation and not enough exhalation. Especially not enough *release* to *allow* the exhalation. It is helpful to encourage the patient to (silently) say 'ahh' during exhalation. This encourages a release of tension.

It is important for patients to learn that there is no need to struggle for the next breath, but to simply allow it to come. Monitoring the response with the capnograph readings of ETCO$_2$ can help both patient and therapist to determine which intervention is improving matters. Often it is best to begin in supine where there are no competing postural demands for the musculature.

Dissociative overbreathing

When overbreathing to dissociate is more pervasive, and is related to past trauma, improving ETCO$_2$ values with breathing interventions may result in the resurfacing of unwanted memories and emotions requiring collaboration with a mental health professional. This concept is discussed more fully in Chapter 6.4.

CONCLUSION

Capnography can assist in designing specific, individualized treatment and management strategies. Having concrete, objective information to work with provides clarity to both the practitioner and the patient, improving the efficiency and effectiveness of the intervention. By providing real-time information about the success (or lack thereof) of any breathing intervention there is confidence instilled in the successful strategies, facilitating a sense of mastery.

Case history

One young boy used breath to dissociate when anxious about being called upon by the teacher – essentially becoming 'absent', not attending to the teacher's questions. The outcome however added to future anxiety rather than diminishing it, as the teacher became frustrated with the boy's lack of response. He himself, his teacher and his parents were all at a loss to explain what happened to him at these times, in class. When connected to the capnograph, and going through a 'think test' where he imagined himself in his classroom being asked a question, it became clear that he changed his breathing at such moments, causing him to become significantly hypocapnic, allowing him to dissociate from an uncomfortable situation. He confirmed that he experienced the same feeling he had while being asked questions in class. Once he was able to identify his altered breathing as the source of the behaviour he could use the capnograph readings to retrain his breathing and learn the difference between the type of breathing that 'spaced him out', and the type that kept him focused.

Another example involved a person who realized that she used to use breath to dissociate in childhood, in response to repeated stints of enforced bed rest due to a recurrent childhood illness. She dealt with her frustration about not being able to go outside to play with her friends, by changing her breathing and essentially 'blissing out'. The habit of overbreathing in response to frustration followed her into adulthood and resulted in angry outbursts that challenged her relationships – which by all accounts were far from bliss full! With capnography training – specifically intentional overbreathing, she was able to identify and associate the change in breathing chemistry with her unwanted emotional response. She was then able to reverse the change in breathing and thereby learn to control her outbursts.

REFERENCES

Benchetrit, G., 2000. Breathing pattern in humans: diversity and individuality. Respiration Physiology 122, 123–129.

Bernardi, L., Sleight, P., Bandinelli, G., et al., 2001. Effect of rosary prayer and yoga mantras on autonomic cardiovascular rhythms: comparative study. British Medical Journal 323, 1446–1449.

Callaham, M., 1989. Hypoxic hazards of traditional paper bag rebreathing in hyperventilating patients. Annals of Emergency Medicine 18 (6), 622–628.

Fried, R., 1999. Breathe well, be well. John Wiley & Sons. Toronto ON.

Levitsky, M.G., 2007. Pulmonary physiology, sixth ed. McGraw–Hill, Toronto ON.

Litchfield, P., 2012. Respiratory fitness and dysfunctional breathing workshop. Santa Fe, NM.

McLaughlin, L., 2009. Breathing evaluation and retraining in manual therapy. Journal of Bodywork and Movement Therapy 13, 276–282.

Thomson, W.S.T., Adams, J.F., Cowan, R.A., 1997. Clinical acid–base balance. Oxford University Press, New York, NY.

Walsh, M., Takeda, C., Takahashi, A., et al., 2006. Volitional hyperventilation during ramp exercise to exhaustion. Applied Physiology, Nutrition, and Metabolism. 31, 211–217.

Chapter | **8.1** |

Breathing patterns in longstanding pain disorders: a somatocognitive approach to evaluation and therapy

Gro K. Haugstad, Tor S. Haugstad

CHAPTER CONTENTS

ABSTRACT

Longstanding pain is associated with alterations in static and dynamic motor patterns of respiration. We have developed and validated a method for assessment of motor behaviours including breathing movements (the *Standardized Mensendieck Test, SMT*), and a therapy modality that integrates physiotherapy and cognitive psychotherapy (*somatocognitive therapy*) in order to optimize these motor patterns. In a randomized, controlled clinical intervention study of women with chronic pelvic pain (CPP) we have demonstrated that this intervention leads to great improvements in motor patterns of breathing and other elements of motor behaviour. We are currently investigating the effect of this intervention in other pain disorders.

BACKGROUND

Clinical exposure to patients with longstanding pain inadvertently brings to attention that their pattern of respiration is altered. Since these motor patterns to the eyes of the trained observer are rather striking, we have searched for tools for the practical evaluation of such patterns, applicable in clinical settings. The effect of the altered pattern of motor activity can be assessed by measuring the chemical consequences thereof for the composition of the blood or the exhaled air (pH, pO_2, pCO_2). However, when looking for instruments that describe the movements proper, we came to draw from the Scandinavian tradition of body examinations (see below). Since these instruments are based on psychodynamic theories, and are rather extensive and time consuming for practical clinical work, we found that there was a need for a new instrument that could be used to assess quality of movements according to principles derived from functional anatomy, and in keeping with a theoretical framework based on the cognitive abilities of the conscious mental domains. Such an instrument should allow therapists who are thoroughly trained in observation and visual analysis of the quality of movements, to rate the different static and dynamic motor patterns, not only of breathing, but also of posture, gait and overall motor behaviours. Scandinavian countries also benefit from several decades of exposure to the Mensendieck tradition (Mensendieck 1954) of comprehensive assessment of motor behaviours, and in Norway this tradition has developed into a school of physiotherapy that approaches such assessment as well as physical therapies in a rigorous, standardized way (Klemmetsen 2005, Halvorsen 2009). Thus, it came ready at hand to develop the Standardized Mensendieck Test (SMT) for the assessment of posture, gait, movement, sitting posture and breathing (Haugstad et al 2006).

The therapeutic approach derived from the Mensendieck tradition combines elements of physical therapy (postural adjustments, breathing regulation, feedback on movement patterns) and elements of self-perception and body awareness. The procedure is a sequence of learning and training that includes developing new motor patterns, in conjunction with full attention of being in one's own body, and integrating these movement patterns in the common activities of daily living. The goal is to improve the functionality of these patterns, through improved body awareness, in combination with learning new habits of movement and breathing. The originator of this approach, Bess Mensendieck, was a contemporary of Sigmund Freud, studying under the same mentor, the founder of the Paris School of Neurology, Professor Jean-Martin Charcot. While Freud later developed his theory mainly around the mental faculties of the unconscious self, Mensendieck was fascinated by the works of Guillaume-Benjamin-Amand Duchenne (Mensendieck 1937), who demonstrated how the central and peripheral nervous systems controlled muscular activity, and thus motor patterns. She was aware of the mental aspects of the effort it takes to change ingrained motor patterns, and that these efforts were often underestimated. In the Mensendieck tradition, this focus on voluntary control of motor behaviours has been quite clear from the original works of Bess Mensendieck. However, the mental parts of therapy may at some points in time have caught less attention than the biomechanical and anatomical aspects of the tradition. In our opinion, it is the integration of mind and body that are so characteristic of this tradition within physical therapy, and it is this integrative approach that we have sought to bring to attention in our work within the field of psychosomatic medicine. Thus, in order to underscore the cognitive aspect of Mensendieck therapy, and bring the mental aspects of the therapeutic approach into conscious attention, we prefer the term 'somatocognitive therapy' as the label of the treatment approach we have applied in our clinical work (Haugstad & Haugstad 2011).

Somatocognitive therapy can thus be understood as a hybrid between physiotherapy and psychotherapy. As such, it is a short-term body-oriented therapy, concentrating on the situation here and now – not focusing on the possible historical roots of the symptoms. The goal is to achieve new body awareness through explorative treatment with functional goals linked to the activities of daily living. The authors were first acquainted with cognitive psychotherapy through Aaron Beck's collaborator, Arthur Freeman (Freeman & Greenwood 1987), who visited Modum Bad

Psychiatric Hospital (Vikersund, Norway), in 1987 as this form of therapy was first introduced into the treatment of anxiety states, firstly for phobic anxiety. It occurred to us that the rigorous and systematic approach to psychotherapy advocated by Freeman and Beck had strong similarities with the Mensendieck tradition of physiotherapy, as it had been developed over the years in the Oslo school (Halvorsen 2009). However, a series of amendments had to be made to amalgamate the two therapy traditions. This work was undertaken together with Professor Ulrik Malt at the University of Oslo, in the Department of Psychosomatic Medicine at Rikshospitalet in the 1990s. The intention of our work has been to develop instruments with the aim of evaluating and treating patients with longstanding pain states and complex disorders, such as gynaecological pain, low back pain, chest pain and widespread pain.

Pain severely affects breathing patterns (Kvåle et al 2002, Haugstad et al 2006). Thus, it came as no surprise that breathing patterns received low scores in a clinical population of pain patients. In our studies, breathing patterns were also among the motor behaviours that benefited the most from the somatocognitive intervention.

THEORY

Mensendieck physiotherapy also contains in origin many of the fundamental principles later developed in theories of motor learning (Fitts & Posner 1967, Gentile 1998, Higgins 1991, Carr & Shepherd 2010, Facchini et al 2002, Hodges & Franks 2002, Flanagan et al 2003). The focus is on cognitive awareness of experience in one's own body, and the process of learning new motor patterns in contrast to old habits (Soukup et al 1999, Kendall et al 2000, Haugstad 2000, Kirste et al 2002, Klemmetsen 2005). New motor patterns are developed through three phases:

1. The cognitive phase, where the conscious awareness of the patient is directed towards sensory input from visual, tactile and proprioceptive stimuli regarding their own body, and compared to ideal mentations with regard to the quality of new patterns being sought;

2. The associative phase, where a consciousness gradually develops that integrates the new ideal patterns with new sensory input from the body; and

3. The automatized phase, where the new and more efficient or functional motor patterns are utilized without conscious thought, and gradually integrated into behavioural patterns in the activities of daily life. Thus, important basic elements are sensory awareness of one's own body, conscious cognition of new ideomotor patterns and integrations of the new experience into everyday functions (Mensendieck 1954).

The first step, and prerequisite of all therapy, is to develop a good working alliance with the patient, without which therapy will be futile (Lambert et al 2004). This can be rapidly achieved in the first encounter with the patient, once the therapist opens to empathic listening to the case history of the patient. The treatment session can then continue by describing a possible explanation for the reported symptoms, and a dialogue thus develops between the therapist and the patient with regard to body experiences (see below). The therapist teaches the patient about the mind/body relations, and explains pain mechanism, in line with the principles of essential cognitive pain education that Lidbeck recommends (2002). Again, the therapist's empathic attitude is of decisive importance to develop the necessary therapeutic alliance with these patients, who have often suffered a great deal (Nerdrum 2000, Kåver 2012).

The generation of movements is initiated by mental efforts, and in therapy this needs to be brought to conscious attention by mentally rehearsing the movement ahead of time, before the physical execution of the movement proper. Thus, the training programmes start with the teacher and pupil imagining (sketching) the movement to be practised (Mensendieck 1937, 1954). In physiologic terms, this preparation for movement involves several areas frontal to the primary motor cortex (Facchini et al 2002, Flanagan et al 2003). This form of ideomotor preparation of the movement proper, called 'motor templates', has been shown to enhance motor learning (Fitts & Posner 1967, Flanagan et al 2003). The focus on the cognition preceding movement, as well as the focus on practising new motor patterns in the activities of daily life, can also be said to be more in keeping with cognitive therapy, developed by Ellis, Beck, Freeman and others (Beck 1976, Freeman & Greenwood 1987).

An additional important aspect of Mensendieck therapy is the focus on the state of tension of a specific group of muscles or agonist. The patient's awareness is guided towards increase of tension in the muscle (maximal contraction), and the decrease of tension (maximal relaxation). This awareness of tension and relaxation is also sought to be integrated into the movements of daily living, much in keeping with the principles of applied relaxation (Öst 1987).

Similar to patients in cognitive therapy, the patients treated by a Mensendieck therapist are always assigned graded tasks to be practised several times each day, preferably while performing the activities of a normal life (Mensendieck 1937, 1954). Thus, the new motor programmes are sought to be automatized and internalized in the patient, including the pattern of tension and relaxation of agonist and antagonist muscle groups.

Mensendieck physiotherapy trainees are taught in a systematic way to be aware of their own bodily experience, thus developing a high level of body awareness themselves, an awareness always sought to be transferred to the pupil or the patient (Mensendieck 1954, Soukop et al 1999, Haugstad 2000, Kendall et al 2000, Klemmetsen 2005, Haugstad et al 2006). We view this as being a very valuable part of physiotherapy training. Unless the therapist himself has been trained in conscious experience of proprioceptive signals from their own body, it is hard to imagine that such consciousness might be transferred to the patient.

Somatocognitive therapy

In somatocognitive therapy the primary goal is for the patient to achieve new body awareness through explorative treatment with functional goals linked into the activities of daily living. As sessions evolve, the therapy necessarily leads to the disclosure of repressed emotions. This is not the primary goal of the therapy, but on the other hand, emotions should be given room and be received by the empathic therapist. The therapist and the patient are seen as equally important partners in exploring the experiences of the patient. As in cognitive therapy, the therapy session is three-phased:

1. The patient recounts from his or her experience since the last session, reports on homework done, and possible new experiences or insights evolved through the new movements that have been practised in the activities of daily living.

2. Learning new active movements in a graded task assignment – again to be practised several times each day, not as separate exercise sessions, but well-integrated in the activities of the day, such as while walking to the bus, sitting in the office, lying down in bed, watching the television, while eating and performing chores. This may influence muscle relaxation, respiration, the flexibility of joints, muscles and ligaments, straining workloads on muscles and joints, extero- and proprioception, awareness of their own body, and reduced fear of movement (kinesophobia) (Vlaeyen et al 2007). It is of utmost importance that the training is started in a gentle manner, and that exercise does not exceed the patient's capacities in any way. These patients often have a long history of suffering from aches and pains, which traps them in a passive lifestyle with fear of movement. An abrupt change to vigorous physical activity may result in physiological responses characterized by increased pain, due to mechanisms such as long-term potentiation (LTP) and wind-up (Staud et al 2005). Often manual release of the tensed muscles may be given, with a dual purpose: first, it improves the circulation of blood to the relevant muscles and leads to new tactile experiences; secondly, it leads to release of endogenic substances like oxytocin (Meyer-Lidenberg 2008), that are known to promote relaxation and foster bonding between therapist and patient. The

second part of the therapy session is always concluded with a brief session of Applied Relaxation.[1]

3. New assignments are given as homework for the patient, again underscoring that the most important part of therapy takes place during the intervals between therapy sessions. The therapist constantly checks that the patient understands the significance of each step, and that the working alliance is upheld.

Development of a Standardized Mensendieck Test (SMT)

A Standardized Mensendieck Test (SMT) was developed to evaluate posture, movement, gait, sitting posture and breathing patterns of patients with chronic pelvic pain, based on the Mensendieck principles of observation and analysis of motor function (Table 8.1.1). To validate the test and to make a comprehensive body examination of a defined group of patients, it was applied in this study of women with chronic pelvic pain (Haugstad 2000). In the context of this chapter we shall focus mainly on the evaluation of breathing movements.

Breathing

Breathing patterns were observed by asking the participants to lie down on the bench with the legs straight. We told the participant that we were observing her in the supine position. In the second observation in this subtest, we asked the subject to flex her knees from the supine position, with the plantar surface on the bench, and we asked her to lift up her pelvis, keep it in this position for 5 seconds and again lower the pelvis. At the same time we observed the respiratory response that occurs as a reflex after completion of this movement. The very last observation and movement in this subtest was to look at breathing with the patient in the supine position as we instructed her to 'Lift the arms up and place them over your head, resting on the bench, keep them there for a short while, then lift them again, and place them along side the body on the bench.' Here we also observed breathing responses after completion of the movement.

Video records were then blinded and analyzed. Each element of the test was assigned a score from 0 to 7, where 0 is the least functional movement and 7 the score for an optimal performance (see Haugstad et al 2006 for greater details).

[1]Applied Relaxation begins with training in Progressive Muscle Relaxation, which is gradually developed into a cue-controlled relaxation coping skill, and systematically applied during *in vivo* exposure to feared situations. Although essentially a form of modern behaviour therapy, Applied Relaxation has also been used in combination with cognitive restructuring as part of a cognitive-behavioural therapy (CBT) approach (see also Öst 1987).

Table 8.1.1 Standardized Mensendieck Test (SMT)

Posture	Score	Movement	Score
Global/line of gravity		Vertical arm lift	
Ankle		Sagittal arm swing	
Knee		Diagonal arm swing	
Pelvis		Balance/hip flexion	
Back		**Average**	
Shoulder		**Sitting posture**	**Score**
Neck		Global	
Average		Support	
Gait	**Score**	Pelvis	
Global		Back	
Foot roll		**Average**	
Propulsion		**Breathing**	**Score**
Rotation		Global	
Average		Armlift	
Movement	**Score**	Pelvic lift	
Global		**Average**	
Frontal arm lift			

The Standardized Mensendieck Test (SMT) scores the motor patterns with regards to posture, movement, gait, sitting posture and breathing. See Methods for explanation. For further details, see Haugstad et al (2006).

Elements used in breathing therapy in a somatocognitive session

The first patient encounter is usually the session where the patient is thoroughly examined by the therapist. As described above, most of the patients with longstanding pain display an affected pattern of respiration (i.e. low scores) in the SMT test. We also observe the respiratory pattern throughout the clinical session, when the patient engages in dialogue with the therapist, during undressing and dressing in the session, and we look for clinical signs which may affect breathing such as an epigastric incision or the use of the accessory breathing muscles (the scalenes and the sternocleidomastoid muscles).

The next step is to establish a working alliance with the patient, i.e. that the patient accepts that his or her breathing pattern is affected, and that this is of relevance to the symptoms constituting the patient's complaints. The empathic therapeutic attitude is of great importance in all forms of therapy. In the past decade, the working alliance has emerged as possibly the most important conceptualization of the common elements in diverse therapy modalities. The working alliance is the product of the patient's and the therapist's conscious determination and ability to work together (Hall et al 2010, Bordin 1979).

In order to establish this kind of mutual relationship with the patient, it is important to direct the patient's attention to how their breathing pattern is affected, and how the motor patterns of a healthy respiratory practice are conducted. To this end, we use diverse simple means, such as an anatomical chart displaying the muscles used during the respiratory cycle of inspiration and expiration, mirrors where the patient can observe himself while the therapist brings to his attention the patterns he is using, all the time using open, Socratic questions, like: 'What do you see now?', 'What do you feel now?' or 'Do you feel that you can fill your lungs to the very bottom, so that your abdomen expands?' The therapist can also demonstrate on his/her own body how he or she is performing when it comes to breathing movements.

We often start with the patient in a sitting position, bringing the patient's attention to how his sitting position is, i.e. it should be a relaxed position, with the soles of the feet both resting on the floor. The patient is asked to place his hands, one over the costal rim and the other over the abdomen and feel the movement of the thorax and abdomen during the respiratory cycle (see Fig. 6.2.1). If their breathing is affected, the patient may relate that they cannot feel any movement of these parts of their body. Since they are lifting their upper thorax and their shoulders, the abdomen is often retracted rather than being expanded during inspiration. Then, the therapist may place his hands on the sides of the lower part of the chest of the patient, and exert a gentle pressure, asking the patient to expand the chest against the forces exerted on it, while asking the patient to inhale. The mechanical force exerted on the chest will bring the patient's attention to the part of the body he should move (by means of somatosensory awareness of that part of the body), and so it is easier for the patient to exercise an intentional movement of a part of the body they have more or less been unaware of. The patient may also be asked to lift his shoulders towards his ears, or tilt the position of the pelvis thus forming a lumbar lordosis, and at the same time take a deep breath, while both the patient and the therapist is assessing how the abdomen expands to accommodate for volume shift from the retracting diaphragm. While performing these simple movements, the patient will often experience and complain of spells of dizziness that may frighten the patient. If this happens, the therapist reassures the patient that this is a totally acceptable and even normal experience, derived from the fact that the respiratory pattern has been frozen in a dysfunctional

manner, and now that this pattern is challenged, and by all the performances of deep inhalation, this may have led to an exaggerated lowering of carbon dioxide levels in the alveolar air. The patient is told that he can continue the exercise in a gentle manner several times a day, during breakfast, at work, in front of the TV set, etc., and experiment by using the old and the new muscular patterns of breathing (for example deep tidal breaths in combination with relaxation in sitting postion, standing and lying postion).

Likewise, breathing exercises can be taught with patients in the supine position, asking the patient to lift the lower back and lower it again while breathing, retracting one leg by the hip, rotating outward in the hip, and extending the leg again, all while inhaling and exhaling. Initially, the therapist may assist the movement, thus demonstrating to the patient how it should be conducted (see Klemmetsen 2005).

At the end of a session, the patient will be given assignments or homework, of exercises and experiments to be performed several times daily, during activities of daily living, reporting back to the therapist in later sessions from the motor experiences, concurrent thoughts that may appear, emotions that emerge and other somatic sensations that develop (such as dizziness, fatigue, changes in patterns of pain and sleepiness, etc). The patients should be prepared by the therapist for such experiences to occur, thus pre-empting the fears that such phenomena might otherwise evoke.

As the therapy progresses, we again review the results from the SMT test, looking at the patient's stance and gait, and gradually start working with the breathing pattern in these positions. This is often difficult to accomplish, and the therapist often has to resort to well-known reflexes tied to the respiratory pattern, such as exercises with rotatory movements of the spinal column in its different segments, stretching of the body with arms above the head, all the time drawing the patient's attention to how this influences the patterns of breathing. Until a functional breathing pattern becomes automatic, the patient may need repeated reminders of how he is performing. At the end of each therapy session, we always include progressive relaxation (Jacobson 1938), adding to the traditional techniques that focus on respiration and breathing patterns as an integral part. As in cognitive therapy, the home assignment tasks are graded, in the sense that the movement patterns that have to be practised several times every day, integrated in the activities of daily living, gradually increase in complexity, much like a piano teacher would add complexity to the scales, triads, études and music until automated mastery is gained.

The progressive steps from the simple to the more complex represented by the development in therapy described above is in accord with the Norwegian body-oriented therapy tradition as developed after the encounters of Wilhelm Reich and Trygve Braatøy in Norway

(Haugstad & Haugstad 2011), as it is also described by Lillemor Johnsen (1981). Johnsen relates to this progression in psychodynamic terms, with reference to Braatøy, as she describes how 'muscular tensions (are) a physical aspect of the patient's defence against unrelieved impulses.' Braatøy 'introduced the supine position in the treatment of neurotic patients in order to bring about the relaxation of posture necessary for giving the treatment its effect.' Again, 'he proposed an actively sensing attitude on the part of the physiotherapist, that he adapt and coordinate the approach to the musculature to the respiratory rhythm of the patient.' This is in keeping with our experience, that in order to facilitate an improvement in the motor patterns of breathing, it is necessary to start working with the patterns evoked by respiratory reflexes is the supine position. Braatøy and Johnsen also underscore their observation that anxiety states are expressed in stereotypic motor behaviours, involving posture and breathing. However, in our therapy we are not focusing on the tensed muscles as representing unsolved unconscious emotional conflicts, and we usually encourage the use of the tied muscles themselves as a means towards muscular release. Sometimes a direct muscular release is necessary, first by gently stroking the area, then by transverse rubs on the muscles involved. The use of mirrors in therapy in order to give the patient feedback on his tensed motor patterns (along with observations of the results from the SMT), in addition to being in harmony with the tradition from Mensendieck, is also in keeping with a widespread practice among physiotherapists using mirror therapy in the management of problems of posture and movement (Watson 2011).

Some results from studies using somatocognitive therapy in populations of pain patients

In an RCT study of 40 patients with chronic pelvic pain (CPP) recruited from the Department of Gynaecology at Rikshospitalet, Oslo University Hospital, patients were assessed for posture and movement patterns with the SMT. All subscores were found to be significantly lower in the patients (p levels < 0.01) than those of the healthy controls (Haugstad et al 2006). The largest differences in scores between the two groups were found for gait, movement and breathing. The subscores were 54% lower for pelvic rotation in the gait group of scores and 52% lower for pelvic lift in the respiration group and diagonal arm swing in the movement group, respectively, compared with the healthy controls. The least difference between the patients and the controls were found in the subscores for posture. The greatest deviation from normal pattern was found for tests that posed a demand on balance and coordination. In the test for hip flexion, the patients had great difficulties when trying to stand on one leg for 10 seconds, scoring 38% below the healthy controls. Further, their ability to coordinate the movements of both arms and both legs in

the sagittal (33%) and diagonal arm swing tests (39%) were well below the healthy controls. The ability to not give in to gravity was found to be reduced in the patients compared to controls, when testing their ability to lift extended arms to shoulder height, and let them fall down. When examining gait we observed a careful gait with short steps and almost no foot propulsion, and a markedly reduced hip extension in the propulsion phase. The typical findings in respiration are high costal breathing with almost no movement in the lower thorax or in the abdominal area (Haugstad et al 2006, appendix). In the evaluation of respiration the scores differed 52% from the healthy controls. The movement pattern may be ascribed to what we call a typical pelvic pain protection pattern (PPP). The patients protect their pelvis in gait, movement and in respiration.

After 90 days of treatment the CPP patients in the Mensendieck somatocognitive therapy group (MSCT) had significantly improved scores in all subtests of the SMT. The patients receiving standard gynaecological treatment only (STGT) for the most part did not show any significant changes of scores. The best treatment response in the STGT + MSCT group was found in the case of scores for respiration. The second group of functions that improved considerably was movement. The patients demonstrated the largest improvement in the movement function tests designed to demonstrate coordination, and the ability to relax. The average SMT score values after treatment were 4.37 ± 0.38 (up 19.3%) for posture, 4.13 ± 0.38 (up 26.1%) for movement, 4.13 ± 0.39 (up 24.8%) for gait, 4.67 ± 0.36 (up 27.9%) for sitting posture, and a considerable increase to 4.72 ± 0.37 (up 58.4%) in the scores for respiration.

The patients' subjective experience of pain was assessed by means of a visual analogue scale (VAS). Before treatment, the patients randomized into the group receiving standard gynaecological treatment scored an average of 6.68 ± 0.29 (average ± standard error). After the treatment period of 90 days, the average VAS score was 6.16 ± 0.50, a reduction by 7.8% (non-significant). The patients in the Mensendieck somatocognitive therapy group scored an average of 5.60 ± 0.40 at baseline. After the 90-day treatment programme, the average score was 2.89 ± 0.40, down by 48.4 %.

When the patients were evaluated with a new SMT and VAS 9 months after the end of treatment, patients in the group receiving standard gynaecological treatment showed no significant change in motor performance. At one year follow-up, the tendencies for the performance of the motor functions on a general level was an increased deterioration, even significantly for some of the subtests in the STGT group (Haugstad et al 2008).

By contrast, the patients receiving Mensendieck somatocognitive therapy demonstrated improved scores after treatment. Moreover the effect of therapy lasted for the 9 months follow-up period, and most functions even improved further after the end of therapy. The scores 9 months after treatment were 4.66 ± 0.30 (up 4.0 %, non-significant change from end of treatment) for posture, 4.85 ± 0.33 (up 13.0 %, p < 0.02) for movement, 4.54 ± 0.39 (up 10.0 %, p < 0.001) for gait, 5.01 ± 0.36 (up 7.2%, non-significant change from end of treatment) for sitting posture, and a considerable increase to 5.36 ± 0.35 (up 13.5%, p < 0.05) in the scores for respiration.

The largest change 9 months after treatment was seen in the respiratory response to lifting and lowering the arms from the supine position ('armlift' – see the test manual, appendix of Haugstad et al 2006). Score for this function increased from 4.68 ± 0.31 to 5.50 ± 0.39 (up 20.2%, p < 0.01) (Haugstad et al 2008).

Preliminary results from ongoing studies on patients with neck and shoulder pain, low back pain, provoked vulvodynia and widespread pain (fibromyalgia) show the same tendency to large improvements in breathing patterns, sometimes occurring concurrently with relief from pain, sometimes well ahead of relief from experienced pain.

CONCLUSION

We suggest that this pattern of further improvement of function during the follow-up period in this RCT study is due to a learning effect. The patients have learned to move in a more natural and relaxed manner. The pelvic protection pattern is thus changed to a more functional and flexible use of the pelvis that promotes blood circulation and lymphatic drainage.

Perhaps most importantly the pattern of breathing is changed, with active use of the diaphragm, and thoracic and low abdominal expansion during inspiration. The aim is that these new patterns will be automatized and integrated in the patient's new image of their own body. These new motor skills are, in turn, utilized without the patient's conscious awareness, and they are gradually interwoven as natural parts of their new daily performance.

Thus, in our opinion, somatocognitive therapy may prove a useful interventional tool when it comes to treating breathing pattern disorders.

REFERENCES

Beck, A.T., 1976. Cognitive therapy and the emotional disorders. International Universities Press, New York.

Bordin, E.S., 1979. The generalizability of the psychoanalytic concept of the working alliance. Psychother Theor Res Pract 16, 252–260.

Carr, J.H., Shepherd, R.B., 2010. Neurological rehabilitation – optimizing motor performance. Butterworth–Heineman, Oxford.

Facchini, S., Muellbacher, W., Battaglia, F., et al., 2002. Focal enhancement of motor cortex excitability during motor imagery: a transcranial magnetic stimulation study. Acta Neurol Scand 105, 146–151.

Fitts, P.M., Posner, M.I., 1967. Human performance. Brooks/Cole Publishing Company, Belmont CA.

Flanagan, J.R., Vetter, P., Johansson, R.S., et al., 2003. Prediction precedes control in motor learning. Curr Biol 13, 146–150.

Freeman, A., Greenwood, V., 1987. Cognitive therapy. Application in psychiatric and medical settings. Human Sciences Press, New York.

Gentile, A.M., 1998. Implicit and explicit processes during acquisition of functional skills. Scand J Occup Therapy 5, 7–16.

Hall, A.M., Ferreira, H., Maher, C.G., et al, 2010. The influence of the therapist–patient relationship on treatment outcome in physical rehabilitation: a systematic review. Phys Ther 90, 1099–1110.

Halvorsen, G., 2009. Mensendiecks historie. Vett & Viten, Oslo.

Haugstad, G.K., 2000. Utvikling og validering av en standardisert, kvantifisert Mensendieck test. Anvendelse av testen ved fysioterapiundersøkelse av kroniske smertepasienter. Master of Sciencies, Faculty of Medicine University of Oslo.

Haugstad, G.K., Haugstad, T.S., Kirste, U.M., et al., 2006. Reliability and validity of a standardized Mensendieck physiotherapy test (SMT). Physiotherapy Theory and Practice 22, 189–205.

Haugstad, G.K., Haugstad, T.S., Kirste, U.M., et al., 2008. Continuing improvement of chronic pelvic pain in women after short-term Mensendieck somatocognitive therapy: results of 1-year follow-up study. Am J Obst & Gyn 199, 615. e1–615.e8.

Haugstad, G.K., Haugstad, T.S., 2011. Therapies and motor function

assessments in longstanding pain syndromes: the effect of somatocognitive therapy in a randomized, controlled intervention study of women with chronic pelvic pain. In: Bennett, J.P. (Ed.), 2011 Physical therapy. Theory, practices and benefits. Nova Science Publishers, Inc., New York.

Higgins, S., 1991. Motor skills acquisition. Physical Therapy 71, 123–139.

Hodges, N.J., Franks, I.M., 2002. Modelling coaching practice: the role of instruction and demonstration. Journal of Sports Sciences 20, 793–811.

Jacobson, E., 1938. Progressive relaxation. University of Chicago Press, Chicago.

Johnsen, L., 1981. Integrated respiration theory/therapy: the breathing me. Birth and rebirth in the fullness of time. Publishing of the University of Oslo, Oslo Norway.

Kåver, A.K., 2012. Allianse Den terapeutiske relasjonen i KAT. Gyldendal Akademisk, Oslo.

Kendall, S.A., Brolin-Magnusson, K., Søren, B., et al., 2000. A pilot study of body awareness programs in the treatment of fibromyalgia syndrome. Arthritis Care and Research 13, 304–307.

Klemmetsen, I., 2005. The Mensendieck system of functional movements. Vett & Viten AS, Oslo.

Kirste, U.M., Haugstad, G.K., Leganger, S., et al., 2002. Chronic pelvic pain in women. Tidsskrift Nor Lægeforen 122, 1223–1227.

Kvåle, A., Johnsen, T.B., Ljunggren, A.E., 2002. Examination of respiration in patients with longstanding musculoskeletal pain. Reliability and validity. Adv Phys 4, 169–181.

Lambert, M.J., Bergin, A.E., Garfield, S.L., 2004. Introduction and historical overview. In: Lambert, M.J. (Ed.), Bergin and Garfield's Handbook of Psychotherapy and Behavior Change. Wiley & Sons, New York.

Lidbeck, J., 2002. Central hyperexcitability in chronic musculoskeletal pain: a conceptual breakthrough with multiple clinical implications. Pain Res Manag 7, 81–92.

Mensendieck, B.M., 1937. The Mensendieck system of functional exercises, volume I. The Southworth-Anthoensen Press, Portland, Maine.

Mensendieck, B.M., 1954. Look better feel better. Harper & Brother, New York.

Meyer-Lidenberg, A., 2008. Impact of prosocial neuropeptides on human brain function. Prog Brain Res 170, 463–470.

Nerdrum, P., 2000. Training of empathic communication for helping professionals. Doctoral dissertation. Oslo University.

Öst, L.G., 1987. Applied Relaxation: description of a coping technique and review of controlled studies. Behaviour Research and Therapy 25, 397–407.

Soukup, M.G., Glomsrød, B., Lønn, J.H., et al., 1999. The effect of Mensendieck exercise program as secondary prophylaxis for recurrent low back pain. A randomized, controlled trial with 12-month follow-up. Spine 24, 1585–1591.

Staud, R., Vierck, C.J., Robinson, M.E., et al., 2005. Effects of the N-methyl-D-aspartate receptor antagonist dextromethorpan on temporal summation of pain are similar in fibromyalgia patients and normal control subjects. J Pain 6, 323–332.

Vlaeyen, J.W.S., Crombez, G., Goubert, L., 2007. Science and psychology of pain. In: Breivik H, Shipley M, (Eds.) Best practice and research compendium. Elsevier, Edinburgh.

Watson, M.J., 2011. Traditional Mirror Therapy (TMT) in the physical therapy management of movement and postural control problems. In: Bennett, J.P. (Ed.), Physical therapy. Theory, practices and benefits. Nova Science Publishers, Inc., New York.

Chapter | 8.2 |

Buteyko breathing method

Rosalba Courtney

WHAT IS THE BUTEYKO METHOD?

The Buteyko Method is primarily a system of breathing training that teaches patients to control their tendencies to overbreathe or hyperventilate. It is based on the theories of the late Ukrainian physician Dr Konstantin Buteyko who believed that carbon dioxide deficiency was a major cause of many chronic diseases. He claimed that his programme of breathing retraining, which aims to raise carbon dioxide, could purportedly benefit up to 150 diseases.

The Buteyko Method made its way to Australasia, Europe and the United States in the 1990s. In these countries the Buteyko Method became best known as a treatment for asthma and was also considered to be helpful for individuals with chronic obstructive pulmonary disease, chronic mouth breathing, sleep apnoea and stress-related disorders.

Research studies on the effectiveness of the Buteyko Method

There have been at least six published clinical trials on the Buteyko Method for asthma (Burgess et al 2011). These studies show that people learning the Buteyko Method are able to substantially reduce their medication with no deterioration in their lung function, and in fact improve their asthma control. These positive research findings have led to a degree of endorsement by health and government authorities in Australia and by the British Thoracic Society who in 2008 endorsed the recommendation of this method for asthma patients. Other research into the Buteyko Method includes one formal case study on sleep apnoea (Birch 2004) and some limited research exploring therapeutic mechanisms (Courtney & Cohen 2008, Al-Delaimy et al. 2001).

Techniques of the Buteyko Method

The Buteyko breathing method encourages breath control as part of daily life, particularly at the onset of asthma or other breathing-related symptoms. However, particularly in the early stages of training, patients are taught a structured daily routine of breathing exercises and

Table 8.2.1 Typical Buteyko Method practice session

Procedure	Description
Step 1 – Beginning Control Pause (CP)	The patient gently inhales and then exhales through the nose and then holds their breath until the point that they feel either 1. The first clear and distinct desire to breathe <u>or</u> 2. An involuntary movement or jerk coming from the diaphragm
Step 2 – Three to five minutes of relaxed reduced-volume breathing or slow breathing	The patient gradually reduces their breathing until they feel a light lack of air. They sustain this while staying relaxed.
Step 3 – Maximum Pause (MP). The MP may be substituted with a CP if MP is contraindicated due to presence of kidney disease, epilepsy, hypertension or other severe chronic illness	The Maximum Pause begins with a gentle inhalation and exhalation. Then the breath is held as long as possible but not to the point of severe discomfort.
Step 2 and Step 3 are then repeated up to 5 times	
Final Control Pause	Same as Step 1

breath-holding techniques, lasting 20 to 40 minutes. A typical routine is shown in Table 8.2.1.

Reduced-volume breathing

The main breath control technique of the Buteyko Method is reduced-volume breathing, where the individual tries to decrease minute volume and raise alveolar CO_2 by reducing tidal volume, i.e. the size of the inhalation and exhalation phase of each breath.

It is particularly important that patients relax during reduced-volume breathing to counteract their body's natural tendency to increase respiratory rate as a response to decreased tidal volume. It has been found that some patients, particularly those who suffer from anxiety, can overcompensate when they try to reduce tidal volume by increasing respiratory rate to the point that minute volume increases rather than decreases (Mueller et al 2005). In these types of patients other breathing control and relaxation strategies may be necessary to raise CO_2.

Reduced-volume breathing has other benefits apart from raising CO_2. If performed correctly it is likely to be an effective means to reduce hyperinflation of the lungs. Dynamic hyperinflation is a condition where end-expiratory lung volume is increased due to air-trapping and incomplete exhalation. It is common in asthma, chronic obstructive pulmonary disease and, while not well researched, it probably also exists in all other conditions associated with chronic elevation of respiratory drive such as chronic anxiety. Dynamic hyperinflation is a key factor in explaining the extent of dyspnoea, diaphragm dysfunction and disruption of neuromechanical aspects of

breathing control in patients with dysfunctional breathing (O'Donnell et al 2007). The extent to which breathing therapies reduce hyperinflation is probably an important measure of their success in reducing dyspnoea and improving breathing function and breathing control.

Reduced lung volumes also lead to increased pressure inside the lungs, particularly at the end of exhalation when this pressure becomes greater (positive) compared to the atmospheric pressure. Generation of positive pressures inside the lungs may have beneficial effects for patients with chronic respiratory disease by equalizing distribution of ventilation and improving matching of ventilation to perfusion.

Breath slowing

In recent years there has been a tendency for some Western practitioners of the Buteyko Method to teach breath slowing as an alternative means for reducing minute volume and this is sometimes done in conjunction with capnometry biofeedback, where a patient observes the effects of their breathing on their end-tidal CO_2 levels and adjusts their breathing rate to raise the levels (see Chapter 7.7). This is a recent development of the Buteyko Method which may have different physiological and biomechanical effects to reduced-volume breathing. It is not the technique used in most of the research trials on the Buteyko Method and was not the technique used by Dr Buteyko, who advised his students to focus on breathing volume and not breathing rate.

Despite the fact that slow breathing is a new addition to the Buteyko Method protocol it has been shown to have beneficial effects. In some patients breath slowing may be a better way to decrease minute volume and raise CO_2 than reduced-volume breathing. Research has shown that slow breathing decreases chemoreceptor sensitivity and enables the patient to tolerate higher levels of CO_2 (Bernardi et al 2001). Slow breathing has also been shown to be very beneficial for treating asthma (Lehrer et al 2004). It might prove to be a useful addition to the Buteyko Method but should probably not replace reduced-volume breathing. A challenge for practitioners is understanding which patients respond better to breath slowing and which respond better to reduced-volume breathing, and how to balance the use of these two techniques for the best results on patients' degree of relaxation, CO_2 levels and extent of hyperinflation.

Breath-holding techniques

The Buteyko Method also uses post-expiratory breath holding as a means to assess and train an individual's breathing. The two types of breath holding are:

1. The Control Pause (CP) and
2. The Maximum Pause (MP).

The Control Pause is used at the beginning and at the end of a session to assess breathing. The Maximum Pause is used to train breath-holding capacity and as a treatment tool to control symptoms.

The Control Pause is an essential part of the Buteyko Method, and many practitioners of this method believe that it indicates both the level of health and the degree of hypocapnia. Recent research suggests that the Control Pause does not give a precise indication of a patient's CO_2 levels but it is nevertheless a good indication of dyspnoea threshold and ventilatory drive (Courtney & Cohen 2008). A longer Control Pause at the end of a practice session is a sign that ventilatory drive from chemical and non-chemical drivers of respiration has decreased and that the tolerance for dyspnoea has increased. This is a very desirable outcome for the individual with hyperventilation, hyperpnoea, hyperinflation and breathlessness. People who regularly practise the Buteyko Method generally find that the Control Pause gets longer and can continue to lengthen after weeks, months and even years of practice.

The Maximum Pause, where the breath is held to more or less maximum tolerance, is used to train breath-holding ability. It is also used to relieve symptoms such as blocked nose and acute bronchospasm. During the Maximum Pause, carbon dioxide levels momentarily increase, enabling the body to reverse carbon dioxide gas exchange so that the body reabsorbs carbon dioxide.

Research with athletes has shown that including breath holding to maximum capacity in their training routines resulted in increased production of endogenous antioxidants and higher anaerobic threshold (Joulia et al 2003). Maximal breath-holds also cause splenic contractions with subsequent increased haematocrit and haemoglobin levels and possible immune stimulation effects (Schagatay et al 2005). It therefore seems likely that these types of haematological, immune, metabolic and anti-inflammatory effects also apply in people undertaking regular Buteyko Method training.

At the termination of the Maximum Pause, most people will take at least a few deep breaths before gaining control of breathing volumes again. The increased bronchodilation following a sudden deep breath, called pulmonary hysteresis, is a well-documented physiological phenomenon. Pulmonary hysteresis may in part explain the bronchodilation that many asthmatics observe after performing a Maximum Pause.

A major aim of the Buteyko Method is to see the gradual lengthening of the CP and MP. People using the Buteyko Method are encouraged to aim for a perfect Control Pause of 60 seconds, and some have been known to perform Maximum Pauses of more than 2 minutes.

Establishing nasal breathing

The Buteyko Method places a lot of emphasis on the importance of establishing and maintaining nasal breathing at all times including during exercise, during sleep and even when the nose becomes blocked as a result of having a cold or allergic reaction. It appears that this is an important part of asthma treatment as it has been shown that replacing mouth breathing with nasal breathing, even without other breathing exercises, improves lung function and reduces asthma exacerbations (Hallani et al 2008).

Patients learning the Buteyko Method are taught to clear obstructed nasal passages by using a variety of breath holding strategies, either as a series of Control Pauses or by doing a Maximum Pause while sitting or walking. To effectively clear the nose with breath-holding techniques it is essential that one learns to take the first breath through the nose, keeping the mouth closed until a quiet breathing pattern can be resumed. A common observation of individuals with chronically blocked noses is that the more they breathe through the nose, the clearer and more comfortable it becomes.

Dr Buteyko's carbon dioxide theory

The foundation of the Buteyko Method is Dr Buteyko's carbon dioxide theory which expands on the well-known and generally accepted negative effects of hypocapnia. The key elements of Buteyko's theory are outlined in Box 8.2.1. Some aspects of this theory are controversial and not supported by currently available research. The main areas of controversy relate to:

1. high prevalence of chronic hypocapnia
2. relationship between acute and chronic hypocapnia and symptoms

Box 8.2.1 **Some key elements of Buteyko's carbon dioxide theory**

1. Up to 150 symptoms and diseases are due to the presence of hypocapnia.
2. Chronic hidden hyperventilation is widespread and almost universal, affecting up to 90% of the world's population.
3. Hypocapnia is an important and generally unrecognized destabilizer of physiological systems and psychological states.
4. Depletion of carbon dioxide affects the core processes of energy production in the mitochondria and vital chemical reactions requiring carbon-containing compounds.
5. Pathophysiological processes in chronic illnesses such as asthma, rhinitis, hypertension, heart disease and sleep apnoea are defence mechanisms against chronic hyperventilation:
6. Normalization of carbon dioxide levels explains symptom reduction and improved health in patients who learn and apply the Buteyko Method.

3. role of diseases such as asthma as defence mechanisms to prevent loss of CO_2
4. emphasis on CO_2 as the single most important mechanism underlying the Buteyko Method.

Importance of CO_2 in human health

Carbon dioxide is important in human health and hypocapnia can contribute to a number of pathophysiological processes in several organ systems (Laffey & Kavanagh 2002). It is involved in a number of key physiological reactions including maintenance of pH, oxygen dissociation and key chemical reactions involving carbon compounds. The functions of CO_2 are elaborated in most standard physiology texts, many books and articles on the Buteyko Method as well as in Chapters 1, 3 and 4 of this book, so will not be discussed here.

Prevalence of chronic hypocapnia

Buteyko's views on the universal prevalence of chronic hypocapnia in conditions treated by the Buteyko Method is not supported by research studies available at this time. The English language scientific literature reports that somewhere between 5–10% of people have evidence of chronic hypocapnia (Folgering 1999). Individuals with asthma, panic disorder, sleep apnoea, cardiovascular disorders and other chronic illness responsive to breathing therapy do have a greater tendency to hyperventilate than

normal healthy individuals, but hypocapnia is not consistent, the extent varies between individuals and many individuals with these diseases have normal levels of CO_2 (Courtney 2011, Perna et al 2004). Any clinician who regularly uses a capnometer will find that chronic hypocapnia is not consistently present in patients. However, since hyperventilation tendencies are often only made evident under conditions of physical or psychological stress or during disease exacerbations, it is possible that patients with normal resting CO_2 have unrecognized tendencies to episodic hyperventilation that destabilize biochemical aspects of breathing homeostasis.

Relationship between hypocapnia and symptoms

It is well established that hypocapnia affects many body systems and can compromise health, however the relationship between hypocapnia and symptoms is not linear or highly predictable. A series of studies in the early 1990s found that there was an inconsistent relationship between symptoms of hyperventilation syndrome and both acute and chronic CO_2 deficit (Hornsveld & Garsson 1997). These studies threw doubt on the very existence of this syndrome and by implication on Buteyko's theory that CO_2 is central to symptom production in over 150 different syndromes and diseases. In recent years it has become increasingly clear that the extent of symptoms and the distress they cause patients is not only due to hypocapnia but also clearly influenced by other physiological and psychological factors and by altered breathing pattern (Courtney et al 2011).

In asthmatics the association between hypocapnia and symptoms is probably closer than for other conditions treated by the Buteyko Method. The acute asthma attack is often accompanied by hyperventilation and hyperpnoea and both of these factors can aggravate bronchospasm. It is therefore highly likely that these are important factors in destabilization of asthma in susceptible individuals (Bruton & Holgate 2005). Further research is needed to explore to what degree the extent of asthma symptoms is tied to carbon dioxide status as compared to other mechanisms.

Disease as a defence mechanism against loss of CO_2

One aspect of Buteyko's carbon dixode theory is that asthma is not a disease but a defence mechanism against hyperventilation and that the primary purpose of this disease is to help the body retain CO_2. This explanation of asthma which attributes the complex immune and inflammatory changes of asthma to hyperventilation is an obvious oversimplification. A more moderate version of this theory which says that the hyperventilation and hyperpnoea aggravates asthma is more plausible as there is sufficient evidence showing that both these factors can contribute to bronchoconstriction (Bruton & Holgate 2005).

Do improvements in CO_2 sufficiently explain the Buteyko effect?

The few studies that have tried to elucidate the mechanisms of the Buteyko Method, while not conclusive, have not tended to support Buteyko's carbon dioxide theory (Al-Delaimy et al 2001, Courtney & Cohen 2008). The tight relationship claimed by Buteyko to exist between length of breath-holding time and an individual's end tidal CO_2 has not been confirmed (Courtney & Cohen, 2008) and end tidal CO_2 has not been shown to increase after Buteyko breathing training (Bowler et al 1998). Most of the randomized controlled trials on the Buteyko Method have not evaluated CO_2 levels before and after treatment which makes it difficult to draw firm conclusions until these types of data are available. However, it is unlikely that increased levels of CO_2 are the sole reason for the health improvements seen in patients who learn the Buteyko Method.

Is a more comprehensive theory for the Buteyko Method more useful?

The mechanisms of the Buteyko Method are likely to be complex and to include psychophysiological, neurological and biomechanical mechanisms in addition to biochemical mechanisms centred on CO_2. The prolonged breath holds which are generally repeated every 5 minutes as part of standard Buteyko practice produce mild intermittent hypoxia (IH). IH is known to be an important influence on respiratory motor plasticity. It produces adaptive effects that are salutogenic and increase the body's homeostatic capacity. Beneficial effects of IH include improving the tone of upper airway dilator muscles by increasing the activity of the vagal and hypoglossal nerves, improving oxygen metabolism and antioxidant status, reducing inflammation and increasing stress adaptation.

In asthmatics, the Buteyko Method control pause has a statistically significant positive correlation with extent of thoracic-dominant breathing, but not with carbon dioxide levels (Courtney & Cohen 2008). This suggests that factors affecting breathing pattern (and probably respiratory drive) are at least as important as a patient's carbon dioxide status in explaining dyspnoea threshold. This possibility is strengthened by the finding that improved breathing pattern after breathing training is associated with decreased dyspnoea (Courtney et al 2011).

The particular combination of techniques that are used during Buteyko practice, i.e. relaxed reduced-volume breathing, gentle slow breathing and post-exhalation breath holds may be particularly effective at improving the biomechanics of breathing by reducing dynamic hyperinflation of the lungs. In dynamic hyperinflation, the muscles of respiration, including the diaphragm and accessory muscles, are short and hypertonic. These shortened and partially contracted respiratory muscles are weak and ineffective at responding to signals to breathe sent by the motor cortex at the onset on inspiration. The situation known as afferent re-efferent dissociation is an important contributor to dyspnoea and poor breathing control in patients with asthma and COPD (O'Donnell et al 2007). It also tends to result in upper thoracic breathing patterns and paradoxical breathing. When the volume of air in the lung is reduced, the diaphragm increases its curvature, functional length and strength thus improving neuromechanical coupling and increasing the freedom and ease of breathing.

It is worth noting that breathing at both low lung volumes and involving sudden deep breaths, both of which tend to occur during a standard Butyeko breathing session, can induce bronchodilation. Reduced-volume breathing has been shown to induce bronchodilation through mechanical effects (Douglas et al 1981) and bronchodilation can result from the large-volume breaths that follow the Maximum Pause as a result of pulmonary hysteresis.

Psychophysiological factors

The impact that the Buteyko Method has on psychological factors should also be considered. Affective states such as fear of bodily sensation and sense of control all influence the quality and extent of dyspnoea (De Peuter et al 2004). The Buteyko Method can conceivably reduce fear and help the asthmatic patient have an increased sense of control, because it trains and encourages the patient's willingness to accept and be present with unpleasant sensations.

The Buteyko Method's comprehensive and plausible CO_2-deficiency model of asthma helps the reattribution of symptoms to a controllable cause with clear instructions as to how to beneficially modify the problem. When students voluntarily pursue a slight lack of air sensation during breathing practice, and train themselves to relax while doing so, the relationship to dyspnoea changes from one of fear and avoidance to acceptance, thus empowering the patient and increasing their sense of self-efficacy.

The effects of the two-way interaction between the body and the mind is very evident in asthma. Asthmatics have been found to suffer from much higher levels of anxiety, depression and panic disorder than the average population (Lehrer et al 2002). Aggravation of depression or anxiety is often accompanied by exacerbation of asthma, whereas successful treatment is associated with improvement in asthma. In asthma there is increased activity of the brain's emotional neural circuitry involving structures in the limbic system such as the insula and anterior cingulate gyrus that are part of the brain's fear network. The extent of activation of this neural circuitry predicts the magnitude of lung function decline (Rosenkranz & Davidson 2009). Rosenkranz argues that it is likely that this circuitry is activated not just from psychological causes or external threat, but also as a response to the internal threats generated from physiological responses linked to chronic inflammation and immune system activation. Breathing therapies that increase sense of control and reduce the sense of anxiety and threat conceivably will reduce the activation of this affective neural circuitry with far-reaching implications for the mind–body aspects of asthma.

FUTURE DIRECTIONS FOR THE BUTEYKO METHOD

Despite its success the Buteyko Method is still considered controversial and is not well accepted by the medical and scientific community or widely utilized.

Training of practitioners in the Buteyko Method tends to vary enormously around the world with training courses varying from 2-day courses that focus primarily on techniques to courses lasting several months that provide extensive training in Buteyko theory and business techniques. The shorter courses are generally targeted to health professionals. The longer courses tend to appeal more to people who are not health professionals, often asthmatics who have successfully used the Buteyko techniques to improve their own health. The latter group tend to be averse to any critical analysis of Buteyko.

There are two aspects to the Buteyko Method, the practical techniques and the theoretical basis. The techniques are unique and effective and it should be acknowledged that Buteyko has made a valuable contribution to the field of breathing therapy. However, many aspects of Buteyko's theoretical teachings which are intricately woven into most Buteyko Method training packages are not supported by current research. To gain wider acceptance, Buteyko theory and training of practitioners need to evolve to embrace a more complex model of breathing dysfunction and a broader understanding of the mechanisms of breathing therapy.

The Buteyko breathing method is one of several successful breathing therapies for asthma (Burgess et al 2011). Further research on the mechanisms of Buteyko and other breathing therapies is needed to clarify which patients will benefit most from which particular set of breathing exercises.

It is likely that the best approach to treating conditions such as asthma with breathing therapy is one that is patient centred rather than therapy centred, with treatment individualized to the needs of the patient. For example, it is believed that asthmatics with dysfunctional breathing are the ones most likely to benefit from breathing therapy (Prys-Picard & Niven 2008, Thomas et al 2001). Because breathing dysfunction can take several forms and arise due to different causes, it is important that clinicians measure and evaluate the various dimensions of breathing dysfunction, their causes and patients' responses to treatment so that breathing therapy and other treatment can be modified as necessary to maximize benefits (Courtney 2011).

REFERENCES

Al-Delaimy, W.K., Hay, S.M., Gain, K.R., et al., 2001. The effects of carbon dioxide on exercise-induced asthma: an unlikely explanation for the effects of Buteyko breathing training. Med J Aust 174, 72–74.

Bernardi, L., Gabutti, A., Porta, C., et al., 2001. Slow breathing reduces chemoreflex response to hypoxia and hypercapnia, and increases baroreflex sensitivity. J. Hypertension 19, 2221–2229.

Birch, M., 2004. Obstructive sleep apnoea and breathing training. Australian Nursing Journal 12 (2), 27–29.

Bowler, S.D., Green, A., Mitchell, A., 1998. Buteyko breathing technique in asthma: a blinded randomised controlled trial. Medical Journal of Australia 169, 575–578.

Bruton, A., Holgate, S.T., 2005. Hypocapnia and asthma: a mechanism for breathing retraining? Chest 127, 1808–1818.

Burgess, J., Ekanayake, B., Lowe, A., et al., 2011. Systematic review of the effectiveness of breathing retraining in asthma management. Expert Review of Respiratory Medicine 5, 789–807.

Courtney, R., Cohen, M., 2008. Investigating the claims of Konstantin Buteyko M.D., PhD: the relationship of breath holding time to end tidal CO_2 and other proposed measures of dysfunctional breathing. Journal of Alternative and Complementary Medicine 14, 115–123.

Courtney, R.C., 2011. Dysfunctional breathing: its parameters, measurement and relevance. PhD Research, RMIT University.

Courtney, R.C., Greenwood, K.M., Dixhoorn, J., et al., 2011. Medically unexplained dyspnea partly moderated by dyfunctional (thoracic dominant) breathing pattern. Journal of Asthma 48, 259–265.

De Peuter, S., Van Diest, I., Lemaigre, V., et al., 2004. Dyspnea: the role of psychological processes. Clinical Pyschology Review 24, 557–581.

Douglas, N.J., Drummond, G.B., Sudlow, M.F., 1981. Breathing at low lung volumes and chest strapping: a comparison of lung mechanics. J. Applied. Physiol. 50, 650–657.

Folgering, H., 1999. The patho-physiology of hyperventilation syndrome. Monaldi Arch Chest Dis. 54, 365–372.

Hallani, M., Wheatley, J.R., Amis, T.C., 2008. Enforced mouth breathing decreases lung function in mild asthmatics. Respirology 13, 553–558.

Hornsveld, H.K., Garsson, B., 1997. Hyperventilation syndrome: an elegant but scientifically untenable concept. Neth J Med 50, 13–20.

Joulia F., Steinberg J.G., Faucher M., et al., 2003. Breath-hold training of humans reduces oxidative stress and blood acidosis after static and dynamic apnea. Respiratory Physiology & Neurobiology 137, 19–27.

Laffey, J.G., Kavanagh, B.P., 2002. Hypocapnia. N Engl J of Med 347, 43–54.

Lehrer, P., Feldman, J., Giardino, N.D., et al., 2002. Psychological aspects of asthma. Journal of Consulting and Clinical Psychology 70, 691–711.

Lehrer, P., Vaschillo, E., Vaschillo, B., et al., 2004. Biofeedback treatment for asthma. Chest 126, 352–361.

Mueller, A., Roth, W.T., Conrad, A., et al., 2005. Psychophysiological responses to breathing instructions. 12th Annual Meeting of the Society for the Advancement of Respiratory Psychophysiology. Hamburg, Germany.

O'Donnell, D., Banzett, R.B., Carrieri-Kholman, V., et al., 2007. Pathophysiology of dyspnea in chronic obstructive pulmonary disease. Proc Am Thorac Society 4, 145–168.

Perna, G., Caldirola, D., Bellodi, L., 2004. Panic disorder: from respiration to the homeostatic brain. Acta Neuropsychiatrica 16, 57–67.

Prys-Picard, C., Niven, R.M., 2008. Dysfunctional breathing in patients with asthma. Thorax 63, 568.

Rosenkranz, M.A., Davidson, R.J., 2009. Affective neural circuitry and mind-body influences in asthma. Neuroimage 47, 972–980.

Schagatay, E., Haughey, H., Reimers, I., 2005. Speed of spleen volume changes evoked by serial apneas. Eur J Appl Physiol 93, 447–452.

Thomas, M., McKinley, R.K., Freeman, E., et al., 2001. Prevalence of dysfunctional breathing in patients treated for asthma in primary care: cross sectional survey. BMJ 322, 1098–1100.

Chapter | **8.3**

Feldenkrais® and breathing

John C. Hannon

INTRODUCTION

Physics, particularly the physics of Judo, forms an important foundation[1] in the Feldenkrais method. Moshe Feldenkrais (1904–1984) wrote a book (1942) which impressed Jigaro Kano, the founder of Judo, sufficiently to arrange for top-level Judo tutoring. This occurred while Feldenkrais was earning an engineering degree in Paris and, subsequently, a DSc in physics (Sorbonne). Later, he became a full-time pioneer of what is now known as bodywork and movement therapy. In the 1950s, he taught movement classes in Tel Aviv. These lessons (the Yanai series) show him requesting the students, on almost every page, to notice their quality of breathing and how this illuminates function. Twenty-nine Yanai lessons (see Box 8.3.4, at the end of the chapter) directly address breathing as a tool for maturing movement quality; these will be briefly introduced here.

As we shall see, Feldenkrais believed movement quality was determined by the interplay of posture and breathing. Without the underpinnings of effective posture, breathing is bound to be physically restricted and neurologically inhibited. Without thoracic resilience, postural responses are forced, effete and inefficient rather than rapid and relevant. As Feldenkrais pointed out[2], the waist must be stiffened for the body to efficiently move itself. Why? The heaviest part, the trunk, must move less than its lighter neighbours: the head and limbs. For this, the trunk's two rigid ends (thorax and pelvis) need bracing. Thus, the waist must be an able mediator of forces.

If the waist is too stiff, movement quality and breathing delicacy inevitably coarsen. But without sufficient stiffness, we lose our uprightness. No wonder there are no bare spaces on the ribs. All available surfaces serve to anchor

---

[1]An example of the intensity of his belief (and that this belief predated his bodywork method, Feldenkrais (1944, p. 10–11)): '[Judo is] based upon a single principle ... For Judo is the art of using the body in general. It is planned to improve general well-being and a sense of rhythm, and develops co-ordination of movement. ... [t]he senses of time and space are so much bettered by Judo practice... Judo should be considered as a basic culture of the body.' (p. 111) 'Judo is the science of the economy of body energy.' Lastly, on p. 27 he points out a relaxed body does not mean absolutely relaxed muscles. Instead, it means stiffening muscles as much as is needed for an action at the moment it is done.

[2]Feldenkrais (1949, p. 54) and, p. 115, '...there are as many breathing mechanisms as distinct attitudes of the body. In proper development, breathing follows a definite rhythm, unhampered by the position of the body. All effort by the limbs necessitates rigidity of the trunk. This is increased to the maximum when the ribs are fixed and the breath is held in the position of inspiration. However, in proper body mechanics, the breathing rhythm is not interrupted, even in violent efforts. When the pelvis is held properly the lower abdomen feels full and forward, the rigidity required for efficient use of the arms is obtained while diaphragmatic breathing is maintained evenly and effortlessly.'

the muscles or connective tissues of the lungs[3], limbs, spine and abdomen. The thorax (the body's largest skeletal volume) gives rise to myriad points of leverage. The elliptical cross-section of the thorax provides an unstable equilibrium in any resting posture. As Figure 8.3.2 shows, leverage and unstable equilibrium are used in Functional Integration® (Feldenkrais' form of manual therapy, also known as FI) to provide a smooth flow of momentum.

A golf ball illustrates these equilibrium states. When the ball sinks into a hole, it is stable; when it rests on a tee, unstable. In both situations, the ball is in equilibrium but it has more potential energy when unstable. More importantly, a small force liberates this energy. In addition, the ball may move in any direction. Most Feldenkrais lessons aim at replacing an unsuspected stiffness with an unstable equilibrium. This poised yet mercurial state frees up breathing. Feldenkrais felt easy breathing required free motion from the thorax, throat, neck, shoulders, abdomen and lower back.

Feldenkrais' Awareness Through Movement® (ATM) lessons predict behaviour. These predictions can be used to construct testable hypotheses to guide research. As Green & Green (1977) commented, Feldenkrais trained himself to become a biofeedback instrument. He also trained himself, after sensing subtle movement patterns, to find ways to help clients feel these patterns themselves. He believed if his students knew what they were doing, they could rid themselves of inefficient movement patterns. In turn, this would allow them to move as they wished.

Moving as we would like is difficult; modern living taxes our posture and breathing. Sitting is the most prevalent awake posture yet chair design often seems aimed at convenient stacking or a spurious sense of luxury. Feldenkrais suggested ways to breathe well while sitting; and how to improve breathing while standing and walking. There may be public health benefits in his approach.[4] He noted:

The well adapted person feels right only when he does the right thing – the ill-adapted feels right while

---

[3]The intricacies extend even into the lung where three fibre systems interact during breathing. Weibel (2009) describes the components: 'The axial fiber system anchors in the hilum and reaches to the alveolar ducts and the acinal sacs; it creates a branched axial scaffold by forming the airway walls. The peripheral fiber system originates in the visceral pleura's connective tissue and manifests as a hierarchical system of interlobular septa in the periphery of the acini. Lastly, the septal fiber system anchors in both the axial and peripheral fiber systems, forming within the alveolar walls close to the capillary network.'

[4]Feldenkrais (1949, p. 163) notes his method aims at re-education not treatment: '… it is a question of teaching and learning and not of disease and cure.' As might be expected from this quote, Feldenkrais practitioners do not treat or diagnose; they counsel their students to obtain confirmation from their physicians that the lessons are appropriate. Professional Practitioner Training usually consists of four years of classes totalling 40 days/year. ATM lessons, lectures, demonstrations and FI tutorials form the training's backbone. The Feldenkrais Guild of North America and the International Feldenkrais Federation are good places to start for more information.

Box 8.3.1 **Awareness as defined by Feldenkrais**

Feldenkrais believed the delay between thought and action is the basis for awareness.[*] He defined awareness as consciousness and knowledge united; an experienced rather than taught capacity. Mehling et al (2009) suggest body awareness cuts two ways; a ruminative self-focus may be maladaptive, while focusing on immediately experienced feelings may be advantageous. Feldenkrais' suggested learning is stimulated by posing problems solvable only with heightened awareness. This he specified as both an internal attentiveness to the body's workings and an external comprehension of social and spatial interactions. He believed movement to be the basis of awareness; particularly breathing movements.[†] In his view, effective learning harnesses work and play in equal amounts; with self-directed and satisfying discoveries arising out of curiosity. His way has little room for will power, anxiety, shame, imitation or compulsion. He said: 'What I'm after isn't flexible bodies, but flexible brains. What I'm after is to restore each person to their human dignity.' (Verin 1981).

---

[*]Feldenkrais (1977, p. 45).
[†] Feldenkrais (1977, p. 16) made an interesting point: 'Most of what goes on within us remains dulled and hidden from us until it reaches the muscles. We know what is happening within us as soon as the muscles of our face, heart, or breathing apparatus organize themselves into patterns, known to us as fear, anxiety, laughter or any other feeling. … We do not become aware of what is happening in our central nervous system until we become aware of changes that have taken place in our stance, stability, and attitude, for these changes are more easily felt than those that have occurred in the muscles…'

---

doing the wrong thing. The fact that he knows it, does not help him any more than the neurotic is helped by knowing that his behaviour is abnormal.[5]

Despite the length of time his lessons have been in print, his ideas have not been tested to stringent scientific standards.

EMBODIMENT

Interestingly, Feldenkrais' ideas can be shaped into testable hypotheses. He explicitly aimed to develop the interoception likely to enhance what Gadow (1980) described as 'cultivated immediacy'. Gadow encouraged the development of embodiment in health care. She noted that patients experience their bodies quite differently than their practitioners do and that 'body and self, though inseparable, are not identical.'

---

[5]Feldenkrais (1949, p. 120).

Mehling et al (2011) recommend a developmental model of embodiment to help understand body awareness-enhancing therapies. In a review of bodywork research in general, Mehling et al (2005a) recommended the need for credible placebos and measures of patient expectations. In addition, they outlined ways of minimizing bias. Mehling et al (2005b) in a pilot study of patients with chronic low-back pain found comparable changes in measures of pain and disability in breath therapy and physical therapy; they suggested breathing therapy improved proprioception.[6]

By using Mehling et al's protocol, Feldenkrais' speculations can be tested. For instance, he predicted restricted sternal and lowest rib movements in people with lower back pain. Box 8.3.2's transcript explores sensing the breathing apparatus; alternate nostril–mouth breathing and how coughing, swallowing and repeated exhaling promote swift involuntary and uninterrupted inhalation. Here, Feldenkrais makes five testable predictions:

1. Normal breathing function is cancelled by faulty habits of standing/sitting/head position.
2. Chest immobility provokes upper abdominal expansion during inhalation.
3. The CO_2 reflex[7] makes proper inhalation automatic, easy and immediately learned.
4. Powerful exhalations normally protrude the lowest part of the abdomen.
5. Stuffy noses clear with repetitions of mouth inhaling followed by exhaling through a single nostril.

INTEROCEPTION

Exteroceptors, such as the eyes and ears, register distant events. Interoception refers to the discernment of inside events. Often a sizeable gap separates personal experience of interoception from modern science's findings. Consider these four statements.

- Banzett et al (1997) found subjects able to feel the inflation of a single pulmonary lobe.
- Burton et al (1977) Hospital patients ventilate well but with scarcely visible muscular activity.
- Loh et al (1977) During quiet supine early inspiration, diaphragmatic descent can be entirely passive.
- Moses (1954) remarked the self-assured person makes use of 'harmonious, balanced co-ordination and a relaxed operating diaphragm.'

Does interoception inform readers to allow self-assessment of such statements? One way of self-assessment is through ATMs. Each of the above statements can be personally validated with the lessons cited in this chapter. As Torday & Rehan (2009) note: 'it takes a process to decipher a process.' An ATM is such a process; one that contributes to what Feldenkrais called the sixth sense – sensing a difference that makes a difference.[8]

For instance, one Yanai lesson[9] is performed almost motionless. After inhaling and following the air in, students imagine the inner contours of the entire upper respiratory tract. Then they explore the oral cavity using a finger. Next, they repeat the process using the tongue. They imagine the oral cavity getting wider in all directions. Subsequently, they imagine the low abdomen doing the same. They imagine both volumes simultaneously and then the chest expanding in all directions as well.

Feldenkrais[10] warns people (no matter how hard the lesson) not to look at their watches or fall asleep. He states that learning to think and to clearly imagine is important. Even more detailed 'examination by imagination' occurs.[11] Another lesson[12] immobilizes the teeth/tongue/lips while practising nasal vocalizations to discover the palate lifts in speech.

Feldenkrais felt if people knew what they were doing, they could do what they want. Here, he shows people, at first, they cannot know what they are doing. He also shows them that within minutes of practice (by paying attention) they can improve function. Such differences are discovered through awareness. Box 8.3.1 summarises Feldenkrais' definition of awareness.

CONTOURS OF BREATHING

Another lesson[13] pays attention to the chest while moving the feet. In it Feldenkrais states:

The bulk of the work, in a kinetic sense, is in the pelvis. All these circles make light movements of the

---

[6] The Yanai lesson #290 (hopping with limp toes) links faulty proprioception with a lack of normal spinal movement. When the head floats on the atlas and axis, even small spinal perturbations can be sensed (and posture adjusted appropriately) before the body actually begins to fall. Feldenkrais predicts, if the breath is unimpeded, balancing on one leg will not be difficult.

[7] Chaitow et al (2002) note the central role of respiration is to maintain balanced concentrations of oxygen and carbon dioxide. Increased arterial carbon dioxide levels increase motor control signals to activate inhalation. Feldenkrais described the CO_2 reflex this way: 'Do not busy yourself with the inhalation, but with the exhalation. The human system is built so there is a certain amount of residual air in the lungs that one cannot exhale even when trying. The lungs themselves do not have muscles and the ribs are not flexible enough to decrease the volume of the chest sufficiently. You cannot exhale the last half liter of air from the lungs. If you wait a little bit, the human being is designed so the CO_2 ratio contained [in] that half liter of air increases rapidly. Once it reaches a certain ratio, the system, by itself, begins breathing in the right way.' (Yanai #17, p. 98).

[8] Feldenkrais (1949, p. 110)
[9] Yanai#23.
[10] Yanai Volume 1A: p.142
[11] Yanai#126
[12] Yanai#5
[13] Yanai#111

spine between the shoulder blades and at the base of the neck. … This is why it affects the chest.

Here he affirms the mechanical connectivity of the chest and spine.

This connectivity is seen throughout his lessons; for instance, a lesson[14] develops sternal flexibility. Another lesson[15] explores moving the legs like frogs. He predicts only those who completely rest their spines can make their two legs truly move together; when one leg moves faster, the other must stiffen itself, spine and chest. Another

lesson[16] helps students (while sitting[17]) sense their scapular relationship to the C7 vertebra while breathing. This ends with the scapula sliding at will.

Lengthening the spine[18] is an important part of his lesson strategies. For instance, a lesson[19] has nine postural variations to change the way the student 'presses the air'

---

[14]Yanai#217
[15]Yanai#117

[16]Yanai#136
[17]Another lesson (Yanai#316) predicts proper sitting requires working abdominal muscles and relaxed chests. The thoracolumbar vertebrae require flexibility and the sternum cannot become mobile enough without the posterior aspect of the lower ribs widening. Yanai#319 describes a characteristic of movement excellence: good organization means the muscles activate in proportion to their mass; large muscles work more and small muscles work less.
[18]Feldenkrais (1977 p. 91)
[19]Yanai#179

Box 8.3.2 A sample Feldenkrais ATM lesson

To give a flavour of his style of lesson, here is a ruthlessly pruned extract from a 45-minute lesson entitled Breathing.* All of his movement instructions are in bold type; my comments are in square brackets. This extract is abbreviated; refer to the actual lesson transcript for a better sense of his teaching and consult with your physician before beginning his lessons.

[The students are lying on blankets; knees bent and shoulder-width apart (soles of the feet resting on the floor). Feldenkrais has previously had them place their hands on their chests to 'listen' for movement].

'… You will discover that there are three different things to listen for. First there is the lower part of your abdomen, next there is the upper part of your abdomen that is near your stomach, and finally there is your chest. As silly as it may seem, many people do not move their chest when they breathe. Not all of your ribs attach to your chest bone, but the action of the ribs, joints, and muscles that hang on the sternum, are cancelled by faulty habits of standing and sitting or by improper positioning of the head. Often this structure does not participate in breathing except in severe cases when the person runs or is tired, then this area despite the stubbornness of the person, begins to move.

Pay attention if you can feel your chest lifting[†] from the floor, or not. It needs to lift your hand from the floor a significant amount. Do not lift it on purpose; only pay

attention if it is lifting. See if you can feel your sternum move.

You will find that when the chest is immobile, the upper part of your abdomen under the floating ribs makes an effort when breathing. This area opens a little and makes a light movement. The person lives on that tiny amount of air. [He now has the students place their **hands on the lowest part of the abdomen** to feel for upward lifting during inhalation].

'How does one arrange for his breathing to be well organized? It is very difficult. To our delight, inherent in the structure of the human body there is something that permits humans to learn this easily. Something permits humans to improve their breathing constantly without undergoing special difficulties.' [He explains how the lungs' residual air rapidly changes its CO_2 ratio, reflexively prompting a healthy inhalation. He instructs: **'exhale all air from your lungs and hold your breath 10 seconds and re-exhale. Then breath-hold two more seconds and re-exhale.'**

[The resulting inrush of air is extraordinarily different than previous inhalations. He predicts those who do not fully exhale never fully feel respiration. He observes that if this exercise is done well, it is awkward enough that almost everyone coughs. Since no one is coughing he asks them to repeat the process by letting out more air and waiting].

---

*Yanai#17.
[†]For more detail on this important distinction: Feldenkrais (1977, p. 100–1) 'Now you will learn to recognize the movements of the ribs, diaphragm, and abdomen that make up your breathing. Proper adjustment of these movements is necessary in order to breathe deeply and easily. You will be able to recognize the difference in the length of the periods of breathing in and out, and to realize that the process of breathing adjusts itself to the posture of the body with respect to gravity. The lower ribs move more than the upper ones and contribute more to breathing. You will finally see that breathing becomes easier and more rhythmical when the body is held erect without any conscious effort, that is, when its entire weight is supported by the skeletal structure. … Many people breathe without letting their breastbone move relative to the spine. Instead of increasing the volume of their chest in accordance with its structure, they hollow their back, that is to say raise the entire chest from the ground, including the lower part of the back, so that its interior volume is increased only by the movement of the floating ribs. See whether your spine presses on the ground for the entire length of the chest as the latter expands and the breastbone moves away from the spine. Do not attempt to force the spine down; make no effort. Simply fill the lungs with air, watch for the chest to rise, and see whether the spine is pressed against the floor at the same time.'

Box 8.3.2 **A sample Feldenkrais ATM lesson – cont'd**

[Feldenkrais requests them to **'cough while feeling with the hands'.** He explains the normal out-pushing of the lowest part of the abdomen accompanies chest-shrinking. He points out that, in all but resting activities, correct breathing has the exhalation pushing out the lower abdomen. He reminds the audience how a cow's 'Moo' and a lion's roar moves their lower bellies; he summarizes that natural breathing always features lower abdominal protrusion.[‡] He then has the students **open their mouths widely while exhaling (and pushing out the lower abdomen). After exhaling, close the mouth (tongue resting on the bottom dental arch), swallow saliva and let air enter the lungs without interruption**].

'The intention of this lesson is not to learn a new way of breathing, rather you are returning to your body its ability to breathe the way it was designed. You are not teaching your body how to breathe. After swallowing your saliva, your lower abdomen opens as air enters your lungs.' [He describes how this deglutition reflex prompts involuntary inhalation. During swallowing, the abdominal muscles are unnecessary, so they relax. He asks them to **repeat this process 30 times** and notice the sinking of the lower abdomen. Then, he has them **inhale through**

the mouth and exhale via the nose** while noticing any differences].

'You do these movements so your body can learn to feel, discern, and use its members according to necessity. You will see that your body alters and becomes wiser. It begins to breathe as it needs according to the situation.' [He tells the students to **inhale through the mouth and exhale through the nose**. He comments stuffy nasal passages make exhalations shorter than the inhalations. He asks the students to **manually close one nostril and exhale through the other while inhaling through the mouth**. He predicts that, with practice, both nostrils will function. Normal function means no noise during quiet breathing].

[He asks them to switch nostrils. Another variation has them start by exhaling through the mouth and switch halfway to exhale through the nostrils. Continue this until able to do three or four exchanges in one breath. Then, roll over, and in the prone position, repeat the entire process until able to do three or four exchanges in a single breath].

[He finishes the lesson by asking the students to put a hand on the abdomen and one on the chest (as they did in the beginning of the lesson) and see if the chest raises and lowers with increased clarity].

[‡]Regarding aberrant function, Feldenkrais' Yanai#126 lesson predicts normal breathing (lower abdominal protrusion) is lost if the neck shortens while the tongue stiffens onto the palate. And Yanai#172 helps students determine if they habitually stop their breathing following their inhalation or their exhalation.

into different portions of the chest wall. Eventually the students feel[20] what it is to relax the spine.

Time is another variable Feldenkrais considered. One series[21] divides the breathing cycle into four parts: inhale, pause, exhale, pause. Students tap and measure out equal lengths of time. Then they breathe in equal segments: inhale–hold–exhale–hold. It is hard to fit a breath to a predetermined time interval; also, challenging positions make the breath ragged. Students become aware that by slowing their movements and minimizing their efforts, the raggedness disappears and previously clumsy movements become more refined.

Another series[22] minimizes inhalation[23] effort. Diaphragm action lengthens the lung (sensed as 'something going up and down at the same time'). Feldenkrais predicts lung tissue will not mould to inflexible ribs. He also predicts people unable to bend their thorax have inflexible lungs because the self-image is deficient. He specifies normal (supine) inhalation where the third and fourth lumbar vertebrae press onto the floor. Then, the diaphragm begins to pull the ribs, next the floating ribs widen

and only at the end of inhalation do the sternum and clavicle participate.

An exercise has interlaced fingers lifting the head to get neck-thorax muscles to relax. He notes: 'Without practice there is not perfect breathing,[24] ... without knowledge there isn't better ability.' Box 8.3.2 captures some of Feldenkrais' thoughts on breathing.

Feldenkrais also gave lessons with the students standing; in one[25] he predicts proper head position can occur only if inhalation occurs while shifting weight onto a heel. Further, exhalation must be delicate and occur only when the weight is fully shifted to the other leg. Another lesson[26] predicts a 'floating movement' during a standing turn only when the abdominal rather than the spinal muscles work. This turning is fast but the breath must be free 'the middle part of the chest is backward and the chest is hanging[27].' Another lesson[28] reiterates why the chest should hang completely from the spine.

A kneeling lesson[29] helps students to discover that releasing lumbar lordosis (while kneeling with the head bowed) permits the chest to hang freely from the spine. This, in turn, allows the muscular skirt of the diaphragm to work evenly.

[20]Feldenkrais (1949, p. 101) remarks the neck and lumbar vertebrae act as sense-organs.
[21]Yanai#180,185,186,187,188,189,191
[22]Yanai#201,202,203,204
[23]Yanai#435 predicts 'clarity of speech [and] lucidity of voice' (p. 2958) will follow with decreased inhalation effort.

[24]Yanai 5A:p.1379
[25]Yanai#274
[26]Yanai#236
[27]Yanai 6B:p.1874
[28]Yanai#283
[29]Yanai#329

STUDENT EXPERIENCES

Student experiences of the Feldenkrais approach are too manifold for discussion here; in every instance, the learning is individualized. To give a sense of the journey students make, the experience of Feldenkrais in fine-tuning his theory may prove helpful. Feldenkrais (1965) recounted a soccer injury (knee cruciate ligament) aggravated by his escape from the German invasion of Paris in 1940. A surgeon advised him surgery was necessary. Feldenkrais, concerned at the poor odds of success, never had the surgery.

*Before I had trouble with the knee I had thirty years' experience with it. I spent a lot of time using the knee properly, but eventually I forgot that old, good way … I found out that I was holding the ground, that I was afraid of slipping with the knee. I was actually making it slip, but I didn't realize it.
I began using the knee correctly and I found it easier … Well, after the knee was all right, I slipped on a banana skin and the whole thing was undone.*

That gave me a shock … I discovered that at the moment of the fall I forgot about my theory and did the wrong thing. I slipped like any normal person would … Each person has an impression of his own manner of speaking, walking, and carriage which seems personal and immutable – the only possible way – and he identifies with this image. His

judgment of the spatial relationships and movements of his body seems innate, and he believes it is possible to change only the vitality, intensity and capability of them … The difficulty in changing a physical or mental habit is due partly to heredity and individuality, but mostly to the necessity of displacing an already-acquired habit … If one simply thinks of his accustomed manner as an alternate term for 'self-image', one comprehends the difficulty in perfecting a particular action. The self-image's habitual configuration is to a certain extent compulsive; the person could not act otherwise. He substitutes a habitual action for the proposed exercise without being conscious of not doing what he wished.

… Good movement is more complex than it seems. First of all, it should be reversible. For instance, if I make a movement with my hand it would be accepted as good, as conscious, clear, and willed movement if I can at any point of the trajectory stop, reverse the movement, continue, or change it into something else … The next important [thing] is that the body should be maintained in a state of action where it can start a movement without preliminaries. For instance … if I can stand so that I can, without preliminaries, rise, stoop, move forward, backwards, right and left, and twist myself – then elementary demands of good posture are fulfilled. This is also true for the voice and the breath … The crucial work consists in leading to awareness in action, or the ability to make contact with one's own skeleton and

---

Box 8.3.3 **Feldenkrais (1977) on breathing**

- 'Good breathing … means good posture, just as good posture means good breathing' (p. 166). 'Breathing is incomplete in any part of the chest that is not fully flexible' (p. 171). Also, Yanai#5A:p.1383.
- Chest stiffening occurs in people with poor body alignment. Although costly to the body economy, the stiffening compensates for the spinal disorganization by providing a path to transmit forces.*

- Normal supine inspiration initiates with the 3rd and 4th lumbar vertebrae lifting. During inspiration, all thoracic vertebrae rest while the chest expands and the sternum lifts.[†]
- Feldenkrais predicted poor breathers will estimate different (and inaccurate) distances of their chest thicknesses.[‡]

---

*Feldenkrais (1977) noted force transmission is best when passed lengthwise through the spine and limb bones. With poor body position, the chest stiffens to channel the force transmission generated by the large pelvic muscles. Without the chest stiffening, the force would be absorbed into the poor body alignment. With good posture, the force is well directed and the chest need not stiffen (p. 90).

[†] Feldenkrais (1977) defined the respiratory role of the crural diaphragm. He also describes an aberrant pattern existing when the sternum remains fixed relative to the spine. In this condition, the spine hollows as the entire chest is raised. Lung volume increases by action of the lowest ribs but the rest of the chest stiffens (pp. 101, 168).

[‡] Here are his directions: Eyes closed, indicate chest thickness by spreading hands the appropriate distance. Measure this with the hands aligned both vertically and horizontally. Try it. (Feldenkrais 1977, p. 23). Feldenkrais (1965) describes the process: 'For example, keeping your eyes closed, try to represent with your hands the thickness of your chest, first with your hands in back and front, then by separating them laterally, and finally vertically. You will be amazed to see that your judgment changed with the positions of your hands and that for each attempt you produced a different result. The variation is often as much as one hundred percent.
When this deviation between the conception of the self-image and the objective (or 'real') facts is nearly one hundred percent, the behaviour of that part of the body is generally defective. For example: someone who holds his chest in a position of exaggerated exhalation will find that according to his self-image the chest seems two or three times thicker than it is in reality. Inversely, someone who holds a position of extreme inhalation will find the self-image underestimates the chest thickness.'

muscles and with the environment nearly simultaneously … The gradual reduction of useless effort is necessary in order to increase kinetic sensitivity, without which a person cannot become self-regulating … That's why I get the students down on the floor. Unless the necessary muscular tension is reduced, they couldn't detect any changes.

MANUAL THERAPY

FI and ATM are two sides of the same coin. Once the underlying principles are understood, exercises and manual therapy can be improvised to match the student's needs. Still, there are many useful tips to be learned. Karzen (2009) is an excellent resource[30] for understanding Feldenkrais' method of manual therapy. Props can help a student to relax. Figure 8.3.1 suggests some prop placements. Hannon (2006) outlines this topic in greater detail. Figure 8.3.2 demonstrates how unstable equilibrium may be harnessed in FI.

[30]He helped edit Feldenkrais' last two books as well as directing/filming almost all of the existing videotapes of his private lessons. Karzen presents Feldenkrais giving 5 FI lessons to a young child with cerebral palsy. Included is an untouched version and one with voice-over with Karzen's comments.

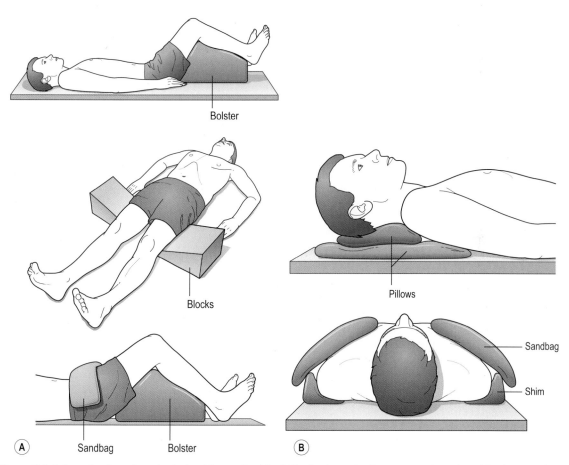

Figure 8.3.1 Props for the spine, chest, shoulders and pelvis. **A** The lumbar spine is encouraged to relax with a large and wide bolster placed under the knees. Foam blocks wedged under the ilia to rotate the pelvis may reduce the lordosis. Look for T11–T12 ribs opening laterally on inspiration. Occasionally, sandbags (duration about 5 minutes) placed obliquely across the upper thighs near the groin crease, helps release the psoas major. **B** The cervical lordosis may need its own pillow to encourage relaxation. If the head and shoulders incline anteriorly, a long, wide and flat pillow (extending head to inferior scapular angle) may aid in easing the breath. In addition, wedging the scapular spine anteriorly with foam blocks plus sandbags across the AC joint and pectoralis minor may increase inspiratory sternal elevation. Rule of thumb: pleasant increase in inspiratory excursion with the bridge of nose level with floor.

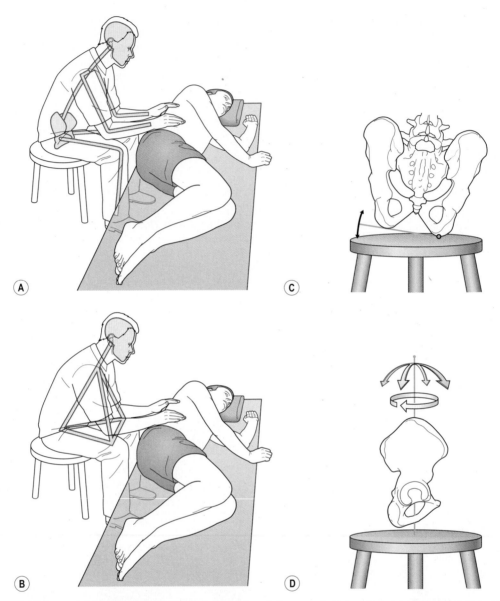

Figure 8.3.2 Using unstable equilibrium in a Feldenkrais session. **A** An example harnessing unstable equilibrium to generate a smooth flow of momentum from practitioner to client. **B** Notice the stable tetrahedron produced by the practitioner's posture and the client's back. Stability reduces random touch and introduces stillness. When the practitioner leans forward, the tetrahedron produces a client-based unstable equilibrium by mildly rocking the client's pelvis and thorax on their elliptical cross-sections. Carefully managed, this helps stiffen the client's trunk. Practitioner-generated selective pushing (heels on floor; elbows on thighs) creates a second (practitioner-based) unstable equilibrium with a small but complex movement. First of all, the practitioner's trunk is stiffened by increasing intra-abdominal pressure using easy and full breathing. **C** The unstable equilibrium is fitted to clinical necessity by slight pelvic tipping onto an ischial tuberosity. **D** Pivoting on the ischium (while hinging at the hips) fine-tunes the unstable equilibrium. A smooth flow of momentum arises from the practitioner's arms, legs and trunk permitting the trunk to gently fall towards the client. Thus, the practitioner exploits gravity to steer the client. The practitioner's hands apply a steady and soft traction/twist force to fix the client's spine and increase breathing ease.
Reprinted with permission from: Hannon, J.C., 2001. The physics of Feldenkrais® Part 5: unstable equilibrium and its application to movement therapy. Journal of Bodywork and Movement Therapies 5 (3), 207–221. *Continued*

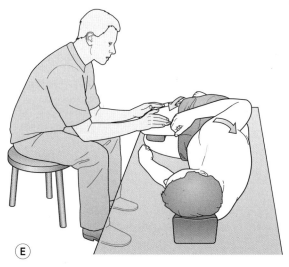

(E)

Figure 8.3.2, cont'd. **E** A spatial therapeutic lens is created by yoking together each unstable equilibrium. The contours of this lens are controlled by manual forces, client placement and positioning of the practitioner's body weight. This lens, suitably directed, may focus the rhythmic power of the client's own breath (along with gravity) to achieve beneficial therapeutic outcomes. *Reprinted with permission from: Hannon, J.C., 2001. The physics of Feldenkrais® Part 5: unstable equilibrium and its application to movement therapy. Journal of Bodywork and Movement Therapies 5 (3), 207–221.*

CONCLUSIONS

The Feldenkrais approach presents many testable predictions. For instance, breathing and posture are cognate. The cited ATM lessons can be mined for testable hypotheses. This chapter recommends future researchers consider the Mehling et al experimental methodology recommendations. Also, since the lessons are designed to clarify interoception, individuals can personally put these predictions to the test.

Central to this approach is the idea of unstable equilibrium. His manual therapy creates this through leverage, and sometimes props. The manual therapy and the lessons Feldenkrais developed share a three-fold task: get the waist to stiffen the trunk appropriately; ensure unimpeded head and breathing functions and, with awareness through movement, perfect the self-image.

Please consult www.whywasteyourbreath.com to access two short videos illustrating simple methods for the encouragement of breathing ease. One demonstrates prop placement and the other shows the use of unstable equilibrium in manual therapy.

ACKNOWLEDGMENTS

Many thanks to Chris Fernie for his technical assistance with the Yanai lessons.

DISCLAIMER

The author is a Guild-certified Feldenkrais Practitioner.

Box 8.3.4 Sample Feldenkrais ATM lessons focused on breathing

These Feldenkrais ATM lessons are referenced in the text. Full texts of each are available in Feldenkrais 1994–2004, and can be identified by the year, volume and page numbers listed here.

Yanai#5 – Equalizing the nostrils. [1994] 1(A):25–9.
Yanai#17 – Breathing. [1994] 1(A):97–102.
Yanai#23 – Palate, mouth and teeth. [1994] 1(A):137–43.
Yanai#111 – Painting with the soles of the feet. [1994] 3(A):727–33.
Yanai#117 – Frog movement with the leg and the arch. [1994] 3(A):773–9.
Yanai#126 – The mouth and head cavity. [1994] 3(B):837–44.
Yanai#136 – Looking at the back while sitting. [1994] 3(B):901–9.
Yanai#172 – Stopping the breath. [1996] 4(A):1155–61.
Yanai#179 – Breathing (To weld by breathing). [1996] 4(B):1209–14.

Yanai#180 – Breathing rhythmically [#1]. [1996] 4(B):1215–21.
Yanai#185 – Lying on the feet, part 3 and breathing rhythmically #2 (Breathing in 4 parts). [1996] 4(B):1251–8.
Yanai#186 – Breathing rhythmically [#3] (the left side). [1996] 4(B):1259–64.
Yanai#187 – Breathing rhythmically [#4] (on both sides). [1996] 4(B):1265–71.
Yanai#188 – Twisting the spine and breathing rhythmically [#5]. [1996] 4(B):1273–80.
Yanai#189 – Directed [intentional breathing] [Breathing rhythmically #6]. [1996] 4(B):1281–7.
Yanai#191 – Pressing to the floor and breathing [Breathing rhythmically #7]. [1996] 4(B):1297–1303.
Yanai#201 – Gluing in the lungs, part 1. [1997] 5(A):1369–75.

Box 8.3.4 Sample Feldenkrais ATM lessons focused on breathing – cont'd

Yanai#202 – Gluing in the lungs, part 2. [1997] 5(A):1377–85.

Yanai#203 – Gluing in the lungs, part 3. [1997] 5(A):1387–93.

Yanai#204 – Gluing and bending the back; Gluing in the lungs, part 4. [1997] 5(A):1395–1401.

Yanai#217 – On the side, the sternum becoming flexible. [1997] 5(A):1481–7.

Yanai#236 – Rotation on an axis [1999] 5(B):1621–7.

Yanai#274 – Introduction to walking 1 [1999] 5(A):1869–75.

Yanai#283 – Continuation on one leg [1999] 6(B):1933–9.

Yanai#290 – Standing on one leg with a hop [1999] 6(B):1985–91.

Yanai#316 – End standing, continuation [2000] 7(A):2163–8.

Yanai#319 – Continuation, the head on the upper arm [2000] 7(A):2185–90.

Yanai#329 – Standing on the knees [2000] 7(B):2245–50.

Yanai#435 – Alternately stomach up/down in the breathing [2001] 9(B):2957–62.

REFERENCES

Banzett, R.B., Shea, S.A., Brown, R., et al., 1997. Perception of inflation of a single lung lobe in humans. Respiration Physiology 107 (2), 125–136.

Burton, G.G., Gee, G.N., Hodgkin, J.E., 1977. Respiratory care: a guide to clinical practice. J.B. Lippincott, Philadelphia, pp. 260.

Chaitow, L., Bradley, D., 2002. The structure and function of breathing. In: Chaitow, L., Bradley, D., Gilbert, C. (Eds.), Multidisciplinary approaches to breathing pattern disorders, Churchill Livingstone. Harcourt Publishers, Limited, London, pp. 25.

Feldenkrais, M., 1942 (2009). Hadakajime: the core technique for practical unarmed combat. Genesis II Publishing, Longmont, Colorado.

Feldenkrais, M., 1944. Judo: the art of defence and attack. Frederick Warne & Co., London.

Feldenkrais, M., 1949. Body and mature behaviour: a study of anxiety, sex, gravitation and learning. International Universities Press, New York.

Feldenkrais, M., 1977. Awareness through movement: health exercises for personal growth. Harper & Row, New York.

Feldenkrais, M., 1994–2004. The Feldenkrais Method: awareness through movement lessons. Dr. Moshe Feldenkrais at Alexander Yanai. Volumes 1A-11B, Published by the International Feldenkrais Federation, Paris.

Feldenkrais, M., 1965. Image, movement and actor: restoration of potentiality. In: Beringer, E. (Ed.), 2010 Feldenkrais M: Embodied wisdom: the collected papers of Moshe Feldenkrais. North Atlantic Books, Berkeley, pp. 93–112.

Gadow, S., 1980. Body and self: a dialectic. J Med Philos 5 (3), 172–185.

Green, E., Green, A., 1977. Beyond biofeedback. Delacorte Press, New York, pp. 106–109.

Hannon, J.C., 2001. The physics of Feldenkrais® Part 5: unstable equilibrium and its application to movement therapy. Journal of Bodywork and Movement Therapies 5 (3), 207–221.

Hannon, J.C., 2006. Wartenberg Part 3: Relaxation training, centration and skeletal opposition: a conceptual model. Journal of Bodywork and Movement Therapies 10 (3), 179–196.

Karzen, J., 2009. Erin learns to walk better: 5 lessons in Functional Integration® with Dr. Moshe Feldenkrais. [5 DVDs] www.feldenkraishawaii.com.

Loh, L., Goldman, M., Davis, J.N., 1977. The assessment of diaphragm function. Medicine (Baltimore) 56 (2), 165–169.

Mehling, W.E., DiBlasi, Z., Hecht, F., 2005a. Bias control in trials of bodywork: a review of methodological issues. J Altern Complement Med 11 (2), 333–342.

Mehling, W.E., Hamel, K.A., Acree, M., et al., 2005b. Randomized, controlled trial of breath therapy for patients with chronic low-back pain. Altern Ther Health Med 11 (4), 44–52.

Mehling, W.E., Gopisetty, V., Daubenmier, J., et al., 2009. Body awareness: construct and self-report measures. PLoS One 4 (5), e5614. doi:10.1371/journal.pone.0005614.

Mehling, W.E., Wrubel, J., Daubenmier, J.J., et al., 2011. Body awareness: a phenomenological inquiry into the common ground of mind-body therapies. Philosophy, Ethics, and Humanities in Medicine 6.6. http://www.peh-med.com/content/6/1/6 (Accessed June 2013).

Moses, P.J., 1954. The voice of neurosis. Grune and Stratton, New York, pp. 89.

Torday, J.S., Rehan, V.K., 2009. Lung evolution as a cipher for physiology. Physiol Genomics 38 (1), 1–6.

Verin, L., 1981. The teaching of Moshe Feldenkrais. In: Kagan, G. (Ed.), The body works: a guide to health and balance. Transformations Press, Berkeley, pp. 83–86.

Weibel, E.R., 2009. What makes a good lung? The morphometric basis of lung function. Swiss Medical Weekly 139 (27–28), 375–386.

Chapter | 8.4

Pilates in the rehabilitation of breathing disorders

Warrick McNeill, Suzanne Scott

Pilates is a system of movement which takes its name from its creator, Joseph Hubertus Pilates, born in Germany (1883–1967), who originally called his system 'Contrology'. Pilates believed that the body should be actively regulated and controlled by the mind, redressing what he saw as the results of chronic physical inactivity from an increasingly urbanized way of life. Latey (2001, 2002) further describes his history and philosophy in detail.

'Breath' is one of the 6 central tenets of Pilates, along with Concentration Control, Centre, Precision and Flow

(Friedman & Eisen 1980). Pilates should be considered as an aid to the rehabilitation of those presenting with breathing pattern disorders caused by movement disorders of the neuromusculoskeletal system, sub-optimal postures, disease processes affecting the physiology of the breathing system or of psychological origin.

A doctor or therapist can refer a client with a breathing pattern disorder to a Pilates studio or teacher, but only when an adequate working diagnosis has been established and the Pilates teacher is informed. As a profession, Pilates has received negative criticism in the *New York Times* and elsewhere, questioning its efficacy for clients with lower back pain.[1,2] Pilates exercises include 'spinal movement', often loaded, so inappropriate spinal motion in a client with a low tolerance to that direction of spinal motion can provoke pain. The authors believe a negative reaction to a Pilates class can occur because of inadequate training of the Pilates teacher, a referral from a doctor or therapist without communication of risk factors, a lack of knowledge on the referrer's part as to what is taught within the Pilates environment, or the inadvertent, or deliberate withholding of information from the Pilates teacher by the client themselves. When deciding whether to refer a client with a breathing pattern disorder to Pilates, an understanding of the system by the referrer is essential. The referral itself should outline the problem, its risk factors, and the aims of the referral. Ongoing communication for reassessment and evaluation reasons should also be considered. Once rehabilitative goals are attained it is common for clients to continue to attend Pilates classes for general wellbeing or postural fitness reasons.

---

[1]www.nytimes.com/2009/06/21/magazine/21FOB-physed-t.html?_r=1&scp=1&sq=&st=nyt (Accessed June 2013)
[2]http://www.dailymail.co.uk/health/article-2161301/Pilates-make-bad-worse-Experts-agree-help-reduce-pain-improve-posture-hidden-dangers.html (Accessed June 2013)

A Pilates teacher's skill set

An appropriately trained and certified Pilates teacher is a keen observer of posture and dynamic movement, their skill set includes a vast repertoire of exercises, an ability to see movement patterning faults, and skills to convey, by verbal or physical (handling) cues how to recruit a more appropriate movement or stability pattern without allowing movement or muscular substitutions. They need to be able to respond, instantly, for safety, therapeutic or somatic reasons, and modify, ramping up or down load, changing the client's position to affect the base of support, and modifying movement complexity – not only to a single client in a one to one situation but often in a group environment. They need to apply the principles of Pilates to the form of the class while creating a balanced exercise routine that targets specific goals and also provides a well-structured class.

Pilates' writings and principles

Pilates' two written treatises, the first published in 1934, 'Your Health: A Corrective System of Exercising That Revolutionizes the Entire Field of Physical Education' and the second in 1945, 'Return to Life through Contrology', are evidence of his desire to promote his beliefs to the wider world. His strongest diktat quotes Schiller, 'It is the mind that builds the body'.

The 'Pilates Principles' were not formally established in his writing and they were distilled from his work

Table 8.4.1 The Pilates Principles (after Freidman and Eisen)

Principle	Description
Concentration	Close attention must always be applied to the detail of all parts of movement. No part of the body is unimportant
Control	All parts of the body need to be controlled during the movement
Centre	The centre – the powerhouse, the focal point of the Pilates Method, the area between the bottom of the rib cage and the line across the hip bones, the starting place for building the foundations of the body
Flowing movement	Movement should not be stiff or jerky, not too rapid or slow, it should be smooth and evenly flowing
Precision	Correct movement every time you exercise
Breath	Full and thorough inhalation and exhalation

and teachings and first codified in a published format in 1980 by Friedman and Eisen, and their interpretation of the principles is summarized in Table 8.4.1. Latey (2002) further updated the principles for the new century.

Pilates: a system, an art, not yet truly a science

There are broadly two styles of Pilates – the hagiographic 'Classic Pilates', keeping the system close to the way Pilates himself taught it – usually fast and dynamic, and 'Modern' (Latey 2001), or 'Evolved Pilates' which allows for change in the system as research evidence from medical and motor control science into Pilates is applied within the Pilates environment.

Pilates is difficult to research experimentally, being regarded as an 'art' with non-standardized execution. There are as yet few papers of high quality (Bernardo 2007), but evidence of what could be called 'the science of Pilates' is emerging.

JOSEPH PILATES ON BREATH

Pilates often used the concept of 'breath' as a symbol of the connection between mind and body. He believed that exhaling completely, assisted by abdominal muscular contraction or with body weight assisting compression, allows the following inhalation to maximize oxygenation of the blood. 'One should 'squeeze' every atom of air from your lungs until they are almost as free of air as a vacuum' (Pilates & Miller 1945). As knowledge of breathing pattern disorders, particularly hyperventilation, has become available since Pilates' day, it is important that a Pilates teacher is alert to signs of disordered breathing and adapts breath cueing accordingly for those at risk.

The mechanics of breathing in Pilates

Despite the diversity in approach between Pilates teachers, the choreography of breath with movement is fundamental to the method. There is an emphasis on breathing as the amplifier of other elements of the grammar of Pilates, particularly the principles of centre and alignment.

An exemplar of how a client may be taught to breathe within the Pilates repertoire should include an emphasis on the laterocostal expansion of the thoracic cage during the inhalation phase, and use of the exhalation phase to facilitate tensioning through the anterolateral abdominal wall. The teacher–client dialogue encourages the experiential embodiment of the breath as the carrier of movement, and uses verbal and tactile cueing to facilitate changes in habitual patterns of breathing.

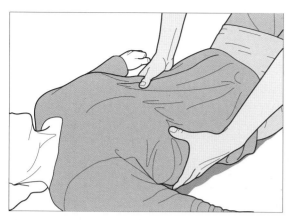

Figure 8.4.1 Laterocostal breathing facilitated by the teacher.

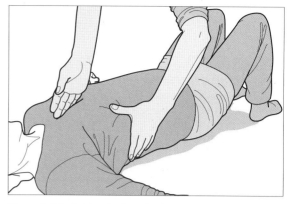

Figure 8.4.2 Teacher-facilitated inferior gliding of the rib cage during exhalation.

Teaching Pilates laterocostal breathing

- The client is instructed to lie supine, with a cushion supporting the head as required according to postural tendency (such as a thoracic kyphosis).
- The teacher places the palms of both hands on either side of the thoracic cage and instructs the client to breathe into their hands, to facilitate a laterocostal expansion of the ribs (Fig. 8.4.1).
- The teacher offers commentary and refinements using hands-on facilitation, tailored to the client, encouraging both successful execution and understanding of what is intended anchored in sensory-kinaesthetic, neuromotor cueing.
- Cueing examples:
  Verbal: 'widen your rib cage out to the side as you breathe'
  Visual-verbal: 'imagine your ribs opening out like an accordion'
  Kinaesthetic-verbal: 'feel your ribs moving out to the sides as your lungs fill with air and sense the weight of the rib cage sinking into the mat as you breathe out.'
- If the teacher observes a tendency towards antero-postero breathing (breathing 'front to back'), characterized by the abdomen rising excessively during inhalation or the rib cage moving antero-superiorly, possibly accompanied by thoracolumbar extension, additional cueing and facilitation, aimed at countering this, will be offered:
- Cueing examples:
  Verbal: 'as you inhale breathe into your back and gently press your ribs into the mat' gently resists the thoracic movement antero-superiorly on inhalation, and facilitates downward gliding of the rib cage during the exhalation phase.
  Tactile 2: with the palms positioned at the sides of the rib cage (as above) the teacher facilitates the

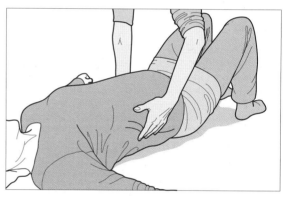

Figure 8.4.3 Teacher-facilitated control of antero-abdominal doming.

exhalation phase guiding the rib cage towards the pelvis with light pressure, so that the rib cage moves postero-inferiorly (Fig. 8.4.2), countering thoracolumbar extension tendency and antero-abdominal doming (Fig. 8.4.3).

- A commonly observed phenomenon is the tendency towards apical breathing, characterized by over-solicitation of secondary respiratory muscles, such as the scalenes, sternocleidomastoid and pectoralis minor, which may present directly as visible symmetrical or asymmetrical activation of these muscles, or indirectly as rigidity or restriction in the carriage of the shoulder girdle. If this is observed, cueing will be altered to address this, with the aim of lessening unnecessary muscle activation to promote a sense of ease and reduction in held tension within the client.
- Cueing examples:
  Verbal: 'Relax your neck – gently turn it side to side as if you were saying 'no' and let your hands feel heavy on the floor.'
  Turning the head reduces the tendency towards rigidity via muscular co-contraction; drawing

attention to the hands is an example of peripheral distraction in order to reduce proximal holding patterns, that may be indicative of habitually elevated tone in secondary respiratory muscles.
Verbal-visual-sensory: 'Imagine your throat softening, let your neck lengthen along the mat and allow the weight of your head and shoulders to melt into the floor.'
Tactile-kinaesthetic: the teacher uses a light, symmetrical, hands-on gesture, sweeping outwards from the sternoclavicular joints towards the acriomioclavicular joints, with the intention of facilitating a widening and releasing (infero-lateral movement) of the pectoral girdle.

Pilates laterocostal breathing – client facilitated

Once the client has experienced laterocostal breathing with hands-on guidance from the teacher, they will typically be encouraged to 'self-sense' and reproduce independently what may be novel movements of the rib cage, using their own hands to replicate the gentle compression and poster-inferior gliding of the rib cage. The teacher may also, through open questions and language mirroring, prompt the client using images, specific verbal and/or kinaesthetic-sensory cues to elicit appropriate performance of the breathing exercise.

If it is an introductory session to Pilates, the client will usually next be directed to extend their awareness of how they are breathing towards sensing the effect on the abdominal wall, and a new cycle of cues will be initiated, in order to integrate breath with centre, prior to movement.

- Cueing examples:
  Verbal: 'as you exhale and the ribs glide down towards your hips, actively draw your abdominals in and back towards your spine.'
  Verbal-visual: 'visualize your ribs being connected to your hips by elastic threads and as you exhale, imagine the threads pulling ribs and hips together, like a corset narrowing the waist.'

If a small cushion or inflated ball is placed between the femurs, the client may be further instructed to access a pelvic floor contraction, via an isometric tensioning of muscles of the medial thigh (adductors) at low (~30%) of maximum voluntary contraction (MVC), in order to integrate the pelvic diaphragm with the respiratory diaphragm (Fig. 8.4.4).

- Cueing examples:
  Verbal-visual: 'Breathe in wide to the back, and as you exhale let your ribs glide down towards your hips and press the inside of your legs gently into the ball, as you draw up inside your pelvis, as if you are narrowing the distance between your hips.'

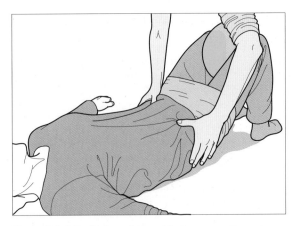

Figure 8.4.4 Facilitation of the adductor connection using a ball.

The above examples of verbal cueing and facilitation are attempts at generalization, so that useful technical information about intention and effect can be extracted. Cueing and hands-on guidance tend to be idiosyncratic and practitioner specific, and presenting a description of 'correct technique' that is universally agreed and followed by all teachers is difficult. In practical terms, verbal-visual cues such as 'tighten your abdominals' and 'pull in, navel to spine' have given way to cues such as 'draw a smile line across your hip bones with your abdominals,' (less accessible, more abstract, arguably more evidentially 'correct'), which aim to create lateral and posteriorly directed myofascial tension, without reducing axial length or narrowing transversely. Such cues may have the additional benefit of reducing stress concentrations at bony sites. According to a biomechanical definition of stress, stress reduction in association with an increase in the surface area over which forces are distributed, is expressed as: stress = force ÷ surface area. This may be of particular benefit in some populations, for example athletes in kicking sports, where a fashion for forceful exhalation accompanying fast, 'sit-up' style exercises, aimed at increasing core-strength, has led to anecdotal evidence of symptomatic changes at the site of the pubic symphysis and/or adductor-groin symptoms, sometimes accompanied by weakening of the pelvic diaphragm, due to repetitive bearing down and rapid, cyclical increases in intra-abdominal pressure.

Pilates breathing, which primarily focuses on integrating a flowing, effortless connection of the breath with the movement of the exercises has, in the authors' experience and practice, been valuable in countering a tendency towards excessive abdominal bracing and rectus abdominis dominance, as a result of inadequate technique when attempting to increase core strength and core stability[3], using abdominal exercise protocols.

Pilates laterocostal breathing and centre

The most direct gain of Pilates breathing is that it facilitates optimal engagement of centre. At a musculoskeletal level this translates as a graded recruitment of some or all of those muscles associated with the dynamic process of centring, most notably the anterolateral abdominal wall, pelvic floor and adductors. Depending on an individual client's movement presentation, and the demands of a particular exercise, other muscles may be cued as an extension of centre, such as the deep lateral rotators of the hip, and more superficial muscles of the posterior hip (gluteus maximus) and pectoral girdle (latissimus dorsi). Directional loading, range of movement and speed of execution will also affect the muscular influences that will be cued to help establish centre dynamically.

In the exercise example below, which is performed in standing, the effect of pressing down on a spring-loaded bar activates the extensors of the glenohumeral joint (GHJ) (latissimus dorsi and teres major), and the resulting increase in thoracodorsal fascial tension can be utilized to encourage axial lengthening, and counter a tendency towards hyperextension in the lumbar spine and forwards sway of the pelvis, which are commonly encountered postural presentations in clients.

Standing latissimus press ('lat press')

The client is positioned facing the frame of the Pilates cadillac, and in neutral wrist alignment is instructed to inhale and on an exhale press down against the spring-loaded roll-down bar. During the next inhalation phase, the client maintains pressure on the bar and on the subsequent exhalation the tension on the bar is gradually released, whilst postural alignment is maintained, with emphasis on axial lengthening of the spine and active tensioning of the abdominals, to counter extension of the lumbar spine and anterior sway or tilt of the pelvis (Fig. 8.4.5).

In the absence of Pilates equipment, the exercise may be performed using a length of Thera-Band™ fixed from above to reproduce resisted GHJ extension.

Cues may be variously directed at using the breath to encourage lengthening in opposition to gravity or towards reducing regional or segmental hyperextension of the lumbar spine.

- Cueing examples:
  Verbal: 'As you press down grow tall through the crown of your head.'
  Verbal-visual: 'As you press down through the outer edge of your hand imagine you are drawing up through your spine, pushing the floor away through the edges of your feet.'
  Verbal-kinaesthetic: 'Feel your tailbone drop and lengthen towards the floor, as your neck lengthens and your head floats up towards the ceiling.'

Variation in Pilates breathing: the four breath and two breath pattern, percussive breathing

The exercise example above illustrates a secondary, important role of breathing in Pilates, that of adding emphasis to, or increasing the duration of, a particular phase of an exercise. In standing lat press, an additional inhalation under spring loading maintains the resisted GHJ extension phase. The purpose of this is, in itself, a variable of Pilates exercise teaching, and may be deployed in a client-specific manner, depending on whether the teaching aim is predominantly musculoskeletal or somatic, in which case an experiential or sensory response may be emphasized. In the example above, this might involve challenging a client with lordotic posture to resist a 'pre-loaded' inclination towards spinal extension on GHJ extension. This may also be useful when working with hypermobile clients, who often present with proprioceptive deficits, possibly due to a reduction in afferent feedback, associated with increased compliance in myofascial and passive tissues. For such clients, the rising tension during the resisted inhalation phase may offer increased afferent feedback to the central nervous system, as more motor units are recruited, and may explain the anecdotally observed improvement in the client's capacity to redirect motor patterning consciously in response to cueing.

This example also demonstrates how, in Pilates, breath with movement tends to alternate with exercise phases of breathing without movement, in order to create a moment of stillness in which the client is directed towards subtle reorganization of habituated motor patterning. Although explanation of mechanisms likely to be involved in such reorganization is lacking, in the authors' opinion, breath patterning is likely to be an important mediator in such processes.

In Pilates cueing language, breath patterns are termed 'two breath', denoting a single inhalation and exhalation phase (corresponding to 'prepare to move' and 'perform the movement' respectively) or 'four breaths', denoting a second inhalation and exhalation phase within the movement sequence, and corresponding to holding a position under isometric muscular activation, prior to eccentrically controlling out of the movement phase or loaded posture.

---

[3]'Core-strengthening' and 'core-stabilization' are terms used frequently to denote exercises performed with or without equipment (such as foam rollers and gym balls) with the aim of promoting proximal strength. In the authors' opinion and experience, these terms are not directly interchangeable with Pilates 'centre', which denotes a more fluid, three-dimensional concept, with sensorimotor and kinaesthetic-somatic emphasis implied within the term.

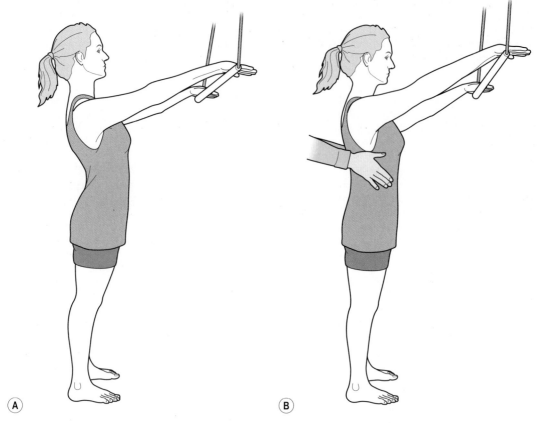

Figure 8.4.5 A An example of a client standing in a lumbar extension posture. **B** Correction of the extension posture using a standing latissimus press with integrated Pilates breathing.

The 'percussive breath' is used with rapid sagittal plane movement at the girdles ('beating' the arms or legs) during the Swimming and The Hundred exercises. The extreme shortening of the inhalation–exhalation phases enables the perturbatory effect of rapid limb movement to be resisted by the isometric tension in global muscles of the trunk. To discourage hyperventilation in the breath-disordered client, a Pilates teacher may choose to avoid this breath patterning till near the end of rehabilitation.

Movement direction and Pilates breathing patterns

The Pilates exercise repertoire contains multidirectional, whole body movement, with a bias towards the sagittal plane and segmental spinal articulation, which is referred to as 'sequential spine movement'. The choreography of the breath may also be influenced by movement direction, with a preference towards inhalation during spinal extension, and exhalation during spinal flexion. The Swan (a Pilates exercise resembling Bhujangasana, the Cobra pose

in Yoga, and McKenzie back exercise therapy), is often performed on an inhalation, with the aim of optimizing spinal extension, using the transitory increase in thoracic volume to augment the backward-bending movement created by extending the arms, as the palms press down into the mat. If a client demonstrates a reduction in spinal extension (as, for example, in age-related stiffening of the spine due to changes in articular and connective tissue characteristics), the choice of an inhalation to initiate the movement phase may enable the client to access moderate, yet significant, increases in range of movement.

In comparison, a client who lacks the ability to stiffen the anterior abdominal wall sufficiently (as in hyperlordotic or athlete sway posture) may be instructed to exhale during spinal extension, to facilitate abdominal muscle recruitment, and offset lumbar extension and anterior pelvic tilt.

Exercises with a component of spinal rotation, such as Spine Twist, may also favour inhalation as rotation is performed, and be accompanied by cues which convey the sensation of 'spiralling up' through the spine and creating axial length as the torso rotates. It is possible to argue that inhalation counters the effect of compression and torsion, so that rotational exercises are better tolerated, although some teachers cue spinal rotation on an exhalation, to facilitate abdominal oblique recruitment, and emphasize anteriorly generated rotational torque.

APPLICATIONV IN TEACHING – REMEDIAL CONTEXTS

Although Pilates is perhaps best described as a somatic movement practice rather than a treatment modality, it may be useful in a number of systemic and musculoskeletal conditions, via application of the breath to create novel musculoskeletal emphases. See Table 8.4.2.

One of the most significant contributions of Pilates to health and well-being, albeit only anecdotally supported at the time of writing, may be attributed to the indirect effects of practising the exercises in a consciously purposed manner. It is this aspect of the system which has led to it being described as thoughtful exercise, a characterization which has some of the connotations of 'mindfulness', a practice in which value is ascribed to being in the moment, and the subject is encouraged to pay attention to sensory information and present time events and processes.

Many of those who regularly practise Pilates often cite its calming influence, and use phrases such as 'it is the still point of my week,' ' I feel so much lighter and calmer after class.' There are many anecdotal examples of clients for whom Pilates practice brings about other changes in self-perception usually associated with reductions in indices of stress and anxiety, such as sleeping better, feeling calmer and having a more positive outlook. Caldwell et al (2009) showed that Pilates does significantly enhance mood, and subjects trend towards a higher sleep quality, and beneficial effects of a Pilates exercise programme on pain, functional capacity and quality of life was shown in patients with post-menopausal osteoporosis (Küçükçakır et al 2012).

Posture in older adults is shown to improve (Kaesler et al 2007) with Pilates practice, as is the dynamic posture of dancers (McMillan et al 1998), and the dynamic balance of healthy adults (Johnson et al 2007).

BREATHING AND STABILITY

Pilates aims to provide stability, initially in the 'centre,' then at the girdles. A balanced recruitment of all the abdominal musculature provides the centre's stability, but only while laterocosto breathing is continuous, allowing

Table 8.4.2 Examples of condition related breathing modification in Pilates

Condition	Pilates modification related to breathing
Emphysema	Encourage a pursed lip resistance to maintain the opening of the airways during the exhalation phase
Asthma	Focus on exhalation, limit inspiratory accessory muscle use
Scoliosis	Breathe in to compressed parts of the thorax and trunk, think of the three dimensions the air can expand into, use a foam roller in some supine exercises to subtly challenge stability while breathing and engage diagonally between the girdles, use breath to lengthen the spine
Low back rehabilitation	Starting in lumbo-pelvic neutral, engage the corset of the low abdominal wall maintaining a gentle steady recruitment while diaphragmatically breathing with a lateral costal focus. Add limb loads to this maintaining the neutral position and breathing pattern while ramping up the abdominal corset activity to balance the limbs load on the centre
Anxiety	A) De-emphasize the breathing component of the exercise if anxiety is related to the performance in class, teach it instead to be a relaxed normal breath, only add Pilates breathing in as the choreography is secure B) Be prepared to devote entire Pilates sessions to breathing alone if anxiety is a part of daily life
Pregnancy	A) For thoracic spine mobility, seated or standing breathing exercises against a ball for proprioceptive feedback B) Relaxation and gentle tensioning of the pelvic floor integrated with breathing

the diaphragm to simultaneously provide respiratory and stability function. This is discussed elsewhere in the text. See Chapter 2.1.

THE FUTURE

The aim of many rehabilitative exercise protocols is to improve unconscious motor patterns associated with dysfunction. Pilates with its goal of 'Health and Happiness' or 'Balance of Body and Mind' (Pilates 1934, Pilates & Miller 1945) uses both motor control exercises and overload training to change the client's neuromusculoskeletal system. Critchley et al (2011), researching the abdominal wall during Pilates matwork exercises, found an increase in abdominal muscular activity while practising Pilates that did not carry over into functional activities. Research aimed at taking desirable effects into life outside the Pilates environment is needed.

REFERENCES

Bernardo, L., 2007. The effectiveness of Pilates training in healthy adults: an appraisal of the research literature. Journal of Bodywork and Movement Therapies 11 (2), 106–110.

Caldwell, K., Harrison, M., Adams, M., et al., 2009. Effect of Pilates and taiji quan training on self-efficacy, sleep quality, mood, and physical performance of college students. Journal of Bodyworks and Movement Therapies 13, 155–163.

Critchley, D.J., Pierson, Z., Battersby, G., 2011. Effect of pilates mat exercises and conventional exercise programmes on transversus abdominis and obliquus internus abdominis activity: pilot randomised trial. Manual Therapy 16 (2011), 183–189.

Friedman, P., Eisen, G., 1980. The Pilates Method of physical and mental conditioning. Doubleday and Company, New York.

Johnson, E., Larsen, A., Ozawa, O., et al., 2007. The effects of Pilates-based exercise on dynamic balance in healthy adults. Journal of Bodywork and Movement Therapies 11 (2007), 238–242.

Kaesler, D.S., Mellifont, R.B., Swete, K., et al., 2007. A novel balance exercise program for postural stability in older adults: a pilot study. Journal of Bodywork and Movement Therapies 11, 37–43.

Küçükçakır, N., Altan, L., Korkmaz, N., 2013. Effects of Pilates exercises on pain, functional status and quality of life in women with postmenopausal osteoporosis. Journal of Bodywork & Movement Therapies 17 (2), 204–211.

Latey, P., 2001. The Pilates Method: history and philosophy. Journal of Bodywork and Movement Therapies 5 (4), 275–282.

Latey, P., 2002. Updating the principles of the Pilates Method Part 2. Journal of Bodywork and Movement Therapies 6 (2), 94–101.

McMillan, A., Proteau, L., Lebe, R., 1998. The effect of Pilates-based training on dancers' dynamic posture. Journal of Dance Medicine and Science 2 (3), 101–107.

Pilates, J.H., 1934. Your Health: a corrective system of exercising that revolutionizes the entire field of physical education. Reprint 1998. Presentation Dynamics Inc, NV.

Pilates, J.H., Miller, W.J., 1945. Return to life through contrology. J.J. Augustin, New York.

Chapter | 8.5 |

Tai chi, Qigong and breathing

Aileen Chan

OVERVIEW OF QIGONG AND TAI CHI

Qigong is a more than 5000-year-old Chinese (Taoist) system of gentle health-enhancing exercises that includes postures, movements, sounds, breathing techniques and meditation. The practice of Qigong aims to cultivate and enhance *Qi*, which is considered in Traditional Chinese Medicine (TCM) to be the vital energy of life.[1] All TCM practice is based on the concept of *Qi*. Tai chi is a martial art that originated in China in the 13th century and can be viewed as a therapeutic form of exercise based on Chinese medicine. Tai chi practice also involves the recognition, development and use of *Qi*. These two separate approaches, Tai chi and Qigong, can be combined as Tai chi Qigong (TCQ), as described in this chapter.

Theoretical basis of *Qi*

According to TCM theory, *Qi* is the fundamental energy that sustains life. All things in the universe, including the human body, are believed to be composed of *Qi*. This vital energy is thought to flow in the body along channels called meridians and collaterals, which connect all the organ systems and tissues. In this hypothesized model, all bodily phenomena are the results of changes and movements in the flow of *Qi*. According to TCM theory, when *Qi* is abundant, flowing freely and in balance, a person usually enjoys good health and longevity. However, when *Qi* becomes unbalanced, stagnant or unable to defend against risk factors, problems of physical, mental or emotional health occur.

   Qi is thought to be stored in energy centres known as *tantiens*. There are three *tantiens*: the lower *tantien* at the navel, the middle *tantien* at the solar plexus, and the upper *tantien* at the imaginary third eye on the forehead. Taoist teachings state that the cultivation of the lower *tantien* is

---

[1] In this text *Qi* (or chi) is considered by the co-editors to be a hypothetical construct, based on traditional views.

the foundation of all Taoist practices (McCaffrey & Fowler 2003). The deep breathing exercise of Tai chi Qigong (TCQ) helps to sink *Qi* into the lower *tantien* for *Qi* cultivation.

Tai chi Qigong (TCQ)

As explained, TCQ is a combination of exercise and meditation. Qigong uses deep, diaphragmatic breathing and coordinates with slow dance-like Tai chi movements. A study by Lan et al (2004) suggests that Tai chi results in a better training effect than Qigong alone, because of its higher exercise intensity. However, Qigong enhances breathing efficiency, during exercise, because of its enhancement of diaphragmatic breathing. Health-oriented Qigong and Tai chi emphasize the same principles and practice elements involving meditative movement that should be considered as one body of evidence.

Body training and breathing training by TCQ

Body training aims for optimal functioning. TCQ exercises are designed to directly or indirectly stimulate *Qi* circulation in specific areas of the body. Postures and movements are designed to strengthen, stretch and tone the body to improve the flow of vital energy. Proper body alignment is considered essential for *Qi* to flow smoothly and at the proper strength through the mind–body energy network. TCQ movements are performed slowly, gently and with mental attention to the breath, body movements and flow of *Qi*. The breath in TCQ not only delivers vital oxygen from the lungs for distribution throughout the body, but is thought, in TCM, to also distribute external *Qi*, gathered from the environment and converted to *Qi* in the body. The deep abdominal breathing is performed slowly and with the mind's attention focusing on the action of the breath. It lowers the diaphragm and activates the lower abdominal muscles by moving them in a constant back and forth motion. One benefit of deep abdominal breathing might involve massage of the internal organs, which is thought to increase the flow of blood and *Qi*. Research has demonstrated that TCQ has beneficial effects on the body – as outlined below, and is becoming a popular holistic modality both in China and in Western countries (Chen et al 2001). The following sections discuss the health benefits of this ancient art.

HEALTH BENEFITS OF TCQ

From the literature, different physical and psychological health outcomes have been identified, the outcomes of which can be grouped into five categories, outlined below.

Balance and fall prevention

Qigong and Tai chi have been shown to produce positive outcomes in balance improvement, postural stability and fall prevention (Yang et al 2007). The results indicated that TCQ could reduce risk factors that lead to falls and could improve balance control of community-dwelling elders.

Cardiopulmonary function

A review of the literature by Taylor-Piliae (2003) showed that simplified forms of Tai chi are ideal for people with impaired health conditions, including those with heart disease and the elderly. Consistent findings were observed in the significant reduction in blood pressure reported in multiple studies, especially when Qigong (Lee et al 2004a) or Tai chi (Wolf et al 2006) were compared to inactive control groups.

Physical function

Declining physical function is the natural process of ageing. An RCT study of a 6-month Tai chi exercise programme indicated its effectiveness in improving 65% of physical functions ranging from daily activities, such as walking and lifting, to moderate–vigorous activities, such as running (Li et al 2001). The results suggest health benefits of Tai chi beyond daily activities of living. They conclude that Tai chi is considered a low-technology exercise, that could prove to be an efficient and cost-effective means of delivering a high-quality, population-based, preventive health-enhancing method.

Psychological health

Psychological factors such as anxiety, depression, stress, mood, fear of falling and self-esteem have also been examined. A decrease in anxiety in participants practising Qigong compared to an active exercise group has been reported (Cheung et al 2005). Depression was shown to improve significantly when comparing a group using Qigong to an inactive control (Tsang et al 2006), and for a Tai chi-practising group compared to usual care group (Mustian et al 2006). General measures of mood were improved significantly for participants practising Tai chi compared to usual care controls (Gemmell & Leathem 2006) and for those practising Qigong compared to a waiting-list control group (Lee et al 2004b).

Quality of life (QOL)

QOL was reported to be significantly improved by Tai chi compared to inactive control group (Lee et al 2007) or active controls (Hart et al 2004), and by Qigong compared to inactive control (Tsang et al 2006).

BENEFITS OF TCQ ON RESPIRATORY FUNCTIONS

It is believed that TCQ is beneficial to the respiratory system since optimal breathing patterns are emphasized in the literature (Taylor-Piliae 2003). Studies have additionally shown that Tai chi can be classified as moderate exercise, as its intensity does not exceed 55% of maximal oxygen intake (Li et al 2001). The Li et al study results showed that Tai chi's slow, deep and diaphragmatic breathing, integrated with body movement and breathing action, are more efficient, when compared with cycling, in terms of ventilatory responses. They confirmed that Tai chi is beneficial for cardio-respiratory function. A study by Chao and colleagues (2002) showed that the average exercise intensity of TCQ is 3.1 MET (metabolic equivalent). This level of intensity is suitable for cardiopulmonary patients. Tai chi involves a series of slow balance movements and breathing promotion to increase energy levels and induce relaxation, which are beneficial and optimal for a person with very low functional capacities. TCQ can improve energy through slow, gentle body movement; controlled rhythmic breathing, relaxation and mindful awareness. TCQ can also increase physical strength and improve well-being, so contributing to the quality of life experienced by clients with chronic respiratory dysfunction. Thus, TCQ is especially appropriate for people with chronic illnesses because of its low intensity, steady rhythm and low physical and mental tension.

Concerns for conducting a TCQ study for people with breathing difficulties

Taking account of the favourable results obtained in previous research studies, TCQ appears to be a suitable intervention to improve physical and psychosocial health among people with respiratory problems. The less healthy physical status among the dysfunctional elderly is another concern when considering a TCQ programme. The applicability of TCQ among this group in the population deserves special attention. Irwin et al (2003) indicated that older people with more severe physical impairments at baseline have revealed the greatest increases in psychological ill-health as measured by SF-36 (a widely used instrument for measuring QOL). Therefore, the concern for the feasibility and beneficial effect of TCQ on a less healthy population is supported. In addition, available information in providing strong claims regarding the effectiveness and applicability of TCQ

on healthy older people, and people with respiratory dysfunction, has been confirmed (Chan et al 2010, 2011).

Exercise intolerance is one of the main factors limiting people with dysfunctional health in performing daily living activities. Anxiety and poor motivation are also associated with exercise intolerance (American Thoracic Society 2006). Inactivity can lead to physical deconditioning that further limits exercise tolerance. Therefore, keeping people physically active is important to reduce the impact of the respiratory deterioration. Regular exercise within limitations imposed by shortness of breath maintains fitness and reduces disability.

Living with a dysfunctional health pattern imposes a certain degree of physical and psychosocial challenge on individuals, such as decline of lung functions, reduced exercise capacity, poor QOL and poor perceived social support. These challenges may lead to poor adjustment to their current status. Because performing regular physical exercise is beneficial to the physical and psychosocial health of a person, TCQ can therefore be considered as a possible means to promote physical and psychosocial health among these people. As the general characteristics of Tai chi and Qigong are suitable for frail elders, the implementation of a TCQ programme in the community is recommended to address this issue.

The TCQ programme for people with breathing difficulties

Most evidence for the physical and psychosocial benefits of TCQ can be generalized to the older population receiving intervention in the form of a TCQ programme within a group-learning environment. To establish evidence for the effectiveness of TCQ in improving physical and psychosocial health among people with breathing difficulties, an experimental TCQ programme has been adopted for people with chronic obstructive pulmonary disease (COPD), a slow progressive disease, usually characterized by coughing, wheezing and sputum production.

This was a randomized controlled study conducted 2 years ago by our team to investigate the therapeutic effect of TCQ on COPD patients (Chan et al 2010, 2011). A total of 206 eligible subjects were randomly assigned to either a TCQ, exercise, or control group. The subjects in the TCQ group completed the 60-minute TCQ practice sessions twice a week for 3 months. The subjects in the exercise group were taught pursed-lip breathing and diaphragmatic breathing techniques. They coordinated breathing with walking as their physical exercise. Return demonstrations of breathing techniques were performed to ensure proper practice. The subjects were advised to perform breathing and walking exercises for 1 hour every day for 3 months. In addition, leaflets with pictures and instructions were provided to facilitate daily self-practise. The subjects in the control group were advised to maintain their routine activities.

Experimental protocol of TCQ programme

The 3-month TCQ programme aimed to help people with breathing dysfunction to develop the skills of TCQ exercise and to incorporate such exercise into their daily living activities. The TCQ programme consisted of 13 movements of breathing regulating Tai chi Qigong (BRTCQ), which were selected and modified from the 18 movements of Tai chi Qigong (Department of Health 2003). This modified 13-form TCQ was designed to make the programme easy to learn and to allow people to master the skills in a short period. The 13-form BRTCQ was chosen to emphasize the elements of breathing, range of motion on upper limbs for enhancing lung expansion, and overall coordination. Participants were required to coordinate their breathing with the movement motions. The modified 13 forms of BRTCQ were approved by two TCQ experts on their validity and feasibility to be used in people with breathing difficulties. They confirmed that these 13 forms were appropriate for the training of breathing and exercise tolerance. Some movements were removed from the original 18 forms, including those forms which put strain on knees which would hurt the already arthritic joints, and those forms with strenuous and low positions were modified to suit frail elders. In fact, side-effects of TCQ are rare and are avoidable by not overworking the body and doing what the participant feels is comfortable.

Mode of delivery of the TCQ training

The TCQ sessions were conducted twice a week on a group basis. Each session lasted for 1 hour. During the TCQ practise sessions participants, led by an experienced TCQ instructor, replicated the motions, postures and speed of movement of the instructor. Participants were encouraged to practise TCQ at home every day. A DVD and TCQ pictures were produced to instruct the practise of the 13 forms of movements and, together with the coordination of breathing patterns, were given to each participant to facilitate self-practise at home. This served as an important reminder in enabling the participants to practise TCQ at home. Figure 8.5.1 illustrates the 13 forms of BRTCQ. Box 8.5.1 contains the self-help session that describes each movement and coordination with diaphragmatic breathing (DB).

DB involves assisted inhalation by contracting the diaphragm, while exhaling slowly as the diaphragm is relaxed. The client is instructed to then expand the abdomen outward during inspiration, and to contract the abdomen during expiration. This manoeuvre increases lung capacity by lowering the diaphragm, allowing air to reach the bottom of the lungs. The reduced respiratory rate leads to increased tidal volume, potentially improving gas exchange in the alveoli, thereby improving blood oxygenation.

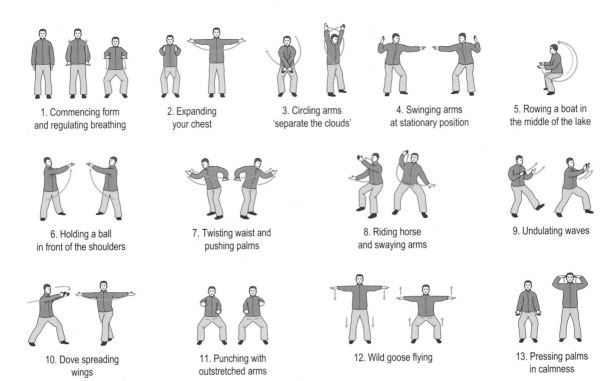

1. Commencing form and regulating breathing
2. Expanding your chest
3. Circling arms 'separate the clouds'
4. Swinging arms at stationary position
5. Rowing a boat in the middle of the lake
6. Holding a ball in front of the shoulders
7. Twisting waist and pushing palms
8. Riding horse and swaying arms
9. Undulating waves
10. Dove spreading wings
11. Punching with outstretched arms
12. Wild goose flying
13. Pressing palms in calmness

Figure 8.5.1 The 13 movements of breathing regulating Tai chi Qigong.

The 13 movements of breathing regulating TCQ (Fig. 8.5.1 and Box 8.5.1)

Box 8.5.1 Instructions for performance of Tai chi Qigong breathing regulating exercises

To begin, you must relax yourself and concentrate on the movements. Do not be distracted by other thoughts. Relax every muscle before starting the movements. Shift your weight to the right leg. Move your left leg apart while keeping your back straight. Look ahead.

Points for attention:

Inhale as you open your arms and exhale as you close.

Inhale as you lift your hands, exhale as you press down.

1. Commencing Form and Regulating Breathing

Raise both arms to the front to about eye level and inhale simultaneously. Then press both arms down and exhale simultaneously.

2. Expanding Your Chest

Raise both arms to the shoulder level and inhale simultaneously. Spread them to the sides, then bring them back to the front and press down while exhaling.

3. Circling Arms 'Separate the Clouds'

Slowly, bend your knees and lower arms to the front. Cross arms at the wrist, with left arm on top. Raise the crossed arms and inhale simultaneously. When the arms are raised to their limits, slowly lower them to the sides and exhale simultaneously.

4. Swinging Arms in Stationary Position

Bring arms to the front and keep then at shoulder level with palms facing each other. Bring the right arm backwards to behind the right ear while looking towards the back. Exhale and push the right hand forward until both palms face each other again. This facilitates the exchange of *Qi*. Repeat with the left arm.

5. Rowing a Boat in the Middle of the Lake

With the palms facing down, lower the arms and exhale simultaneously. When both hands are at the same level on each side, turn palms outwards. Raise both arms and inhale simultaneously. When the arms are raised to their limits, exhale and press both arms down simultaneously.

6. Holding a Ball in Front of the Shoulders

Raise the right arm and lift the heels while inhaling. Exhale while lowering the arm and heels. Repeat with the left arm.

7. Twisting Waist and Pushing Palms

Bring arms back to the body at waist level and inhale simultaneously. Push out right hand at an angle of 45° and exhale simultaneously. Keep fingers upwards. Inhale while bringing the right hand back to the waist. Repeat with the left hand.

8. Riding a Horse and Swaying Arms

Start on the left hand side. Bring left hand to eye level and right hand to waist level. Keep knees steady while turning the body to the right and inhale simultaneously. Repeat with the right hand and exhale while turning the body to the left.

9. Undulating Waves

Shift weight to the right leg. Step forward with the left leg to form a 'bow' step. Raise hands up to shoulder level. Lift the heel of the rear leg while pushing hands forward and exhale simultaneously. Shift your weight back onto the right leg while lifting the left toes, and withdraw both hands to the chest while inhaling simultaneously.

10. The Flying Dove Spreads Its Wings

Shift the weight onto the right leg. Stretch both arms outward to the back and inhale simultaneously. Then shift the weight forward again, bring the arms back to the front and exhale simultaneously.

11. Punching with Outstretched Arms

Shift weight to the right leg. Bring the left leg back to the original position. Punch out the left fist while exhaling then inhale while holding back the fist. Repeat on the right fist.

12. The Wild Goose Flying

Raise both arms at the sides while inhaling. Do not go too high. You don't need to bring the hands together. Keep them at shoulder width, and then lower the arms while exhaling.

13. Pressing the Palms in Calmness

Raise the arms with palms facing upward while inhaling. Bring arms to a level between the mouth and nose. Then lower the arms and palms facing downward. Raise the arms again. Withdraw the left leg. Shift weight to the right leg. Lower the arms.

Now, rub your hands a couple of times, when they are warm, rub them over the face.

Skills mastery of the participants

Ensuring the skills mastery of the participants was essential to guarantee a successful delivery of the intervention. The TCQ instructor assessed the skills mastery of the participants during the class. Any incorrect performance was identified and rectified.

TCQ programme evaluation

Programme evaluation was conducted after the completion of the TCQ programme. The aim was to collect information regarding perceptions of the benefits and the perceived limitations of the TCQ programme. The participants stated the TCQ programme was enjoyable and expressed their desire to continue practising TCQ in the future.

Effects of TCQ on people with respiratory dysfunction

A total of 206 (187 (90.8%) were males and 19 (9.2%) were females) eligible subjects were randomly assigned to one of the three groups: TCQ group (n = 70), exercise group (n = 69), and control group (n = 67). The participants had an age range from 55 to 88, with a mean age (standard deviation) of 72.9 (7.7). The mean duration of COPD was 11.1 (9.6) years. Based on the criteria of the American Thoracic Society (2004), 42.7% of the subjects were at a severe stage of COPD, 41.7% were at a moderate stage, and 15.5% were at a mild stage. No significant differences in demographic data and baseline characteristics were found, except in gender ($P = 0.021$) because fewer women were included in the TCQ group. The confounding effect of gender was therefore controlled as covariate in data analyses.

After the 3-month intervention period, there were significant differences among the three groups in lung functions and exercise capacity. The TCQ group demonstrated a prominent improvement in forced expiratory volume in one second (FEV_1) ($P < 0.001$) and forced vital capacity (FVC) ($P = 0.002$). The exercise group showed no significant differences in lung functions, while the control group demonstrated deterioration in lung functions. Significant improvement in 6-minute walking test (6MWT) was also observed in the TCQ group from baseline to the third month ($P = < 0.001$). Findings revealed the exercise group and the control group remained relatively stable in exercise tolerance during the 3-month study period. The observed increase in 6MWT was not an isolated outcome; rather, it paralleled improvements in FVC and FEV_1, and health related quality of life (HRQL) in particular. Therefore, improvements could be attributed to adaptation to the practice of TCQ exercise.

This study adopted the St George's respiratory questionnaire (SGRQ) to measure the HRQL of COPD clients. The results showed statistically significant improvement in symptoms domain ($P = 0.010$) and activity domain ($P = 0.035$) in the TCQ group when compared to the exercise group and the control group across the study period. Subjects in the TCQ group were able to improve their HRQL, which covered a wide range of disturbances of physiological and psychosocial functions, with no significant declines. Nonetheless, a worsening trend in HRQL was found in both the exercise group and the control group. In view of the progressive decline of physiological and psychosocial functions in COPD clients in the literature, regular TCQ exercises could help clients to improve their functional capacity and slow down the disease progression.

Social support is another resource that may be used by clients with chronic illnesses. Symptom management and social support play an important role in optimizing HRQL (McCathie et al 2002). In the current study, multidimensional scale of perceived social support (MSPSS) was adopted for the measurement of social support. During the first 3 months, subjects in the three study groups did not show any changes in their perceived social support from family, friends and significant others. However, increased self-perceived social support from friends was noted in the TCQ group at the 6-month follow-up assessment ($P = 0.045$). The exercise group and the control group did not show any significant changes in the perceived social support throughout the 3-month study period and in the follow-up evaluation. Practising TCQ in a supportive atmosphere can foster feelings of self-efficacy (Jin 1992). Through continuous practice, the participants gradually develop mastery. In addition to continuous practice, the successful completion of the TCQ programme might have further fostered the sense of self-worth. The self-concept can be viewed from academic perspectives on the actual achievement and competencies; or social perspective viewed by peers, family and significant others; or self-presentation as a result of self-esteem, self-confidence and self-image. Therefore, it is not difficult to explain why the TCQ group reported better health.

It was concluded that TCQ exercise is effective in improving physical and psychosocial functional health in COPD patients. Details of study results of this RCT study have been reported elsewhere (Chan et al 2010, 2011). In addition, the potential for TCQ to be considered favourably in the selection of health promotion programmes included the fact that the costs associated with TCQ intervention were low because no special equipment was needed. TCQ is therefore considered an efficient and cost-effective health service in the community.

SUMMARY

TCQ is a form of exercise that adopts the Chinese philosophy for health promotion and health maintenance. It is an undemanding exercise that may be considered to be a desirable choice for people with respiratory dysfunction. People with respiratory dysfunction experience a wide variation in their level of exercise tolerance. These people are always recommended to perform regular exercises that are suitable and beneficial to them. TCQ is an appropriate exercise to help maintenance of lung functions, which can enhance breathing efficiency during exercise. It is an easy, safe and effective exercise for this group of the population. No injury or discomfort related to the TCQ programme was reported. TCQ was well tolerated and enjoyed by the participants. Participants were able to master the learned TCQ skills within the 3-month intervention period.

Participants also expressed their desires to continue practising TCQ upon completion of the programme. Practising TCQ could be seen as an achievable task for people with respiratory dysfunction. With reference to the feedback from the participants, the TCQ programme was found to be feasible in the community setting. The findings are most relevant in providing guidance for the development of community intervention. In order to increase the application of TCQ in the context of care for respiratory dysfunctional clients, establishing a TCQ training programme to deliver exercise training to these people in the community is expected to have a beneficial effect on their health outcomes.

Understanding the benefits of TCQ in promoting the physical and psychosocial health is of great value in guiding the prescription of an effective intervention to address the health needs of people. TCQ has characteristics that are particularly suitable for older people with respiratory dysfunction. In addition, its easy application in a clinical setting has particular relevance to the current economic situation because health care resources, in terms of both manpower and funding, are few.

REFERENCES

American Thoracic Society, 2004. Standards for the diagnosis and management of patients with COPD. European Respiratory Journal 23, 932–946.

American Thoracic Society, 2006. American Thoracic Society/European Respiratory Society statement on pulmonary rehabilitation. American Journal of Respiratory and Critical Care Medicine 173, 1390–1413.

Chan, A.W.K., Lee, A., Suen, L.K.P., et al., 2010. Effectiveness of a Tai chi Qigong program in promoting health-related quality of life and perceived social support in chronic obstructive pulmonary disease clients. Quality of Life Research 19 (5), 653–664.

Chan, A.W.K., Lee, A., Suen, L.K.P., et al., 2011. Tai chi Qigong improves lung functions and activity tolerance in COPD clients: a single blind, randomized controlled trial. Complementary Therapies in Medicine 19 (1), 3–11.

Chao, Y.F.C., Chen, S.Y.C., Lan, C., et al., 2002. The cardiorespiratory response and energy expenditure of tai-chi-qui-gong. The American Journal of Chinese Medicine 30 (4), 451–461.

Chen, K.M., Snyder, M., Krichbaum, K., 2001. Clinical use of tai chi in elderly populations. Geriatric Nursing 22 (4), 198–200.

Cheung, B.M.Y., Lo, J.L.F., Fong, D.Y.T., et al., 2005. Randomized controlled trial of qigong in the treatment of mild essential hypertension. Journal of Human Hypertension 19 (9), 697–704.

Department of Health, 2003. The 18 movements of Taiji Qigong. [VCD]. Hong Kong: Department of Health.

Gemmell, C., Leathem, J.M., 2006. A study investigating the effects of tai chi chuan: individuals with traumatic brain injury compared to controls. Brain Injury 20 (2), 151–156.

Hart, J., Kanner, H., Gilboa-Mayo, R., et al., 2004. Tai chi chuan practice in community-dwelling persons after stroke. International Journal of Rehabilitation Research 27 (4), 303–304.

Irwin, M.R., Pike, J.L., Cole, J.C., et al., 2003. Effects of a behavioral intervention, tai chi chih, on varicella-zoster virus specific immunity and health functioning in older adults. Psychosomatic Medicine 65, 824–830.

Jin, P., 1992. Efficacy of Tai chi, brisk walking, meditation, and reading in reducing mental and emotional stress. Journal of Psychosomatic Research 36 (4), 361–370.

Lan, C., Chou, S.W., Chen, S.Y., et al., 2004. The aerobic capacity and ventilatory efficiency during exercise in qigong and tai chi chuan practitioners. The American Journal of Chinese Medicine 32 (1), 141–150.

Lee, M.S., Lee, M.S., Kim, H.J., et al., 2004a. Effects of qigong on blood pressure, high-density lipoprotein cholesterol and other lipid levels in essential hypertension patients. International Journal of Neuroscience, 114, 777–786.

Lee, M.S., Lim, H.J., Lee, M.S., 2004b. Impact of qigong exercise on self-efficacy and other cognitive perceptual variables in patients with essential hypertension. The Journal of Alternative and Complimentary Medicine 10 (4), 675–680.

Lee, L.Y.K., Lee, D.T.F., Woo, J., 2007. Effect of tai chi on state of self-esteem and health-related quality of life in older Chinese residential care home residents. Journal of Clinical Nursing: 16 (8), 1580–1582.

Li, F., Duncan, T.E., Duncan, S.C., et al., 2001. Enhancing the psychological well-being of elderly individuals through Tai Chi exercise: a latent growth curve analysis. Structural Equation Modeling: A Multidisciplinary Journal, 8, 53–83.

McCaffrey, R., Fowler, N.L., 2003. Qigong practice: a pathway to health and healing. Holistic Nursing Practice 17 (2), 110–116.

McCathie, H.C., Spence, S.H., Tate, R.I., 2002. Adjustments to COPD: the importance of psychological factors. European Respiratory Journal 19, 47–53.

Mustian, K.M., Katula, J.A., Zhao, H., 2006. A pilot study to assess the influence of tai chi chuan on functional capacity among breast cancer survivors. The Journal of Supportive Oncology 4 (3), 139–145.

Taylor-Piliae, R., 2003. Tai chi as an adjunct to cardiac rehabilitation exercise training. Journal of Cardiopulmonary Rehabilitation 23 (2), 90–96.

Tsang, H.W.H., Fung, K.M.T., Chan, A.S.M., et al., 2006. Effect of a qigong exercise programme on elderly with depression. International Journal of Geriatric psychiatry 21 (9), 890–897.

Wolf, S.L., O'Grady, M., Easley, K.A., et al., 2006. The influence of intense tai chi training on physical performance and hemodynamic outcomes in transitionally frail, older adults. Journals of Gerontology Series A: Biological Sciences & Medical Sciences 61 (2), 184–189.

Yang, Y., Verkuilen, J., Rosengren, K.S., et al., 2007. Effects of a taiji and qigong intervention on the antibody response to influenza vaccine in older adults. American Journal of Chinese Medicine 35 (4), 597–607.

Chapter | **8.6** |

A review of the use of yoga in breathing disorders

Shirley Telles, Nilkamal Singh

YOGA: DEFINITIONS, YOGA AS A LIFESTYLE, AND PRACTICES TRADITIONALLY INCLUDED

In ancient India importance was given to maintaining a state of balance or homeostasis (= *samatvam*, in Sanskrit). The word *samatvam* may be considered synonymous with yoga: *samatvam yoga ucyate*, 'yoga is equilibrium' (*The Bhagvad Gita*, compiled *c.* 500 B.C., Chapter 2, Verse 48). Yoga includes different aspects of a healthy lifestyle such as a particular diet (plant-based and low in saturated fat) and increased physical activity (Taimini 1961). Modification of thought patterns, to achieve a balanced state, is given equal importance in yoga, when needed. This is in line with one of the best known definitions of yoga, given by the sage Patanjali (*c.* 900 B.C.): 'Yoga is the process of gaining mastery over mental fluctuations' (Patanjali's Yoga *Sutras*, compiled *c*. 900 B.C., Ch. 1, V. 2).

TYPES OF YOGA, DESCRIPTIONS FROM TRADITIONAL TEXTS AND CONTEMPORARY KNOWLEDGE

More recently Vivekananda (1863–1902) suggested that yoga is more than physical practices or mental control; it is part of every aspect of life, with the following four types of yoga practices being the traditional categories:

- work done selflessly (*karma yoga*)
- book knowledge as well as the truths of life (*jnana yoga*)
- devotion to a non-deity-specific Supreme force (*bhakti yoga*) and
- spiritual growth (*raja yoga*), also called eight limbed or *ashtanga* yoga, which includes: moral codes of conduct (*yama*), self purification and study (*niyama*), physical postures (*asanas*), breath regulation (*pranayamas*), sense withdrawal (*pratyahara*), concentration (*dharana*), meditation (*dhyana*), and absorption in the self (*samadhi*) (Saraswati 2006). See Figure 8.6.1.

However, more recently there are types of yoga that are frequently named either after the founder or the method. In most cases these can be traced back to the original texts. Examples include Iyengar yoga (named after B.K.S. Iyengar), and Bikram yoga (named after Bikram Choudhury). Examples of yoga practices named after the method include Hatha yoga, where the emphasis is on physical practices, Kriya yoga (popularized by Paramahamsa Yogananda) based on the philosophy of *kriya* yoga from Patanjali's Yoga *Sutras*, Tantric yoga which uses the body as a means for spiritual growth, Mantra yoga (popularized by Maharishi Mahesh yogi), Integral yoga (popularized by Sri Aurobindo), and Vinyasa yoga (popularized by K. Pattabhi Jois).

Hence in recent years these new terms have given rise to a lack of clarity and it is often forgotten that traditionally there are the four types of yoga practices (of *bhakti*, *jnana*, *raja* and *karma* as described above).

IMPORTANCE OF RESPIRATION IN YOGA AND THE YOGA THEORY OF DISEASE

It is believed that if our way of life is contrary to nature's laws, we inevitably lose physiological balance or homeostasis. At some point the body will react by developing a disease. According to yoga texts a person would develop a disease based on their predisposition towards a particular

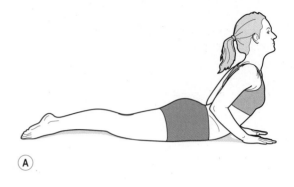

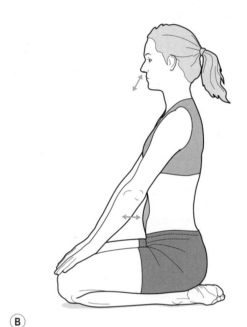

Figure 8.6.1 Yoga practices found useful in respiratory disorders based on clinical observations. **A** A yoga posture, bhujangasana. **B** A yoga breathing technique, kapalabhati.

disease-bearing factor (Telles 2010). For example, the *Taittreya Upanishad* describes five levels of existence: (i) physical, (ii) a level of subtle energy (*prana*[1] or *chi*), (iii) the instinctual mental level, (iv) the intellectual mental level, and (v) the fifth and ideal level, a state of optimal homeostasis and balance.

Imbalances are considered to occur at the instinctual mental level when there is conflict between the instinct and the intellect (Taimini 1961). The first overt manifestation of these imbalances is at the level of subtle energy (*prana* or *chi*), which results in irregular breathing. In Patanjali's Yoga *Sutras* (Ch. 1, V. 31) it is said:

---

[1]In this text *prana* (as with chi in Traditional Chinese Medicine), is seen by the co-editors as a hypothetical construct, based on traditional views.

the manifestations of a distracted state are mental anguish, tremors, rough and erratic breathing, and general nervousness.

If at this stage a person realizes that something is wrong, they may be able to make the necessary physical and mental changes. This is why awareness of internal and external sensations is an important part of yoga practice. If people are aware that their breathing is fast or irregular, and they tend to hold their breath, they would also need to be aware of the relevance of such signs. At this stage corrective measures could possibly prevent disease. However this is speculative.

It is traditionally believed that if imbalances in the mental state continue unchecked, the imbalances in breathing also remain uncorrected. These imbalances can manifest as physical disease. This is the basis for several conditions considered to have a psychosomatic basis (e.g. asthma or gastro-esophageal reflux disease (GERD)).

The reason why some individuals develop a disease of the respiratory system, while in other persons some other system is involved, is believed to be because of genetic predisposition or some inherent weakness or vulnerability of that system (Telles 2010).

This emphasis on respiration and respiratory control is mentioned in other yoga texts as well. *Hatha Yoga Pradipika* (*c.* 300 A.D.) states:

> *when the breath (used interchangeably with life energy) is irregular the mental state is erratic; when the breath is steady, the mental state is steady as well.*

By this practice the yogi attains stability and hence should regulate the breath (*Hatha Yoga Pradipika*, Ch. 2, V. 2).

Yoga breathing or *pranayama*, definition and types

Voluntarily regulated yoga breathing techniques are called *pranayamas* (*prana* = 'vital force' or 'life energy', also conveying 'breath', and *ayama* = 'to prolong', in Sanskrit). In general, the correct way of breathing according to yoga is recognized to be slow, deep and with inhalation and exhalation in a ratio of 1:2 (Singh et al 1990). An exception to this concept of *pranayama* techniques being slow in rate is a yoga technique called *kapalabhati*, which involves active exhalation and breath rates from 60–120 breaths/minute (Ramdev 2009). This practice has been considered a *pranayama* as well as a *kriya* or cleansing practice. *Pranayamas* differ in the way they modify breathing, involving:

1. changes in rate
2. alternate nostril breathing
3. exhalation during which a sound is produced
4. volume changes of breathing
5. breathing with a constricted glottis
6. breath holding, and
7. mouth breathing.

The description that follows covers the methods of practising the different *pranayamas*, the precautions and contraindications, the physiological effects of practising these techniques and their applications in treatment.

THE METHOD OF PRACTISING DIFFERENT *PRANAYAMAS*, PRECAUTIONS AND CONTRAINDICATIONS

All *pranayama* practices are ideally practised early in the morning, or at least 2 hours after the last meal, in a well-ventilated room, with the practitioner keeping the eyes closed, the spine erect and turning their awareness towards the movement of air in the nasal passages.

Pranayama (or yoga breathing) practices involving changes in breath rate

Method: The main technique involving fast breathing is *kapalabhati*, hence this technique alone will be described here. The practice involves the following steps: breathing out forcefully through both nostrils, contracting the abdomen/abdominal muscles while breathing out (initially placing a hand on the abdomen helps to sense the abdominal movements); so that inhalation follows without effort, the rate should not be more than 60 breaths/minute (which is safer than faster rates), and after every 5 minutes of practice, the practitioner should rest for 1 minute.

Precautions and conditions which are contraindications for the practice based on clinical observations are:

1. hypertension
2. coronary artery disease
3. recent abdominal/thoracic surgery, and
4. epilepsy (as it can provoke an attack).

The practice may result in overbreathing (if practised for longer than prescribed), hence it should be avoided in those who have a tendency to hyperventilate (e.g. those with panic attacks). A single case report (Johnson et al 2004) mentioned that *kapalabhati* practice resulted in pneumothorax, without a clear explanation for the reason.

Pranayama involving changes in which nostril (left, right, or alternate) is breathed through

Method: For left, right, and alternate nostril breathing the first step is the same. This step is folding the index and middle fingers so that the tips touch the palm of the dominant hand. For the three practices the right nostril is occluded with gentle pressure from the thumb while for the left nostril gentle pressure from the ring and little fingers is used. The remaining steps differ for the three practices.

Left nostril *pranayama* is called *chandra anuloma–viloma* (where *chandra* = the moon, *anuloma–viloma* = inhale-exhale, in Sanskrit). The next step is occluding the right nostril and inhaling and exhaling exclusively through the left nostril. Right nostril *pranayama* is called *surya anuloma–viloma* (where *surya* = the sun, in Sanskrit). The next step is occluding the left nostril and inhaling and exhaling exclusively through the right nostril. For alternate nostril breathing called *anuloma–viloma* there are additional steps. These are as follows: breathing out through both nostrils; closing the right nostril and breathing in through the left nostril; closing the left nostril and breathing out through the right nostril; breathing in through the right nostril, and finally breathing out through the left nostril. This is one cycle. The practice is continued with repeated cycles.

Precautions and contraindications based on research findings: of the three practices there are contraindications for right nostril breathing alone. This technique when practised by normal volunteers for 40 minutes raised the systolic, diastolic and mean blood pressure with increased peripheral vasoconstriction (Raghuraj & Telles 2008). Hence this technique is to be avoided in those with/predisposed to hypertension.

Pranayama involving exhalation during which a sound is produced

There are two types of *pranayamas* under this category. These are called bumblebee breathing (*bhramari pranayama*) and pleasant chanting (or *udgeeth pranayama* chanting the syllable '*Om*'). The practice involves repeated exhalations with the respective sounds. The methods for both techniques are different.

Method: For *bhramari pranayama*: keeping the shoulders relaxed and raising the arms, flexed at the elbows, the thumbs are used to close the ears by gently pressing on the cartilage in front of the ear. During the practice the index fingers are placed on the forehead, while other fingers are placed on the eyelids and at the base of the nose. The actual practice involves breathing in and out through the nose while making a humming sound like a bumblebee.

Precautions and contraindications: *Bhramari pranayama* is generally considered safe but based on clinical observations is best avoided in tinnitus.

Method: For *udgeeth pranayama*, breathing in deeply, and exhaling, chanting '*Om*' as a single syllable in each exhalation.

Precautions and contraindications: *Udgeeth pranayama* is generally considered safe and there are no known precautions or contraindications.

Pranayama involving increasing the depth of breathing

The depth of breathing is increased in *bhastrika pranayama* (= bellows breathing, in Sanskrit).

Method: *Bhastrika pranayama* involves breathing in fully and deeply through both nostrils followed by breathing out fully through both nostrils. The practice continues with these deep in and out breaths.

Precautions and contraindications: This practice results in overbreathing and hence is best avoided in people who have hyperventilation or anxiety disorders.

Pranayama with breath holding

Certain *pranayama* techniques involve a period of breath holding. In certain *pranayamas*, the duration of breath holding is shorter than either inhalation or exhalation, whereas in other *pranayamas*, the duration of breath holding exceeds that of inhalation or exhalation. Breath holding can follow either an in-breath or an out-breath or both.

Generally breath holding is not recommended for beginners but is practised by experienced yoga masters. The reason for this is that breath-holding *pranayamas*, if practiced incorrectly, can have adverse psychological effects (Naveen & Telles 2003). The technique should be avoided in hypertension, coronary artery disease and in people on any medication for psychiatric conditions. Even advanced yoga practitioners are required to practise these *pranayamas* with certain physiological 'locks' or *bandhas*. There are three such 'locks': a chin 'lock', an abdominal 'lock' and a perineal 'lock'. A study compared the oxygen consumed during long with short breath-holding *pranayamas* (Telles & Desiraju 1991). Interestingly, varying the duration of breath holding compared with inhalation–exhalation made a significant difference to oxygen consumption. Long breath holding was associated with a 19% decrease in oxygen consumption during the practice, whereas short breath holding was associated with a 56% increase in the oxygen consumed. The mechanisms underlying these differences remain to be understood.

Pranayama techniques: breathing in through the mouth

Conventionally correct breathing involves inhaling through the nose. In certain *pranayamas* considered to be heat dissipating, inhalation is through the mouth and exhalation is through the nose.

Methods: There are different techniques, e.g. breathing in through clenched teeth (*sadanta pranayama*), breathing in through the mouth with the tongue folded backwards (*sitkari pranayama*) and inhaling through the mouth with the sides of the tongue folded as if to form a beak (*sitali pranayama*). The general posture and other factors are the same as for other *pranayamas*.

Precautions and contraindications: While these are considered safe practices, breathing in through the mouth can result in the inhaled air being cooler than usual, which could cause a bronchospasm in cold-reactive bronchial asthmatics.

PHYSIOLOGICAL EFFECTS OF THE *PRANAYAMAS* (Fig. 8.6.2)

Pranayama practices involving changes in breath rate

Kapalabhati (= shining forehead, in Sanskrit) as the name suggests, influences brain functions. Following *kapalabhati* practice there was a significant increase in attention based on performance in a cancellation task (Telles et al 2008), and on an increased P300 amplitude in the P300 auditory odd ball task (Joshi & Telles 2009). Attention is a function of the dorsolateral prefrontal cortex (DPFC). This may explain why a separate, functional near infrared spectroscopy study showed increased deoxyhaemoglobin over the DPFC (Telles et al 2012a), with decreased oxy-haemoglobin, and no change in cerebral blood flow during *kapalabhati*, suggesting that the DPFC is active with the practice. *Kapalabhati* practice also improved visual and tactile perception as an immediate effect (Telles et al 2011a). *Kapalabhati* practice also influences other functions suggesting activation. There was a shift in the autonomic balance towards vagal withdrawal (Telles et al 2011b) and an increase in energy expenditure based on recordings

made with an open circuit metabolic analyzer. Another effect of the technique was an increase in alveolar dead space, possibly because the increase in rate decreases depth of breathing (Singh & Telles 2012).

Pranayama involving changes in which nostril is breathed through

An ancient yoga text called the *Swara* yoga text (*swara* = the flow of air through the nostrils in the form of energy) described different and distinct effects of breathing through the right nostril, the left nostril, or through both nostrils alternately. This text states that breathing through the right nostril is supposed to be heat generating, associated with activities such as studying the scriptures, hunting, scaling a fort or mountain and controlling an elephant, horse or chariot (*Shiva Swarodaya*, Ch. 5, V. 114–123). In contrast, breathing through the left nostril is described as heat dissipating, and associated with passive activities such as building a temple, rendering service, cultivating the land and performing religious rites (*Shiva Swarodaya*, Ch. 5, V. 102–113). It has also been mentioned that when breath flows through both nostrils, one should remain quiet (possibly introspective) and avoid any activity (*Shiva Swarodaya*, Ch. 5, V. 128).

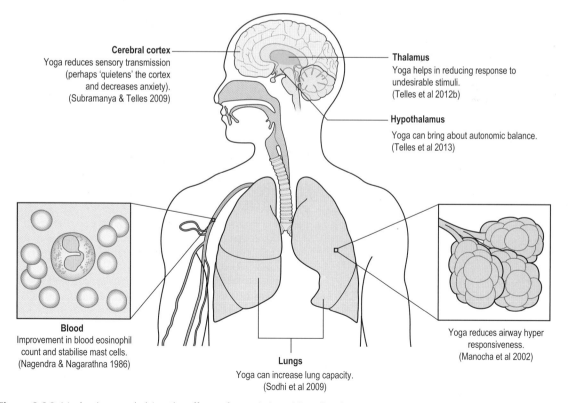

Cerebral cortex
Yoga reduces sensory transmission (perhaps 'quietens' the cortex and decreases anxiety). (Subramanya & Telles 2009)

Thalamus
Yoga helps in reducing response to undesirable stimuli. (Telles et al 2012b)

Hypothalamus
Yoga can bring about autonomic balance. (Telles et al 2013)

Blood
Improvement in blood eosinophil count and stabilise mast cells. (Nagendra & Nagarathna 1986)

Yoga reduces airway hyper responsiveness. (Manocha et al 2002)

Lungs
Yoga can increase lung capacity. (Sodhi et al 2009)

Figure 8.6.2 Mechanisms underlying the effects of yoga in breathing disorders.

Scientific studies have partially corroborated the descriptions of these practices in ancient texts. For example, right-nostril breathing (RNB) over a 1-month period, when practised for 45 minutes, increased oxygen consumption and caused sympathetic activation (e.g. increased peripheral vasoconstriction, systolic blood pressure and heart rate (Telles et al 1996)). Comparing the effects of right, left, and alternate-nostril breathing with breath awareness and no intervention showed that RNB increased systolic, diastolic and mean blood pressure along with peripheral vasoconstriction (Raghuraj & Telles 2008). These effects may be taken to suggest the energizing (based on oxygen consumed) and heat-generating effects of right-nostril yoga breathing described in the ancient texts.

Anuloma–viloma pranayama resulted in a slowing of breath after the practice as well as increased respiratory sinus arrhythmia (Jovanov 2005). In an earlier study it was shown that after practising *anuloma-viloma pranayama* for 4 weeks, volunteers showed a decrease in heart rate and systolic blood pressure both at rest and when they held their breath until the breaking point, suggesting reduced sympathetic activation (Bhargava et al 1988). In a more recent study, the systolic and diastolic pressure decreased after *anuloma-viloma pranayama* practice and the systolic and mean blood pressure were lower after left nostril yoga breathing (Raghuraj & Telles 2008).

Uninostril breathing practices also have lateralized effects on the cerebral hemispheres. These results were based on EEG as well as on performance in tasks specific to a particular cerebral hemisphere, and they suggested that forced uninostril breathing activates the opposite cerebral hemisphere (Shannahoff-Khalsa et al 1991). In contrast, yoga-based uninostril breathing did not show a lateralized effect on performance on hemisphere-specific tasks, as all participants who practised right, left and alternate-nostril yoga breathing showed improved scores in a right hemisphere-specific task (Naveen et al 1997). In addition, the immediate effects of right-nostril yoga breathing on bilaterally recorded auditory-evoked potentials were studied (Raghuraj & Telles 2004). During right-nostril yoga breathing, the peak amplitudes of two of three evoked potential components increased on the right side, with recruitment of greater numbers of neurons on the right side during the practice.

Pranayama involving exhalation during which a sound is produced

Two examples are *bhramari* ('bumblebee' in Sanskrit) *pranayama* and *udgeeth pranayama*. Practising *bhramari pranayama* every day along with left- and alternate-nostril yoga breathing over an 8-week period reduced symptoms in patients diagnosed with anxiety neurosis (Crisan 1996). Patients also showed decreased pulse rate, metabolites of epinephrine and norepinephrine in urine, and also increased skin resistance levels. Paroxysmal gamma waves were observed in eight participants practising *bhramari pranayama* (Vialatte et al 2008). This was described as most probably non-epileptic in origin and was considered a possible neural correlate of the mental state associated with yoga and meditation.

When the immediate effects of chanting 'Om' were compared with the effects of chanting 'one', both practices decreased the heart and breath rates, whereas chanting 'Om' alone decreased skin resistance levels, which was interpreted as a sign of mental engagement with the content of chanting the syllable 'Om' (Telles et al 1998).

Pranayama involving increasing the depth of breathing

The effects of *bhastrika pranayama* were assessed on reflexes (Bhavanani et al 2003). The reaction time (RT) of schoolboys who had practised yoga for 3 months was recorded before and after nine rounds of *bhastrika pranayama*. Following the practise, there was a significant decrease in both visual and auditory RT.

Pranayamas which involve inhalation through the mouth

Certain *pranayamas* involve inhaling through the mouth and exhaling through the nose. Perhaps because air is inhaled through the mouth and does not have the warming effect of passage through the nostrils, these have been called cooling *pranayamas*. In descriptions of these practices, based on the experiences of yoga practitioners, practising these *pranayamas* is reputed to be good for oral health, and may even help to reduce the body temperature of a person with a fever (Ramdev 2009).

APPLICATIONS OF THE DIFFERENT *PRANAYAMA* PRACTICES IN HEALTH AND OTHER DIMENSIONS OF LIFE

Most of the applications cited below are inferred indirectly based on the effects of the *pranayamas* on specific variables and certain task performances.

The possible uses of the *pranayamas* are as follows: *kapalabhati* in obesity (by increasing the energy output) and conditions associated with a poor attention span; *anuloma-viloma pranayama* in people predisposed to/diagnosed with hypertension; *brahmari pranayama* in anxiety disorders; *bhastrika pranayama* to increase the speed of response in people who are slow; short *kumbhak pranayamas* (inhale : hold : exhale : hold = 2 : 1 : 2 : 1) in obesity in contrast to long *kumbhak* (inhale : hold : exhale : hold = 1 : 4 : 2 : 2) in stress management.

STUDIES OF YOGA AS THERAPY

The therapeutic effect of yoga has been studied for many health problems, but this chapter is focused on breathing, and some yoga studies have targeted respiratory disorders. However, the effect of yoga-specific breathing techniques is rarely isolated from other aspects of yoga practice, so firm conclusions about benefits of yoga breathing in particular cannot yet be made.

Studies have indicated significant health and lifestyle benefits when yoga has been applied to individuals with a variety of respiratory diseases, including irreversible chronic bronchitis, pulmonary tuberculosis, bronchial asthma, and older people with chronic obstructive pulmonary disease (COPD).

Several studies that used pulmonary function tests before and after extended yoga practice found increases in exercise tolerance plus higher O_2 saturation and more normal CO_2 levels post-exercise in asthmatic subjects trained in yoga (Jain & Talukdar 1993).

MECHANISMS UNDERLYING THE EFFECTS

Practising *pranayamas* with breath holding lowered chemosensitivity to hypercapnia (Miyamura et al 2002) indicating an effect on the neural control of breathing. *Pranayamas* practised without breath holding improved the functioning of the respiratory airways and muscles involved in respiration (Madanmohan et al 2003). Yoga techniques including *pranayamas* have several beneficial effects on lung capacity and on the small airways.

Apart from the physical effects, the psychological state has a definite impact on respiration. In turn the breath pattern is known to influence the emotions. Breathing in particular patterns which were characterized by the experimenters, participants found it easier to simulate six emotions: joy–laughter, sadness–crying, fear–anxiety, anger, erotic love and tenderness (Bloch et al 1991).

The ways in which yoga may influence the mental state may be speculated upon. Voluntary slow deep breathing stretches the lung tissue, producing inhibitory signals from two sources: by the action of slowly adapting receptors and by hyperpolarizing currents (Jerath et al 2006). These inhibitory signals are believed to synchronize neural elements leading to changes in the autonomic nervous system, characterized by reduced metabolism and parasympathetic dominance. While parasympathetic dominance is generally associated with mental calmness, there are reports that the bronchial hyper-responsiveness in bronchial asthma is due to parasympathetic dominance with low sympathetic activity (Scanlon 1984). Certain yoga practices, contrary to the common impression, do cause parasympathetic withdrawal (Telles et al 2011b). Other *pranayama* practices which involve breathing selectively through one nostril cause sympathetic activation (Raghuraj & Telles 2008). These changes in autonomic activity may underlie the improvement in bronchial asthma following yoga practice.

The effects of *pranayamas* are probably due to interaction between the respiratory centers in the brainstem and the hypothalamus. In panic disorder, dysregulation of both respiratory control systems and the hypothalamic-pituitary adrenal (HPA) axis have been implicated. Previously elevated adrenocorticotrophic hormone (ACTH) and persistent irregularities in the tidal volume due to a high frequency of sighs were found in persons with panic disorder, and regression analyses showed that tidal volume irregularity and frequency of sighs were strongly predicted by ACTH levels prior to any challenge. A feature common to most *pranayama* practices is that they regularize breathing (Saraswati 2006). Whether this in turn influences ACTH is not known, but could be a way in which physiological stress reduction occurs with yoga, particularly yoga breathing. As already mentioned, these are mere speculations and further research is necessary to understand why yoga practice produces the many and diverse effects that are reported.

Particular importance is given to breathing in yoga. Hence this review would be incomplete without this verse from *Hatha Yoga Pradipika* (Ch. 2, V. 16):

> *by the proper practice of pranayama all diseases are eradicated while through the improper practice of pranayama all diseases can occur.*

REFERENCES

Bhargava, R., Gogate, M.G., Mascarenhas, J.F., 1988. Autonomic responses to breath holding and its variations following pranayama. Indian Journal of Physiology and Pharmacology 32 (4), 257–264.

Bhavanani, A.B., Madanmohan T., Udupa, K., 2003. Acute effect of Mukh bhastrika (a yogic bellows type breathing) on reaction time. Indian Journal of Physiology and Pharmacology 47 (3), 297–300.

Bloch, S., Lemeignan, M., Aguilera, N., 1991. Specific respiratory patterns distinguish among human basic emotions. International Journal of Psychophysiology 11 (2), 141–154.

Crisan, H., 1996. Yoga therapy research: a short review. Vivekananda Kendra Prakashan. Chennai, India.

Jain, S.C., Talukdar, B., 1993. Evaluation of yoga therapy programme for patients of bronchial asthma.

Singapore Medical Journal 34 (4), 306–308.

Jerath, R., Edry, J.W., Barnes, V.A., et al., 2006. Physiology of long pranayamic breathing: neural respiratory elements may provide a mechanism that explains how slow deep breathing shifts the autonomic nervous system. Medical Hypotheses 67 (3), 566–571.

Johnson, D.B., Tierney, M.J., Sadighi, P.J., 2004. Kapalabhati pranayama: breath of fire or cause of pneumothorax? A case report. Chest 125 (5), 1951–1952.

Joshi, M., Telles, S., 2009. A nonrandomized non-naïve, comparative study of the effects of kapalabhati and breath awareness on event-related potentials in trained yoga practitioners. Journal of Alternative and Complementary Medicine 15 (3), 281–285.

Jovanov, E., 2005. On spectral analysis of heart rate variability during very slow yogic breathing. Conference proceedings: Annual International Conference of the IEEE Engineering in Medicine and Biology Society 3, 2467–2470.

Madanmohan, T., Jatiya, L., Udupa, K., et al., 2003. Effect of yoga training on handgrip, respiratory pressures and pulmonary function. Indian Journal of Physiology and Pharmacology 47 (4), 387–392.

Manocha, R., Marks, G.B., Kenchington, P., et al., 2002. Sahaja yoga in the management of moderate to severe asthma: a randomised controlled trial. Thorax 57 (2), 110–115.

Miyamura, M., Nishimura, K., Ishida, K., et al., 2002. Is man able to breathe once a minute for an hour?: the effect of yoga respiration on blood gases. The Japanese Journal of Physiology 52 (3), 313–316.

Nagendra, H.R., Nagarathna, R., 1986. An integrated approach of yoga therapy for bronchial asthma: a 3-54-month prospective study. The Journal of Asthma 23 (3), 123–137.

Naveen, K.V., Nagarathna, R., Nagendra, H.R., et al., 1997. Yoga breathing through a particular nostril increases spatial memory scores without lateralized effects. Psychological Reports 81 (2), 555–561.

Naveen, K.V., Telles, S., 2003. Yoga and psychosis: risks and therapeutic potential. Journal of Indian Psychology 21 (1), 34–37.

Raghuraj, P., Telles, S., 2004. Right uninostril yoga breathing influences ipsilateral components of middle latency auditory evoked potentials. Neurological Sciences 25 (5), 274–280.

Raghuraj, P., Telles, S., 2008. Immediate effect of specific nostril manipulating yoga breathing practices on autonomic and respiratory variables. Applied Psychophysiology and Biofeedback 33 (2), 65–75.

Ramdev, S., 2009. Prāṇāyāmā rahasya with scientific factual evidence (Rev. ed.). Divya Prakashan, Uttrakhand, India.

Saraswati, S., 2006. Asana Pranayama Mudra Bandha. Yoga Publications Trust, Bihar, India.

Scanlon, R.T., 1984. Asthma: a panoramic view and a hypothesis. Annals of Allergy 53 (3), 203–212.

Shannahoff-Khalsa, D.S., Boyle, M.R., Buebel, M.E., 1991. The effects of unilateral forced nostril breathing on cognition. International Journal of Neuroscience 57 (3–4), 239–249.

Singh, V., Wisniewski, A., Britton, J., et al., 1990. Effect of yoga breathing exercises (pranayama) on airway reactivity in subjects with asthma. Lancet 335 (8702), 1381–1383.

Singh, N., Telles, S., 2012. High frequency yoga breathing can increase alveolar dead space. Medical Science Monitor 28;18 (7), LE5–LE6.

Sodhi, C., Singh, S., Dandona, P.K., 2009. A study of the effect of yoga training on pulmonary functions in patients with bronchial asthma. Indian Journal of Physiology and Pharmacology 53 (2), 169–174.

Subramanya, P., Telles, S., 2009. Changes in middle latency auditory evoked potentials following two yoga based relaxation techniques. Clinical EEG and Neuroscience 40 (3), 190–195.

Taimini, I.K., 1961. The science of yoga. The Theosophical Publishing House, Madras, India.

Telles, S., 2010. A theory of disease from ancient yoga texts. Medical Science Monitor 16 (6), LE9.

Telles, S., Desiraju, T., 1991. Oxygen consumption during pranayamic type of very slow-rate breathing. Indian Journal of Medical Research 94 (B), 357–363.

Telles, S., Nagarathna, R., Nagendra, H.R., 1996. Physiological measures during right nostril breathing. Journal of Alternative and Complementary Medicine 2 (4), 479–484.

Telles, S., Nagarathna, R., Nagendra, H.R., 1998. Autonomic changes while mentally repeating two syllables – one meaningful and the other neutral. Indian Journal of Physiology and Pharmacology 42 (1), 57–63.

Telles, S., Raghuraj, P., Arankalle, D., et al., 2008. Immediate effect of high-frequency yoga breathing on attention. Indian Journal of Medical Sciences 62 (1), 20–22.

Telles, S., Maharana, K., Balrana, B., et al., 2011a. Effects of high frequency yoga breathing called kapalabhati compared with breath awareness on the degree of optical illusion perceived. Perceptual and Motor Skills 112 (3), 981–980.

Telles, S., Singh, N., Balkrishna, A., 2011b. Heart rate variability changes during high frequency yoga breathing and breath awareness. Biopsychosocial Medicine 5, 4.

Telles, S., Singh, N., Gupta, R.K., et al., 2012a. Optical topography recording of cortical activity during high frequency yoga breathing and breath awareness. Medical Science Monitor 18 (1), LE3–LE4.

Telles, S., Raghavendra, B.R., Naveen, K.V., et al., 2012b. Mid-latency auditory evoked potentials in 2 meditative states. Clinical EEG and Neuroscience 43 (2), 154–160.

Telles, S., Raghavendra, B.R., Naveen, K.V., et al., 2013. Changes in autonomic variables following two meditative states described in yoga texts. Journal of Alternative and Complementary Medicine 19 (1), 35–42.

Vialatte, F.B., Bakardjian, H., Prasad, R., et al., 2008. EEG paroxysmal gamma waves during Bhramari Pranayama: a yoga breathing technique. Consciousness and Cognition 18 (4), 977–988.

Chapter | 9 |

Self-help approaches

Leon Chaitow, Dinah Bradley, Chris Gilbert

INTRODUCTION

In the end, the degree of effort an individual puts into his or her own rehabilitation towards more normal breathing patterns will determine the outcome. Breathing retraining has to be self-applied; it cannot be 'done' to the patient. If patient compliance is to be achieved, self-help strategies – whether involving lifestyle and dietary modification (if appropriate), relaxation, postural and breathing methods, or methods aimed at releasing tense tight muscles – need to be understandable, safe and easy to perform. The methods listed in this chapter conform to these needs. Some derive from well-researched methods (anti-arousal breathing and autogenic training, for example) while others have proved themselves in practice to the satisfaction of one or more of the authors. Although there are many other methods, those presented in this chapter represent a selection that are recommended; they may be reproduced free of copyright for individual patient use.

STRESS SCAN

Check for signs of tension in each area:

HEAD: Jaw, tongue, lips, eyes, forehead. Pressure, heat or pulsations in head?
NECK: Braced? Out of balance?
SHOULDERS; BACK; CHEST: Rapid heart rate?
BREATHING: High? Stopped? Fast? Shallow? Uneven?
ABDOMEN: Tense muscles? Stomach discomfort?
HANDS: Cool? Moist?
OTHER AREAS: Legs, arms, feet, pelvic muscles, thighs.
THOUGHTS AND FEELINGS: Anger, fear, worry, guilt, impatience, insecurity, resentment.

Signs of effective relaxation:

- Muscles and joints looser
- Breathing fuller, slower, lower
- Heart rate slower, less noticeable
- Hands and feet warmer, drier
- Head cooler, less pressure
- Shoulders dropped to a natural position
- Jaw unclenched
- Thinking: better concentration, less pressured, more objective, broader perspective

ANTI-AROUSAL BREATHING EXERCISE

Place yourself in a comfortable (ideally seated/reclining) position, exhale FULLY through your partially open mouth, lips just barely separated.

This outbreath should be performed slowly. Imagine that a candle flame is about 6 inches from your mouth and exhale (blowing a thin stream of air) in such a way as to not blow the candle out. As you exhale, count silently to yourself to establish the length of the outbreath. An effective method for counting one second at a time is to say (silently) 'one hundred, two hundred, three hundred, etc.' Each count then lasts about 1 second.

After exhaling fully, without any sense of strain, allow the next inhalation to be full, free and uncontrolled. By exhaling completely a 'coiled spring' is created so that the next inhalation occurs without effort. Once again, count to yourself to establish how long your inhalation lasts.

Without pausing to hold the breath, exhale FULLY, through the mouth, blowing the air in a thin stream (again you should count to yourself at the same speed).

Many people find a brief (one second) pause at the end of the exhalation helps to establish an unhurried rhythm.

Continue to repeat the inhalation and the exhalation for not less than 30 cycles of in and out (with a one second pause after breathing out).

The objective is that in time – after some weeks of practising this daily – you should, without strain, achieve an inhalation phase which lasts for 2–3 seconds while the exhalation phase lasts from 6–7 seconds. Most importantly, the exhalation should be slow and continuous. It is no use breathing the air out in 2 seconds and then simply waiting until the count reaches 6, 7 or 8 before inhaling again.

By the time you have completed 15 or so cycles, a sense of calm is frequently apparent.

Apart from practising this once or twice daily, it may be useful to repeat the exercise for a few minutes (about five cycles of inhalation/exhalation takes a minute) if you feel anxious or 'stressed'.

NOTE: Once this exercise has been successfully learned, it can usefully be combined with either the Brugger position, or the 'reducing shoulder movement' method, described below.

REDUCING SHOULDER MOVEMENT DURING BREATHING (Fig. 9.1)

Stand in front of a mirror and breathe, and notice whether your shoulders rise. If so, there is a strategy you can use to reduce this tendency.

Before starting one of the breathing exercises (for example, the anti-arousal exercise described above), sit in a chair with arms and place your elbows and forearms fully supported by the chair arms. Slowly exhale through pursed lips, and then, as you inhale through your nose, push *gently* down onto the chair arms to 'lock' the shoulder muscles, preventing them from rising. As you exhale release the downward pressure. Repeat throughout the exercise.

As a substitute for the strategy described above, especially if there is no armchair available, sit with your hands interlocked, palms upward, on your lap.

As you inhale, lightly but firmly push the pads of your fingers against the backs of the hands, and release this pressure when you slowly exhale. This reduces the ability of the muscles above the shoulders to contract, and will lessen the tendency for the shoulders to rise.

Repeat one of these methods – or Brugger's position (see next section) for several minutes morning and evening.

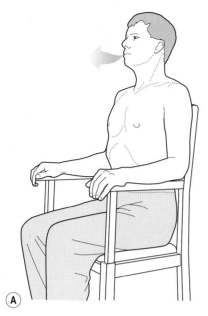
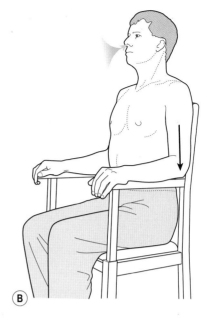

Figure 9.1 Inhalation exercise without shoulder shrugging.

BRUGGER'S RELIEF POSITION (Fig. 9.2)

This position should be adopted for a few minutes, several times a day, especially if you have to spend much of the day seated, for example at a desk or computer.

- Sit very close ('perch') to the edge of your chair, arms hanging down at your side.
- Place your feet directly below your knees and then move them slightly more apart and turn them slightly outward.
- Roll your pelvis slightly forward to produce a very small degree of arching of your low back.
- Ease your sternum (breastbone) slightly forward and up.
- Turn your arms outward so that the palms face forward.
- Separate your fingers until your thumbs face slightly backward.
- Tuck your chin in gently.
- Maintain this posture while you practise four or five cycles of slow breathing to a pattern such as that outlined under the heading 'anti-arousal breathing' (above).
- Repeat this whenever you sense muscle tension during sitting, or if you feel the need for deeper breathing.
- This 'relief' posture ensures that the chest can be as free and open as possible and reverses many of the stresses caused by long periods of sitting.

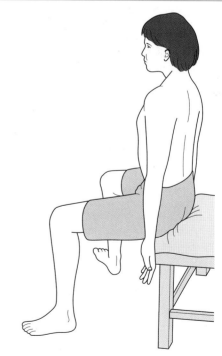

Figure 9.2 The Brugger relief position. *Reproduced with kind permission from Liebenson., C.,1999. Motivating pain patients to become more active. Journal of Bodywork and Movement Therapies 3 (3), 149.*

AUTOGENIC TRAINING RELAXATION

Relaxation exercises focus on the body and its responses to stress, trying to reverse these, while meditation tries to bring about a calming of the mind and through this a relaxation response.

Autogenic training (AT) is a form of exercise which combines the best of both relaxation and meditation. The modified AT exercise described below offers a way of achieving effective relaxation.

Exercise for effective relaxation

Every day, at least once, for 10 minutes at a time, do the following:

- Lie on the floor or bed in a comfortable position, small cushion under the head, knees bent if that makes the back feel easier, eyes closed.
- Practise the anti-arousal breathing exercise (or some other relaxing breathing exercise) for a few minutes before you start the AT exercise.
- Focus attention on your dominant (say right) hand/arm and silently say to yourself 'My right arm (or hand) feels heavy.'
- Try to sense the arm relaxed and heavy, its weight sinking into the surface it rests on. Feel its weight. Over a period of about a minute repeat the affirmation ('My arm/hand feels heavy') several times and try to stay focused on its weight and heaviness.
- You will almost certainly lose focus as your mind wanders from time to time. This is part of the training in the exercise – to stay focused, so don't be upset – just go back to the arm and its heaviness which you may or may not be able to sense.
- If it does feel heavy, stay with it and enjoy the sense of release – of letting go – that comes with it.
- Next, focus on your other hand/arm and do exactly the same thing for about a minute.
- Move to the left leg and then the right leg, for about a minute each, with the same messages and focused attention on each.
- Go back to your right hand/arm and this time affirm a message which tells you that you sense a greater degree of warmth there – 'My hand is feeling warm (or hot).'
- After a minute or so, go to the left hand/arm, then the left leg and then finally the right leg, each time with the 'warming' message and focused attention. If

warmth is sensed, stay with it for a while and feel it spread. Enjoy it.
- Finally focus on your forehead and affirm that it feels cool and refreshed. Hold this cool and calm thought for a minute before completing the exercise. Finish by clenching your fists, bending your elbows and stretching out your arms. The exercise is complete.

By repeating the whole exercise at least once a day you will gradually find you can stay focused on each region and sensation.

Explanation

'Heaviness' represents what you feel when muscles relax and 'warmth' is what you feel when your circulation to an area is increased, while 'coolness' is the opposite, a reduction in circulation for a short while – usually followed by an increase due to the overall relaxation of the muscles.

Measurable changes occur in circulation and temperature in the regions being focused on during these training sessions. Success requires persistence – daily use for at least 6 weeks – before benefits are noticed, usually a sense of relaxation and better sleep.

How to use these skills for health enhancement by visualizing change

- If there is pain or discomfort related to muscle tension, AT training can be used to focus on the area, and by getting that area to 'feel' heavy, this will reduce tension.
- If there is pain related to poor circulation the 'warmth' instruction can be used to improve it.
- If there is inflammation related to pain this can be reduced by 'thinking' the area 'cool'.

The new skills gained by AT can be used to focus on any area – and most importantly helps to allow you to be able to stay focused – to introduce other images, 'seeing' in the mind's eye a stiff joint easing and moving, or a congested swollen area melting back to normality, or any other helpful change which would ease whatever health problem there might be.

AT trainers strongly urge that you avoid AT focus on vital functions, such as those relating to the heart, or to the breathing pattern in the case of anyone with a breathing disorder, unless a trained instructor is providing guidance and supervision.

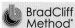 BradCliff Method® **SELF-EFFICACY QUESTIONNAIRE**

RoBE Scale

These questions ask what you are confident to do without being affected by symptoms related to your breathing.

Circle the number that best describes how confident you feel for each statement.

The guidelines are:

not at all confident 1 2 3 4 5 6 7 8 9 completely confident

How confident are you that you can:

do the tasks you need to, without being affected by your symptoms
1 2 3 4 5 6 7 8 9

any tasks that are particularly difficult:_____
_____

talk without being affected by your symptoms
1 2 3 4 5 6 7 8 9

any times this is particularly difficult:_____
_____

enjoy recreational activities without being affected by your symptoms
1 2 3 4 5 6 7 8 9

any activities that are particularly difficult:_____
_____

feel calm and achieve a good breathing pattern when you want to
1 2 3 4 5 6 7 8 9

any time this is particularly difficult:_____
_____

identify what triggers your symptoms
1 2 3 4 5 6 7 8 9

any situation this is particularly difficult:_____
_____

go into situations that might bring on your symptoms
1 2 3 4 5 6 7 8 9

any situations you avoid:_____
_____

improve your symptoms with what you do
1 2 3 4 5 6 7 8 9

improvements you make to your breathing will be useful and valuable
1 2 3 4 5 6 7 8 9

persist at improving your breathing even when it is difficult
1 2 3 4 5 6 7 8 9

MOOD STATE: My mood today
1 2 3 4 5 6 7 8 9
Low   good

My mood last 6 months
1 2 3 4 5 6 7 8 9

© Janet Rowley 2005

RoBE Scale information for practitioners

Rowley breathing pattern disorders self-efficacy scale

Why self-efficacy?

Self-efficacy (SE) is a person's confidence they will successfully perform a task, based on their *self-appraisal* of their skills. SE can predict how likely a person is to succeed, and

by improving their SE we can improve their likelihood of success. An SE scale is useful for showing change – hopefully improvement, in a person's confidence in applying what you have taught them. This scale can also help pinpoint areas that need working on.

Clinical application of the RoBE

The ideal response for each question is the score of 9, and 8–9 is what would be expected in a normal population.

(N.B. Some people always avoid using end numbers, others avoid always making the same response.)

The lower the numerical response by a patient, the less confident they are in the area the question refers to.

When we address such an area we can improve their self-efficacy in that area, and they are more likely to put into practice what you have taught them.

Here are some useful responses for each question if the patient has a low score:

Question 1: confidence doing daily tasks without being affected by symptoms

- Which tasks were you thinking of in particular?
- Why do you think these are difficult – e.g have you tried some of them since coming for treatment and felt you still couldn't successfully control your breathing?
- Are there any other strategies we need to add to help you with these tasks? (this question refers to tasks such as housework, normal employment, shopping, etc., i.e. what they need to do over a normal week)

Question 2: talk without being affected by symptoms

- Were you thinking of any particular situations, e.g. on the phone, presenting to others, or talking with particular people (e.g. intimidating people, or with friends who all talk fast, etc)
- What do you already do to help yourself when you talk?

Question 3: enjoy recreational activities

- Which activities were you thinking of? If it is a physical task is it actually the BPD causing symptoms, or are you just plain 'out of breath' with exertion.
- Is it the physical task or an emotional factor (e.g. anxiety) that seems to be the difficulty?

Question 4: identify triggers

- Are you aware of any triggers? Discuss likely triggers and explore the trickiest situations the patient encounters (this overlaps with the other questions).

Question 5: improve your symptoms with what you do

- Have you experienced any success when you try to improve your breathing? If so, itemize these, put them in writing, give them value.
- Have you felt you couldn't control your breathing despite your efforts at any time? If so, what made you think you'd failed? (e.g. 'because I was still anxious and breathing too fast). Challenge these evaluations, e.g. did your anxiety or symptoms

improve at all? A patient with low SE will place greater emphasis on negative experiences and negative self-feedback, e.g. any pain or discomfort. Look to see if any of the four key factors (described below) were pulling them down.

Question 6: manage your symptoms without introducing medication

- This addresses locus of control, i.e. taking responsibility. If introduced medication is not related to BPD, ignore such medication when answering this question.

Question 7: go into situations that might bring on symptoms

- Avoidance is an expression of low SE. To regain full participation in their previous lifestyle, it is necessary to minimize/eliminate such avoidance.
- What are the situations you might avoid? What is likely to happen (e.g. 'I feel really anxious'); develop strategies to address this (e.g. 'the anxiety in itself is not harmful…').
- Are there mildly difficult situations you could trial first, before the more difficult ones?

Question 8: make useful improvements by improving breathing

- This addresses underlying attitude to treatment. If the patient hasn't bought into the treatment, their compliance and adherence is likely to be low regardless of how you treat.
- 'Why do you think that?' (e.g. 'a friend said it would never work')
- Explain the science (basic physiology) and the art (mind–body connection) and if they still are not convinced, perhaps consider suspending treatment until they wish to continue.

Question 9: persist at improving breathing pattern

- This also addresses attitude and behaviour, as lack of persistence is a feature of low SE.
- Develop a plan of attack, e.g. timetable practise, identify factors likely to discourage them and develop a strategy to counter them, set goals, reward scheme, whatever it takes (there is extensive literature on enhancing motivation and persistence).

Four key factors that enhance self-efficacy

These factors are commonly listed as influencing a person's SE. If we utilize them in our treatment we can enhance SE. It is likely you are already using some of them. The 4th factor is likely least utilized. For example, a patient feels 'down' after practising breathing and assumes it isn't helping – but closer questioning reveals the symptoms have actually decreased, and they have been irrational when assessing physiological feedback.

1. Mastery experience – thought to be the most significant influence on self-efficacy, this refers to a person's experience of success in mastering a particular task.

2. Vicarious experience – drawn from observations of others achieving positive results in similar tasks to one's own.

3. Verbal persuasion – refers to the influence of others' words; particularly those perceived to be creditable and trustworthy.

4. Physiological information gleaned from 'listening to' one's own body, utilizing this information to make an assessment, albeit not necessarily accurate, of one's achievement.

Useful reading

Schwarzer, R. (Ed.), 1992. Self-efficacy: Thought Control of Action. Hemisphere Pub Corp, Washington.

Maddux, J. (Ed.), 1995. Self-Efficacy, Adaptation, and Adjustment: Theory, Research and Application. Plenum Press, New York.

NASAL SALINE IRRIGATION – INSTRUCTIONS FOR PATIENTS

1. Clean a quart (1200ml) glass jar carefully, then fill it with bottled water. You need not boil the water.
2. Use 2–3 heaped teaspoons of rock salt. Do not use table salt as it contains additives.
3. Add one rounded teaspoon of baking soda (pure bicarbonate).
4. Store at room temperature and shake or stir before each use.
5. Mix a new batch weekly.

Use

1. Pour some of the mixture into a clean bowl. Warming it to body temperature may help but make sure that it is not HOT. Try 5-second increments in the microwave.
2. Fill a syringe or bulb irrigator. To avoid contamination DO NOT place bulb or syringe into jar.
3. Stand over the sink or in the shower and squirt the mixture into each side of the nose several times.
4. Rinse the nose up to two to three times daily.

It is normal for drops of water to occasionally drain from your nose for up to 30 minutes after irrigation. You may want to carry tissues with you. If your nose stings or burns, try using half as much salt next time. You may also want to try a different water temperature. Do not use very hot or very cold water.

Xylitol nasal spray recipe

Xylitol is a five-carbon sugar alcohol that is generally believed to enhance the body's own innate bactericidal mechanisms. Increasing evidence indicates that a xylitol nasal spray may also help some patients suffering from chronic rhinosinusitis (Weissman et al 2011). There is considerable variation in how xylitol nasal sprays are made. Some people also add salt to the mixture. This xylitol recipe is derived from Weismann et al 2011.

Mixing the spray

1. Purchase a reusable sinus-spray bottle at a pharmacy and powdered xylitol at a health food store.
2. Mix a cup of warm water (240 ml) with $2\frac{1}{2}$ tsp (12 mg) of powdered xylitol until xylitol is dissolved.
3. Pour the solution into the nasal-spray bottle and store at room temperature and shake before each use.

Using the spray

1. Hold one nostril closed while placing the nasal spray in the other nostril. Breathe in through the nostril while spraying the solution deep into the nose.
2. Repeat with other nostril. Blow your nose gently and use two to three times a day to prevent infections.

Reference

Weissman, J.D., Fernandez, F., Hwang, P.H., 2011. Xylitol nasal irrigation in the management of chronic rhinosinusitis: a pilot study. The Laryngoscope 121 (11), 2468–2472.

RECOMMENDATIONS FOR HYPERVENTILATION

Dr L. C. Lum (whose pioneering work is extensively referred to throughout this book) served for many years as a chest physician at Papworth Hospital in Cambridge.

Lum was very influential, along with physiotherapist Diana Innocenti, in bringing hyperventilation to the attention of the medical and psychological professions. The following pages contain two handouts that he provided for his patients.

FACTORS INVOLVED IN HYPERVENTILATION

L.C.Lum

1. *Early history*. About 80% of hyperventilators give a history of poor bonding with one or other parent, often both. The remainder either have a family history of asthma, bronchitis or emphysema, or have clearly derived the habit of overbreathing from the parents. There is often a history of proneness to fainting in childhood, or of phobic tendencies. Often other members of the family have similar symptoms.

2. *Personality*. The usual personality is perfectionist, and often obsessional, while being basically insecure. I attribute this to the lack of parental bonding. Children need close ties with *both parents*.

3. *Onset on holiday*. It is very common for symptoms to start when on holiday after a period of stress. Hyperventilators seem to keep going while the pressure is on, and crack when it is relieved. (Weekends too are a favoured time for symptoms to start.)

4. *Exacerbation of symptoms at rest*. There seems to be a failure of 'fine-tuning' of respiration, so that breathing changes do not follow accurately changes in activity. For example, in the evening, the breathing does not subside from the level appropriate to daytime activity, to the lower metabolic requirement of watching TV, or trying to go to sleep. A corollary to this is that the commonest situation for developing panic attacks is driving a car (maximum of stimulation combined with minimum of physical effort); next commonest are watching TV and in bed! There are probably physiological analogies with the holiday situation.

5. *Muscle pains*. These are very common, and most often affect the neck, shoulders and upper back. They were attributed to tetanic spasm in isolated muscle fibres as long ago as 1937, and I believe this to be correct, since one can usually locate tender trigger areas in these muscles. Similar tender nodules are usually present at the anterior edge of the parietal muscles when the patient complains of parietal or frontal headache, and at the insertion of the nuchal muscles into the occiput. Less commonly one finds general limb pains, particularly in the legs, associated with a tendency to spasm of whole muscle groups.

6. *Climate and weather*. Hyperventilation is exacerbated by hot (and particularly humid) weather – for the obvious reason of the importance of breathing in heat loss. The influence of hot, humid weather was well documented by American army doctors during the Second World War. Hypoxic stimulation at altitude is also important (the threshold seems to be about 5000 feet). Similarly, effects can be seen with marked changes in barometric pressure as with the approach of frontal systems. The development of the painful muscular nodules of HV is probably how Farmer Giles predicts weather changes by his 'rheumaticks'. The turbulent weather in the UK at the end of 1987 provoked many exacerbations, and such severe panic attacks in some patients that I had to put them in hospital.

7. *Low blood sugar*. It is common for symptoms to occur or to get worse before lunch and in the late afternoon, since even a moderately low blood sugar can gravely exaggerate the symptoms of hyperventilation. The diet needs specific modification.

8. *Crying*. Hyperventilators often complain of emotional lability, and are prone to tears. In the laboratory after a session of breath testing, it was common for patients to begin crying, without knowing why. This is due to loss of cortical inhibition due to cerebral hypoxia.

9. *Menstruation*. Symptoms tend to be worse during the premenstrual week and the early days of the period. Progesterone, the hormone secreted by the ovaries after ovulation, is a strong respiratory stimulant, and can reduce carbon dioxide level of the blood by as much as 25%. Hence, any tendency to overbreathe is made worse during this time. In

addition, the symptoms of premenstrual tension (PMT) – headache, tension, irritability, tendency to tears – are common in HV.

10. *Occupational hazards: the voice.* Singers, actors and wind instrumentalists are particularly vulnerable. It has terminated many operatic careers. One of the greatest dramatic sopranos of the 20th century, Rosa Ponselle, always suffered so severely with stage fright that she retired from opera at the height of her career.

11. *Speech.* Hyperventilators are usually animated, breathless talkers who try to get too many words on one breath. They must be taught to slow down, use shorter phrases, with a small sip of air between phrases, rather than a large gulp between long sentences.

12. *Allergy.* There is a high incidence of allergic phenomena – e.g. eczema, asthma, rhinitis and hay fever – in hyperventilation states. Hyperventilation causes certain blood cells to produce an excess of histamine, a substance which causes allergic reactions.

See also: Hyperventilation syndromes: physiological considerations in clinical management. In: Timmons, B. H., Ley, R. (eds) 1994. Behavioral and psychological approaches to clinical management. Plenum, New York, pp. 113–23.

FAULTS IN HYPERVENTILATION AND CORRECTIVE EXERCISES

L.C.Lum

1. BREATHING TOO FAST (normal rate is 10–14 breaths per minute; hyperventilators are usually nearer 20, and often much higher)
2. IRREGULAR AMPLITUDE OF BREATHS
3. IRREGULAR RHYTHM
4. FREQUENT SIGHS OR YAWNS
5. HABITUAL SNIFFING AND COUGHING
6. FAST BREATHLESS TALKING

The above faults are all associated with excessive use of the upper thorax. Hyperventilators often do not use the diaphragm at all. Habitual diaphragmatic breathers do not suffer from chronic hyperventilation.

7. GENERAL TENSION OF THE WHOLE BODY

This shows up particularly in the muscles of the neck, just at the base of the skull, the shoulder muscles, and anywhere down the back on either side of the spinal processes. However, any muscles of the body or limbs may be affected. Chronic tension causes painful knots of muscle in spasm. Particularly liable to be affected are the locations listed above, muscles over the temples (which cause migraine-like headaches), muscles in the chest wall, particularly under the left breast or alongside the breast bone, around the shoulder, elbow and wrist joints. These are more common on the left side, but often affect the right side of the chest. However, virtually any muscle in the body may be affected. The usual result is an aching pain, sometimes stabbing. Occasionally a whole muscle may go into spasm, causing severe cramp-like pains.

Diaphragm exercises

NOTE: These exercises are designed to overcorrect the faults. The hyperventilator's respiratory center has become 'set' to keep the $PaCO_2$ at an abnormally low level; the very slow rate teaches the hyperventilator to resist the inspiratory drive.

Inhalation with the diaphragm *actively* pushes out the front wall of the abdomen. Exhalation is completely *passive*. The lung empties itself as a balloon does. NO exhalatory effort is required. One just relaxes, and lets the air fall out.

There must be no pause between inhalation and exhalation. As you begin to let the air come out, feel yourself relax, and continue to relax during the count before the next breath, resisting the desire to sneak in a small breath during this time. You should aim at getting the number of breaths down to between six and eight breaths a minute. Time yourself with a clock, and teach yourself how many counts it takes to achieve this. You may not be able to slow your breathing down this much at first. Eight is what you should aim for initially; eventually get down to six.

Practise sessions

You should do five or six sessions (minimum four), each lasting 10 minutes, every day. These should be in the semi-recumbent position. You should not attempt to do anything else (e.g. watch TV, listen to music or the radio) during this time. It is helpful to do similar breathing before getting up and when settling down to sleep, but *do not count these as practise*; you don't learn much when you are half asleep.

Standing practise

Stand with the feet apart, weight more on one foot than the other (change the weight from time to time). Let the arms hang loosely across the front of the abdomen, with one hand loosely holding the other arm above the wrist, so that the forearms feel the movements of the abdominal wall. The shoulders should be down, and the whole attitude appear relaxed. You can do this for a few minutes at a time whenever the opportunity occurs, e.g. when shopping.

Periodic reminders

Develop the habit of paying attention to your breathing frequently (4–6 times an hour), by reminding yourself to take a couple of breaths with the diaphragm. Usually, this should be when you change from doing one thing to doing another (e.g. using the phone, in jobs around the house, in reading or writing, between paragraphs and pages).

Cultivate relaxation at all times

Watch your body language. Does your attitude reflect tension or relaxation? Most overbreathers are in a chronic state of tension which shows in the way they sit, stand, walk, hold a pen or drive a car – in fact their every attitude and movement.

Learn the relaxed way of sitting, standing and walking, and get the habit of asking yourself, 'What message is my body language sending out?' Whenever you change activity, action, or posture, your first thought must be to do it in a relaxed way.

Hyperventilators are invariably fast, breathless talkers. They put too much effort into voice, facial expression, and gesture. They speak in long sentences without pausing for breath and then have to take a gasp before the next sentence. Learn to break up your speech into small phrases of a few words each. Learn the trick of taking a short sip of air (with the diaphragm) after each short phrase. Talking on the telephone usually increases overbreathing. It is useful to make a tape of your voice on the telephone and in ordinary conversation round the house. This will help you to identify harmful mannerisms.

Walking rhythm

Hyperventilators' breathing is always fast and irregular. The rhythm of the feet provides a regular beat with which to coordinate your breathing. Walking at your normal pace, take two steps for breathing in, two for breathing out, and hold your breath for two steps. (This pause is shorter than the pause during practise, because walking requires twice as much air as sitting.) Do not worry about diaphragm breathing at first. First of all get the rhythm right. When you can do this easily, start to train yourself to breathe with the diaphragm while walking. It is difficult to learn two things at the same time.

Walking to eliminate body tension

The natural rhythm of the body requires that, as one leg goes forward, the opposite arm should swing forward. A limber, relaxed gait requires that the shoulder should also swing forward with the arm. This is known as 'contrary body movement' in dancing. What happens to the back muscles is that, as one shoulder is pulled forward by the muscles on one half of the back, the same muscles on the opposite side must relax (this is a physiological law). Consequently, during walking the back muscles alternately contract and relax, instead of being tense all the time. When you have mastered this method of walking you will soon find that the painful nodules in the back and neck disappear.

Try to walk as if you were pleased with yourself. Remember that body language is a two-way affair: if you make yourself move as if you were relaxed and pleased with yourself, you will begin to feel that way.

Index

Index